THE COMPLETE GUIDE TO

STRENGTH AND CONDITIONING TRAINING

Morc Coulson and Matt Brown

BLOOMSBURY SPORT

LONDON · OXFORD · NEW YORK · NEW DELHI · SYDNEY

BLOOMSBURY SPORT
Bloomsbury Publishing Plc
50 Bedford Square, London, WC1B 3DP, UK
Bloomsbury Publishing Ireland Limited,
29 Earlsfort Terrace, Dublin 2, D02 AY28, Ireland

BLOOMSBURY, BLOOMSBURY SPORT and the Diana logo
are trademarks of Bloomsbury Publishing Plc

First published in Great Britain 2026

A catalogue record for this book is available from the British Library

Library of Congress Cataloguing-in-Publication data has been applied for

ISBN: PB: 978-1-3994-2136-2; eBook: 978-1-3994-2135-5

2 4 6 8 10 9 7 5 3 1

Typeset in ITC Galliard by seagulls.net
Printed and bound in China by C&C Offset Printing Co., Ltd.

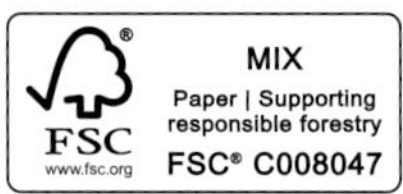

To find out more about our authors and books visit www.bloomsbury.com
and sign up for our newsletters

For product safety related questions contact productsafety@bloomsbury.com

CONTENTS

Scan the QR code below to access a YouTube playlist of accompanying video demonstrations.

Look out for individual QR codes throughout the book that will take you to relevant videos depending on which section you are working on.

INTRODUCING STRENGTH AND CONDITIONING

Strength and conditioning (S&C) is made up of two key words: 'strength' and 'conditioning'. Within the profession these words act both in union and as separate entities that have clear definitions:

- **Strength** – Developing an individual or team's strength and *power* outputs to support and improve sport-specific performance.
- **Conditioning** – Preparing an individual or team to cope with the physical demands of their sport while developing *neuromuscular* robustness to injury.

When the terms are combined there is no universally accepted definition of S&C, but it usually refers to the practical application of sports science to enhance movement quality to improve performance and reduce risk of injury.

S&C involves a wide range of training methods and is not just reserved for athletes: it can be used by anyone, as it can help to improve performance of activities of daily living, such as gardening and DIY. What's more, there are many suggested benefits from S&C in addition to improved performance and reduced injury risk. These include:

- Increased resting metabolism
- Improved *body composition*
- Improved *flexibility*
- Improved heart and lung health
- Increased bone strength
- Improved mood and sleep quality

S&C is a rapidly evolving discipline within the highly competitive sports performance industry. Since prac-

titioners must be prepared to deliver programmes to clients on the spot or at short notice, it is essential that they have a sound foundation of scientific knowledge that supports practical expertise.

What is an S&C practitioner?

The main role of an S&C practitioner is to develop the physical capabilities of clients while minimising their risk of injury.

To do this, there are a wide range of skills that a practitioner must develop to provide a holistic service. For example, in addition to devising appropriate training programmes, practitioners must have a clear understanding of the role nutrition plays to help clients recover from training or competition, aid with adequate muscle growth and repair and minimise risk of injury and illness.

In addition, many practitioners within the S&C industry are freelance or self-employed business owners, which means they must be confident about health and safety policy and risk assessments to ensure the safety of the people they train.

What is the difference between an S&C coach and a personal trainer?

There are many differences between a strength and conditioning coach and a personal trainer:

- A personal trainer is usually qualified to level 3 whereas an S&C coach is usually qualified to level 4 with a sports science undergraduate background.
- An S&C coach will normally create individualised long-term training programmes, whereas a personal trainer often creates more generalised ones for shorter periods of time.
- An S&C coach will have a more focused approach to evidence-based fitness testing that can be used to inform programme development.
- S&C coaches liaise with a wider range of external professionals, such as sports coaches, team managers, medical staff, physiotherapists and dieticians.

About this book

The aim of this book is to provide a clear and informative guide to S&C to enhance and embed further learning for those working in the sector as well as anyone who is studying to pursue a career within it. It covers the fundamental principles of the discipline – such as the components of fitness, training principles, sample programmes, periodisation and performance testing – as well as additional topics

and skills that S&C practitioners must understand and perfect so that they can succeed in the profession. It also provides a practical insight to enable practitioners to incorporate these skills into their programme delivery. At the start of each chapter there is a list of areas covered. The book in its entirety covers most of the occupational standards for strength and conditioning.

As part of this practical insight, we have created a bank of videos showing how to do a range of exercises that are typical of an S&C programme. These demonstrations provide further context and reinforce the concepts outlined in the book. We will also provide QR codes throughout the book to signpost where these additional resources are provided.

There are five main sections:

- **Part 1: Client consultation (chapters 1–3)** This section takes a look at how S&C coaches gather client information before devising a programme, using screening, needs analysis and goal setting.
- **Part 2: The fundamentals of strength and conditioning (chapters 4–13)** This section examines the overarching components and principles of fitness, then breaks them down chapter by chapter to examine them in more detail: what they are and how the body responds to them, what factors can affect adaptations, suitable training methods, training variables, and sample programmes.
- **Part 3: Testing the components of fitness (chapters 14–23)** This section first explores what performance assessment involves, including its benefits, where it can take pace, associated methodology and terminology, data collection, protection, analysis and feedback, the role of *validity* and reliability, and the relevance of assessments to programme training and future testing. It then provides chapter-by-chapter detailed advice on how to test each of the components of fitness.

- **Part 4: General training strategies (chapters 24–28)** This section covers more general topics associated with S&C coaching, including manipulation of training variables, fatigue and recovery strategies, practitioner skills, motivation, and legal and ethical considerations.
- **Part 5: Nutrition for strength and conditioning (chapters 29–31)** This section takes a brief look at some aspects of nutrition, such as what nutrients are and why they are needed, nutritional deficiencies and energy balance.

Using the material provided within this textbook, practitioners will be able to:

- Understand what a client requires within an S&C programme by using strategies such as needs analyses, goal-setting techniques and effective communication techniques.
- Design comprehensive S&C programmes tailored to clients and the sport they compete in.
- Have the ability to perform rigorous, evidence-based and scientifically sound testing protocols to assess performance levels of individuals or teams.
- Develop data analysis, visualisation and feedback skills to evaluate the effectiveness of training programmes and how to report this back to the client and relevant support staff.
- Gain a broad knowledge base of the peripheral topics that support S&C practitioners within their role, including sports nutrition and recovery strategies.

To do this, we have developed a navigation tool called the S&C road map to help you through the process.

THE S&C ROAD MAP

In order to develop S&C programmes, practitioners can follow a logical process known as the S&C road map (*see* fig. 0.1). Part 1 of the road map starts with

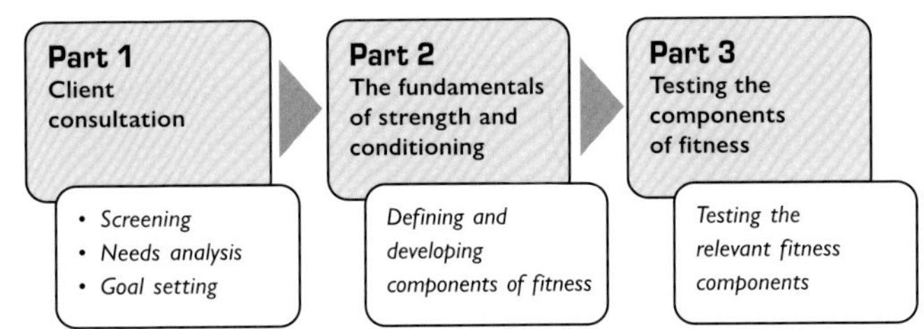

Figure 0.1 S&C road map

an initial client meeting (known as a consultation) in which information is gathered that will help the practitioner to develop a tailored training programme. Part 2 is where the practitioner uses their knowledge and experience to consider which components of fitness (described later in the book) to include in the programme. Part 3 is a guide on how to test the components of fitness to establish the client's fitness levels in the relevant components. All of this informs programme development.

How to use this book

In order to gain the most value from this textbook, readers should:

- Read the introduction to each section and chapter to gain insights into how each will benefit S&C practitioners.

- Use the 'take-home messages' at the end of each chapter to reflect and consolidate the learnings from the chapter.

- Use additional material where provided (such as videos) to enhance learning and add context to the text.

- Use the Glossary to assist with definitions of any technical terms. Glossary terms are highlighted in bold italics when they are first mentioned in the text.

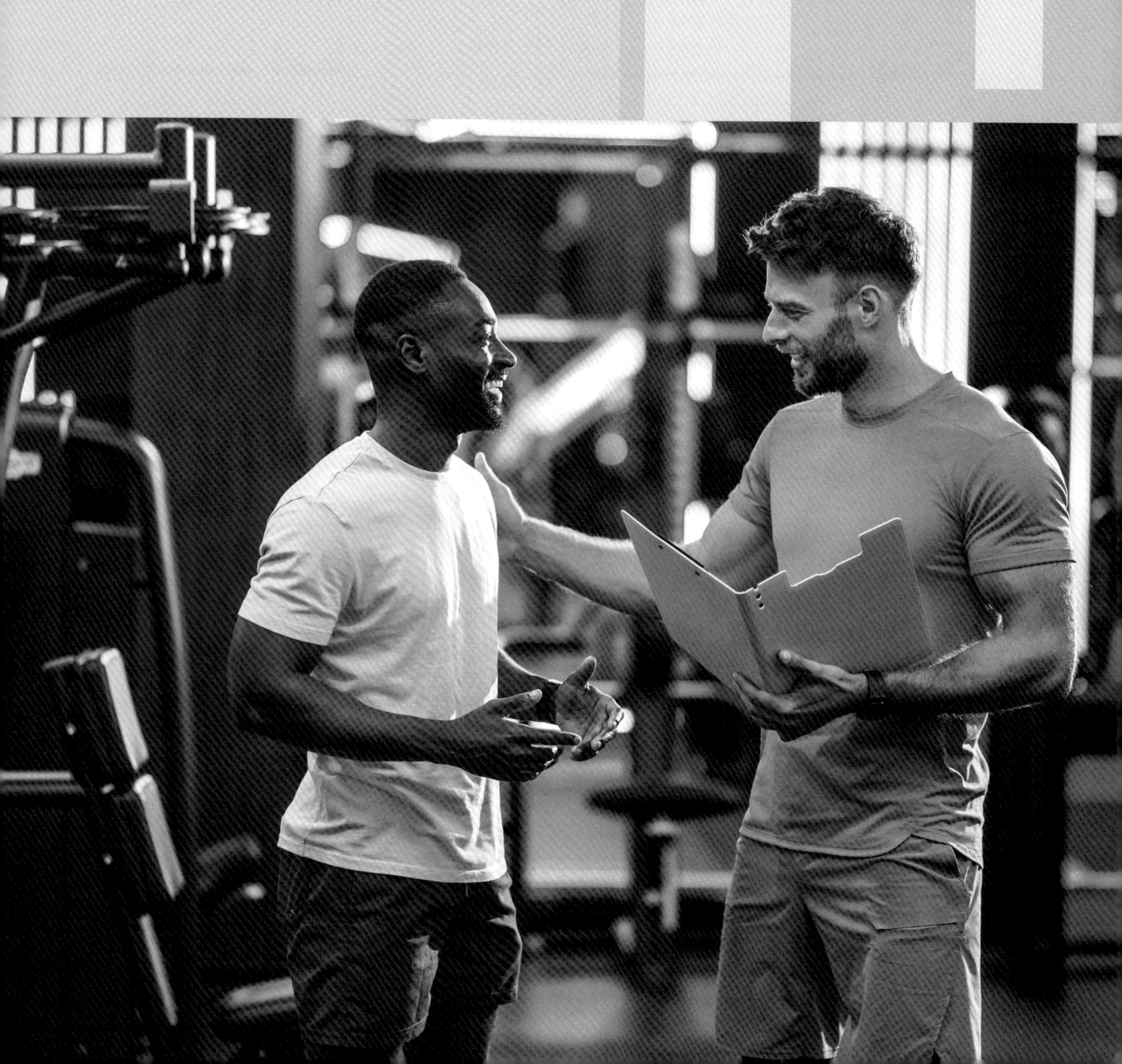
1

THE COMPLETE GUIDE TO

STRENGTH AND CONDITIONING TRAINING

PART **ONE**

CLIENT CONSULTATION

An initial consultation between an S&C practitioner and a client is important for gathering information and setting out boundaries.

Practitioners should tell potential clients during the very first consultation about their role and the limitations of what they can offer as a service within the boundaries of their expertise. This is known as a scope of practice and is essentially the roles and responsibilities the practitioner is qualified to undertake based on their skills and qualifications.

If the client is happy with the scope of practice, the practitioner can move on to the next three stages: carrying out health screening to establish whether it is appropriate to provide training to the client, performing needs analysis to identify and assess the specific demands of a client's sport or event or their desired outcomes, and goal setting.

To find out more about scope of practice, please visit UKSCA's official guidelines, which can be found here: uksca.org.uk/blog/11.

//Screening

The areas covered in this chapter are:

- An explanation of the consultation process specific to strength and conditioning programme planning

- Evidence-based pre-exercise health screening methods such as **PAR-Q** and PAR-Q+ for use by S&C practitioners

- Recognised **risk stratification** tools

- The relevance of data protection and client confidentiality

Introduction

Having completed the scope of practice discussion, you should carry out a process known as health screening. This will enable you to know if you are able to work with the client within your scope of practice or if referral to an appropriate professional is required. This chapter deals with the necessary information you are required to gather using evidence-based methods typically employed in the S&C environment.

Screening

Before a client starts an exercise programme it is important to identify if there are any health issues that might impact the programme. This process is known as preparticipation health screening (or just screening). The purpose of screening is to identify:

- If a client should receive medical clearance before undertaking an exercise programme
- If a client has a clinically significant disease(s), whether they may benefit from a medically supervised exercise programme
- If the client has medical conditions that may mean they cannot do the programme

HOW TO PERFORM SCREENINGS

There are several ways to perform screenings. Below, we look at two of the most common in S&C practice:

1) Pre-exercise questionnaires

As a screening tool for use by S&C practitioners, the American College of Sports Medicine (ACSM) recommend the use of the Physical Activity Readiness Questionnaire (PAR-Q), which was developed by the

PAR-Q AND YOU

Please read the following questions and answer each one honestly.	Yes	No
1 Has your doctor ever said that you have a heart condition and that you should only do physical activity recommended by a doctor?		
2 Do you feel pain in your chest when you do physical activity?		
3 In the past month, have you had chest pain while you were not doing physical activity?		
4 Do you lose your balance because of dizziness, or do you ever lose consciousness?		
5 Do you have a bone or joint problem that could be made worse by physical activity?		
6 Is your doctor currently prescribing drugs for your blood pressure or heart condition?		
7 Do you know of any other reason why you should not do physical activity?		

If you answered YES to one or more questions:
Talk to your doctor BEFORE you become more physically active or have a fitness appraisal. Discuss with your doctor which kinds of activities you wish to participate in.

If you answered NO to all questions you can be reasonably sure that you can:
- Start becoming much more physically active. Start slowly and build up gradually.
- Take part in a fitness appraisal. This is a good way to determine your basic fitness level. It is recommended that you have your blood pressure evaluated.

However, delay becoming active if:
- You are not feeling well because of temporary illness such as a cold or 'flu.
- You are or may be pregnant: talk to your doctor first.

Note: If your health changes so that you then answer YES to any of the above questions, tell your fitness or health professional. Ask whether you should change your physical activity plan.

'I have read, understood and completed this questionnaire. Any questions I had were answered to my full satisfaction.'

Name:	Signature of witness:
Signature:	Signature of parent/guardian:
Date:	*Note:* This physical activity clearance is valid for a maximum of 12 months from the date it is completed and becomes invalid if your condition changes so that you would answer YES to any of the seven questions.

Figure 1.1 Physical Activity Readiness Questionnaire (Source: Physical Activity Readiness Questionnaire (PAR-Q) 2002. Reprinted with permission from the Canadian Society for Exercise Physiology). (For a blank template, please visit: bloomsbury. com/uk/complete-guide-to-strength-and-conditioning-training-9781399421362)

RISK STRATIFICATION QUESTIONNAIRE

Client name:

D.O.B.:   /   /   Date:

Please answer the following questions to the best of your knowledge:	Yes	No
1 Has there been a heart attack or sudden death before age 55 (father, brother or son) or before age 65 (mother, sister or daughter) in your family?		
2 Are you a current smoker or quit within the previous six months?		
3 Have you been diagnosed with systolic blood pressure 140mmHg or above, or diastolic of 90mmHg or above, on at least two occasions?		
4 Do you have total serum cholesterol of more than 5.2mmol/L, or LDL more than 3.4mmol/L, or HDL less than 1.03mmol/L?		
5 Is your BMI 30kg/m^2 or above?		
6 Are you sedentary?		
7 Is your impaired fasting glucose 100mg/dL or more?		

Sub-total number of 'Yes' answers:

Is your HDL level above 1.6mmol/L? If yes, subtract 1 from the total above.

Total number of 'Yes' answers:

Low risk	**Moderate risk**	**High risk**
Men ≥45: women ≥55 and no more than 1 'Yes' answer	Men ≥45: women ≥55 and 2 or more 'Yes' answers	Those with known cardiovascular, pulmonary or metabolic disease

Figure 1.2 Example of a Risk Stratification Questionnaire (for a blank template, please visit: bloomsbury.com/uk/complete-guide-to-strength-and-conditioning-training-9781399421362)

Canadian Society for Exercise Physiology (*see* fig. 1.1). The current version, the PAR-Q+, is designed to identify potential symptoms of cardiovascular, pulmonary and metabolic disease, as well as other health conditions or injuries that might be aggravated by exercise. It also advises clients to seek medical approval prior to undertaking a programme of exercise where appropriate.

A PAR-Q should be completed before any other information is gathered. If no issues are identified, a programme of light to moderate exercise can be undertaken at an *intensity* relevant to the fitness level of the client. If any issues are identified that are beyond the scope of the practitioner's experience, the client should be referred to a suitably qualified colleague or health professional.

Note: PAR-Qs are only valid for a 12-month period.

2) Risk stratification

A more in-depth screening process can be used to identify those at increased risk of heart disease. This process is known as risk stratification. There are several methods of risk stratification that can be used. However, a typical example such as that in figure 1.2 places clients into one of three categories: low (or apparently healthy), moderate or high risk.

Note: Specific health information is required for this process.

The ACSM suggests those in the moderate category should not be prescribed any vigorous exercise unless medical approval is given and those in the high-risk category should not be allowed to exercise unless supervised by a qualified person, following medical approval.

Note: With all client information, the practitioner must respect confidentiality by ensuring safe storage and private access.

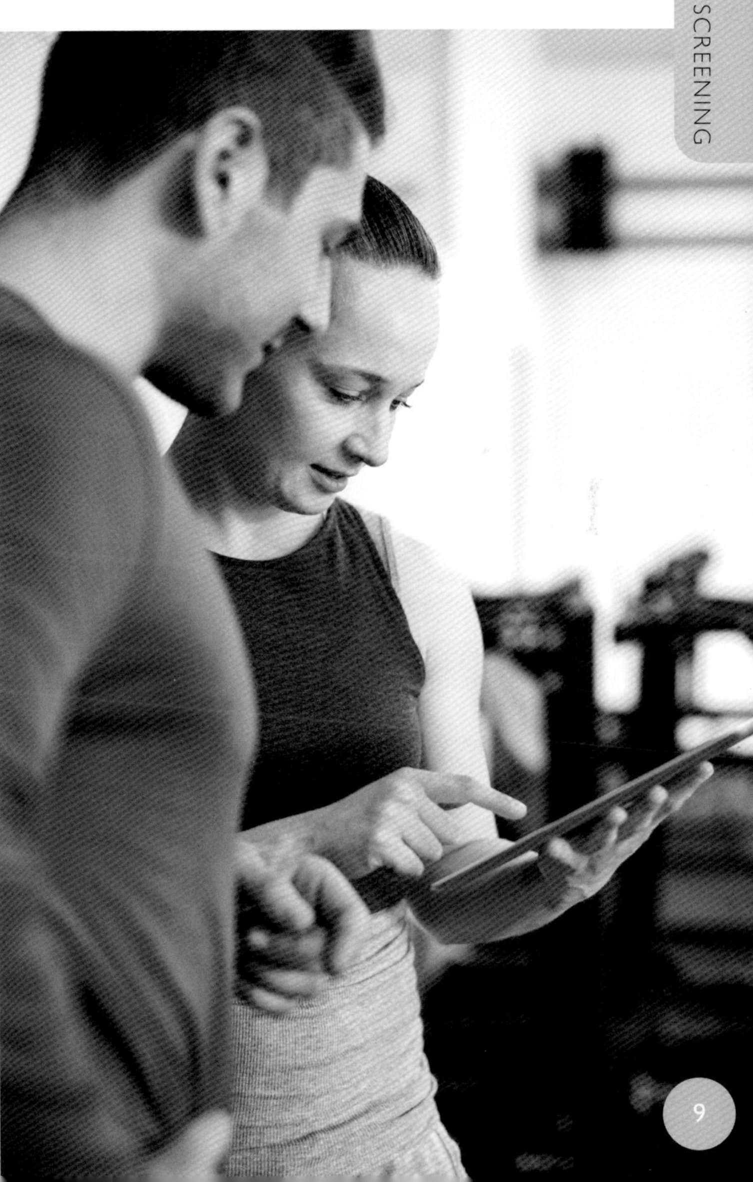

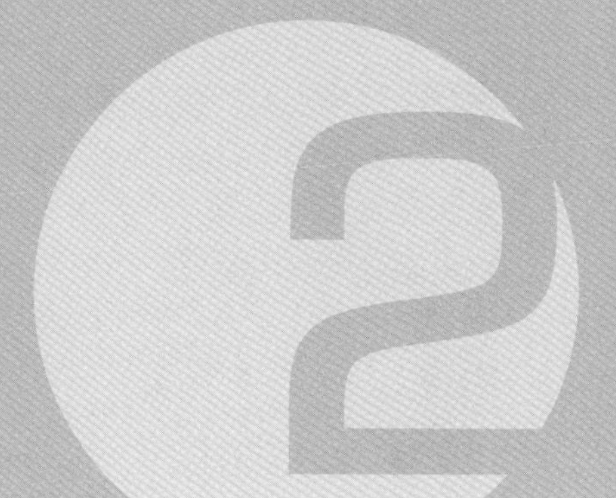

//Needs analysis

> **The areas covered in this chapter are:**
>
> - How to perform needs analysis, including:
>   - profiling of the client
>   - assessing the demands of the client's sport
>
> - How to assess training session considerations, for example using the STEPS model

Introduction

Once the health screening has been completed and the client has the all-clear to proceed, the S&C practitioner should carry out needs analysis before beginning to design the training programme. This involves an evaluation of:

1. Profiling of the client
2. The demands of the client's sport

This, in combination with baseline or normative testing (this refers to the first time any testing is carried out), allows the practitioner to identify a client's strengths and weaknesses in the fitness components that are important for the client in relation to their chosen sport. This information can then be used to develop training programmes that align with the client's goals with a focus on performance enhancement and injury prevention.

How to perform needs analysis

Needs analysis should be based on gathering information shown in table 2.1 to assess the profile of the client and the demands of their sport. The amount of information collected is dependent on many factors, such as the experience of the practitioner and the equipment available. It is advisable to collect as much information as possible so that you can design a tailored training programme.

Having completed the needs analysis process based on the client's needs and the demands of their sport or event you should now go on to consider any requirements related to training sessions that will be developed. It is possible that at this stage you will have an idea of the type of sessions you intend to develop. If not, then considerations can be made when you start to develop the sessions for the S&C programme.

Table 2.1	INFORMATION TYPICALLY COLLECTED IN NEEDS ANALYSIS			
CLIENT ANALYSIS				
Client status	**Training history**	**Training frequency (per week)**	**Training intensity**	**Training type**
• Beginner • Intermediate • Advanced	• Length of training time • Injury history and current status	• Number and type of sessions per week	• Use %HRmax, RPE, %1RM etc.	• Sprint, endurance, strength, power, stability, *plyometrics* etc.
SPORT/EVENT ANALYSIS				
Sport details	**Kinematics**	**An/aerobic**	**Power**	**Muscular**
• Competition schedule • Playing surface • Level (i.e. professional or amateur) • Sport position • Kicking, running, throwing? • Type of equipment used	• Sprinting, jogging, walking (linear, lateral) • Bending, twisting, jumping (unilateral or bilateral)	• Average and maximum *heart rate* (HR), VO_2max, average VO_2, total distance, lactate threshold, *anaerobic power*, repeat sprints, total jumps, number of direction changes	• Force-*velocity* characteristics (i.e. peak force, rate of force development, ground contact time, peak and average power, peak velocity, time to peak velocity)	• Major muscles recruited • Strength, power, hypertrophy, and *muscular endurance* in terms of priority • Common injury sites and causative factors (impact, repetition etc.)

Training session considerations

Once the client and sport/event analysis has been completed, the practitioner must identify specific requirements of the planned training sessions.

A common method to ensure considerations are made during the planning process is to use the STEPS (space, time/task, equipment, people/players, specificity) model. An example of how to use the STEPS model to gather session information is shown in table 2.2.

The STEPS information gathering can be completed in a variety of ways. For example, it may be written and stored to reflect on after the training or it may be planned by a group of other professionals within planning meetings, such as coaches, sports scientists and medics or by parents or guardians. This form of support and input from other people may contribute to the development of the client, by

Table 2.2	STEPS MODEL FOR SESSION INFORMATION GATHERING
Steps	**Category information**
Space	• What space is required for the desired training session? • Are outdoor or indoor facilities required? • Is the space shared, so may also be occupied by other practitioners/users/clients?
Time/task	• How much time is available/required for the training session/drill? • Are there external factors that may impact time availability (e.g. another group or class using the space)?
Equipment	• What equipment is needed to complete the training session/drill? • Is the equipment available for use? Is it shared equipment that may be used by others? • Does the client have familiarity with and know how to use the equipment? Delivering a tutorial on how to use equipment will need to be considered within the 'time' section.
People/players	• How many people/clients will take part in the training session/drill? • Is the training/drill design appropriate for the number of people/clients? • What are the training competencies/experience of the clients? • Do all or some of the people require specific assistance or support to participate in the training session and will this be available to them?
Specificity	• What other factors need to be considered for the training session/drill to be a success? • How do all the above considerations fit in with the aims of the training session? • Does the drill design deliver on the expected aims? • Are additional support practitioners required to assist with delivery?

providing input from a range of professionals with specific areas of expertise.

When you carry out needs analysis you should also consider factors such as client availability and their ability to travel to training sessions. (A template that uses the STEPs model to help you identify training session considerations and can be used can be found in Appendix 1).

By completing the needs analysis, you should have gathered enough information to be able to develop an S&C training programme. However, before you do this you need to agree goals with the client to inform the development. You therefore need to go to the next stage of the S&C road map, which is goal setting.

Take-home messages

- If it is appropriate to continue, needs analysis should be completed. The information it provides will form the foundation for the creation of a training programme.

- The STEPS model can provide a useful framework for gathering the information required for the training session considerations and for designing programmes and training drills.

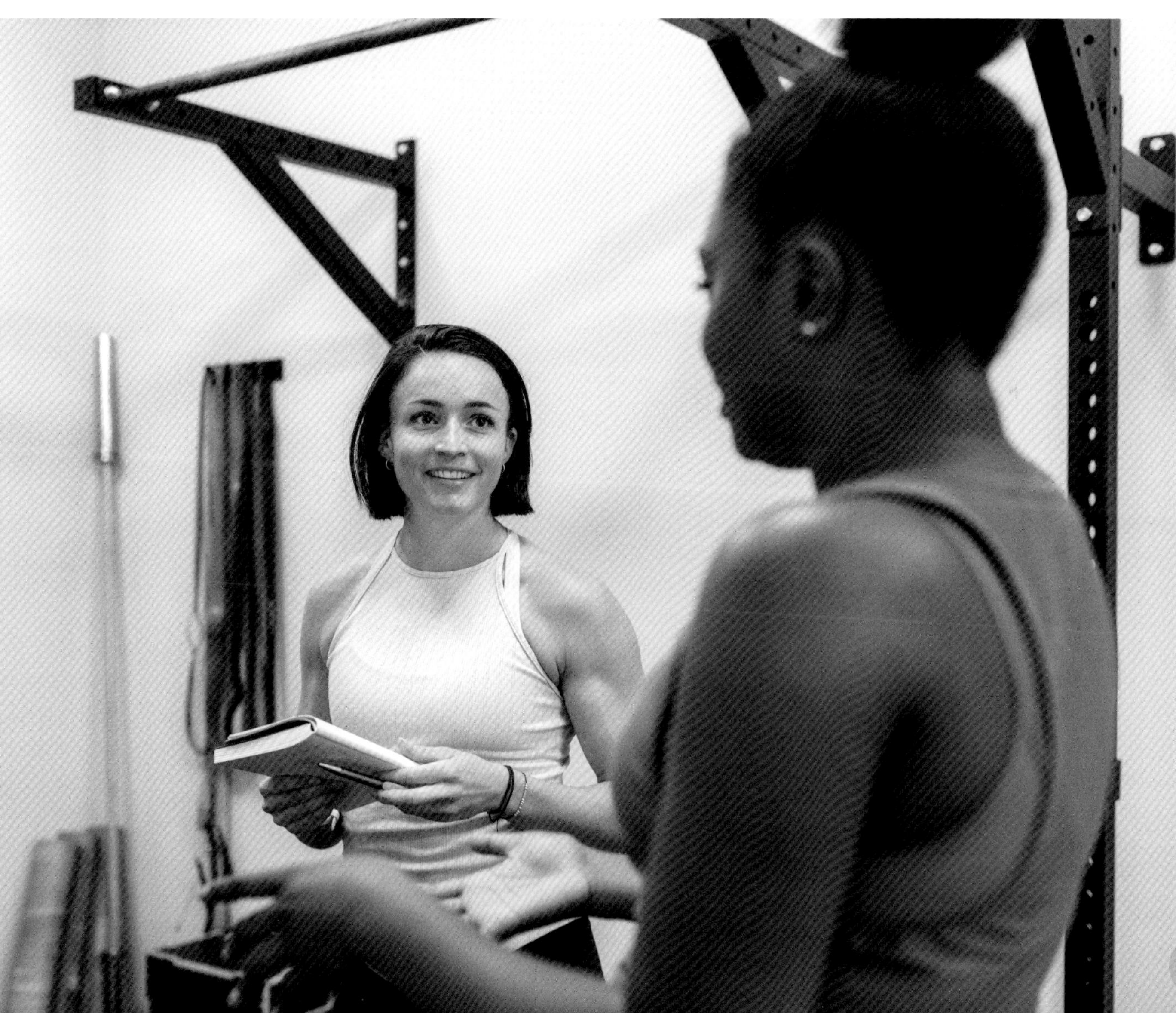

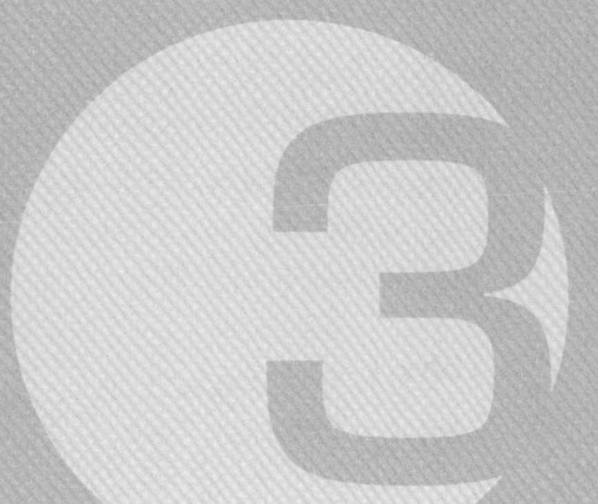

//Goal setting

The areas covered in this chapter are:

- Consulting with the client, focusing on results, goals, client needs and changing circumstances

- Understanding client expectations and aspirations within the training environment

- Goal setting by assessing short-, medium- and long-term goals

- Setting SMART goals linked to a client's needs, wants and motivators

- Classifying goals according to their goal objective, which can be broken down to process, performance and *outcome goals*

- Identifying and overcoming training *barriers*

- The use of individual performance plans within S&C

Introduction

Having completed the needs analysis and training session considerations, you should have a discussion with the client to explore and agree what they want to achieve. The process of setting goals can help to maintain motivation and direction by defining potential objectives. Within an S&C environment it is important to understand the purpose of goal setting and established processes that are used. This chapter deals with a systematic approach to goal setting that can help to identify barriers that clients may have to training and how to overcome them. The chapter also shows how to use more in-depth methods that are more specific to the client and their chosen sport.

Goal setting

Goal setting can be thought of as the overall process whereby specific performance targets are identified and pursued in order to achieve success or an end-state. This is often done to help motivate and improve the self-confidence of the client with a view to improving performance. Goal Setting Theory was first proposed by Locke and Latham as a motivational technique to

Client name:	Practitioner name:	Date: / /
Client – *please write down any goals that you would like to achieve in the …*	**Agreed goals**	
Short term: Take part in S&C sessions.	**Process:** Enrol in twice-weekly sessions for the first month, increasing to three sessions. **Performance:** Keep a training log to track the number of completed sessions. **Outcome:** Planned sessions have become an integral part of the weekly routine.	
Medium term: Lose body fat and gain strength.	**Process:** Complete weekly food diaries while maintaining training logs. **Performance:** Achieve an overall body fat reduction of 2–3% and an increase in overall strength of 5–10%. **Outcome:** To implement consistent dietary changes.	
Long term: Maintain fat loss and strength gain.	**Process:** To modify the training programme at regular intervals to keep the client engaged. **Performance:** Set new targets based on revised goals. **Outcome:** Changes to exercise and dietary behaviours become habitual.	

Practitioner – Identify how you will make the programme **SMART**

- *Specific:* Weight loss and strength gain.

- *Measurable:* Short- and long-term weight loss target in kg and strength gain in RM weight.

- *Achievable:* Increase or decrease based on weekly measurement.

- *Relevant:* In line with current guidelines.

- *Time-bound:* Weekly for the short term, leading to a 30-week medium-term goal with maintenance for the longer term.

Barriers: *Please write down any barriers to taking part in exercise that you can think of:* Worried about my ability. Difficulty getting to sessions.	**Solutions:** Introduce the client to a 'buddy' (another client in a similar position). Explore the possibility of sharing transport.

Figure 3.1 Sample goal setting questionnaire

provide structure for a training programme. In order to simplify the goal setting process, a questionnaire such as that in figure 3.1 can be used. The example is that of a client who has written down suggested short-, medium- and long-term goals.

The first step in the goal setting process would be to agree goals with the client. As can be seen on the questionnaire, these can be organised as short-, medium- and long-term periods.

- **Short term** – These goals are typically set over a period of only a few weeks.
- **Medium term** – These goals are usually set over a period of a few months.
- **Long term** – These goals are set over a longer period of six months to one year but can extend over several years.

GOAL OBJECTIVES

Once short-, medium- and long-term goals have been established and agreed they can be classified in terms of the goal objective. These categories are process, performance and outcome goals, as explained below:

- **Process goals** – This type of goal relates to objectives such as the technique of the client or the strategy employed that underpins performance. For example, development of leg strength to improve running speed.
- **Performance goals** – This relates to discreet standards irrespective of other variables. Performance goals are often expressed in terms of personal achievement or numerical value. For example, a specific time target for a 100-metre sprint. Personal achievement can also be compared to previous performances.
- **Outcome goals** – This type of goal is concerned with the end result and can also be compared to other individuals. For example, winning a particular tournament or event.

Goal setting is not an exact science, so to help you develop and agree goals with the client, a common tool known as the SMART model can be used. The acronym SMART stands for specific, measurable, achievable, relevant and time-bound. This can help you to focus on specific elements of each goal.

Specific – It is important that goals are specific to what the client wants to achieve. For example, a goal of 'increasing *aerobic fitness*' could be made more specific if it was 'to be able to complete a 5km Parkrun'.

Measurable – As goals should be evaluated regularly, it is important that you are able to measure them. For example, this could be by measuring heart rate at a specific running speed to see it there is a decrease over a period of weeks, which would indicate an improvement in aerobic fitness.

Achievable – For many clients, failure to achieve a goal can negatively impact motivation. Try to set goals that are more likely to be reached, as this has been shown to positively impact confidence and motivation.

Relevant – Any goals should align with the event/ sport and the aspirations of the client. For example, focus on *aerobic* endurance to improve a 5km Parkrun time.

Time-bound – It is widely acknowledged that setting time frames in which to achieve goals can help to motivate clients as well as enable the tracking of progress. Typical time frames used are short-, medium- or long-term, as described previously.

Barriers to achieving goals

Once you have agreed and recorded the client's SMART goals it is then important to consider any barriers to achieving the goals that the client may have. Reasons for not adhering to a training programme are known as training barriers. Any barrier that cannot be overcome, such as illness and accidents, are known as real barriers whereas those that can be overcome by using appropriate strategies are known as perceived barriers. Solutions to barriers are known as facilitators or motivators. By identifying a client's barriers, appropriate strategies can be used to help overcome them, as shown in table 3.1.

If your client is involved with a sport or event and has specific goals that relate to this then you can carry out a more detailed process by creating an individual performance plan (IPP), which is commonly used in sporting environments.

Individual performance plan

An individual performance plan (IPP), also known as an individual development plan, is essentially a more detailed process of goal setting that can help develop clients. An IPP usually documents process and performance goals in areas such as physiological, technical, tactical and psychological. Although an IPP can be used for those with general fitness goals, they are more often used for clients with specific performance goals. A typical IPP for a football player can be seen in figure 3.2.

IPPs should be completed at the start of any training programme and be specific to the client. Once goals have been established, each area of the IPP should be developed in order to identify areas that the client should focus on. For example, to identify areas for development of technical skills for football players, a template such as that in figure 3.3 could be used.

An additional example to identify areas for development for a client's movement competency can be viewed in figure 3.4. Once areas for development have been identified and transferred to the IPP, an action plan can then be completed in consultation with the client.

Table 3.1	PERCEIVED BARRIERS AND POTENTIAL SOLUTIONS
Perceived barrier	**Potential solutions**
Time commitments	Design time management strategies, such as the use of a diary for planning.
Injury	Depending on the injury, other parts of the body can still be trained. Non-impact exercise such as swimming could be prescribed.
Cost – facility or equipment	Design training activities that can be done at home. Any clothing can be adapted.
Access – getting to a facility	Consider bus routes. Otherwise, design home-based or outdoor activities.
Age	All fitness levels are relevant. Training can be age/ability specific.
Lack of enjoyment	Use exercise variety and reinforce goals.

These example templates use a subjective ranking scale to rate various aspects of technical performance. If the assessment involves more than one person, then consultation should take place to establish standardisation prior to the assessment. In the example used, three areas have been identified that are the weakest in terms of the technical development score. These have been transferred to the IPP and an agreed action plan has been developed. The same process can also be used for the other areas of the IPP.

At this point you should have completed part 1 of the S&C road map and you should now be ready to develop your client's S&C programme. Part 2 of the

| Athlete name: Player 1 | Practitioner: Team manager | Date: xx/xx/xxxx |
| Playing position/event: Attacking midfielder – football | | Review date: xx/xx/xxxx |

Agreed performance goals:

- To improve metabolic capacity to be more successful in completing position-specific physical demands.
- To improve non-dominant foot use.
- To develop a playing style that complements the tactical model of the team.
- To bring positive energy and a winning mindset to the team.

	Areas for development	Action plan
Physiological	• Develop aerobic capacity. • Improve repeated sprint ability. • Improve ability to shield/protect the ball.	• Incorporate HIIT drills into the training plan to develop the aerobic energy system. • Perform repeated sprints with short rest intervals within the training microcycle. • Commit to an S&C training programme to increase force and power outputs.
Technical	• Left foot long passing. • Left foot crossing. • Closing down.	• Incorporate left foot long balls into technical sessions and inform the coach. • Include extra training sessions to work with a defensive coach on closing players down.
Tactical	• Understand the tactical requirements of my playing position within the team's specific game model. • Develop an understanding of how and when to press the opposition to win the ball in advanced positions on the pitch.	• Learn the game model within tactically focused training drills that provide position-specific information within a controlled environment. • Learn from the technical coaches within drills how to analyse opposition positioning and how to exploit this during a press.
Psychological	• Learn to overcome nerves and pressure so it does not negatively impact performance. • Understand how my actions and mindset can impact those of my teammates.	• Learn how to use techniques such as self-talk to control negative thoughts and use them to fuel performance. • Work closely with the team psychologist to better understand how I can positively impact the performances of my teammates.

Additional comments:

Figure 3.2 Example individual performance plan (for a blank template, please visit: bloomsbury.com/uk/complete-guide-to-strength-and-conditioning-training-9781399421362)

Technique	Score												Areas for IPP
	0	1	2	3	4	5	6	7	8	9	10	10+	
Control													
Feet										x			
Knee					x								
Chest							x						
Head								x					
Running									x				
Dribbling													
Right foot										x			
Left foot			x										
Passing short													
Right foot										x			
Left foot					x								
Passing long													
Right foot								x					Left foot long passing
Left foot		x											
Crossing													
Right foot										x			Left foot crossing
Left foot		x											
Shooting/finishing													
Right foot											x		
Left foot				x									
Heading													
Defending							x						
Attacking									x				
Defending													
Tackling					x								Closing down players
Prevent players turning					x								
Closing down players			x										

Figure 3.3 Example technical development template (for a blank template, please visit: bloomsbury.com/uk/complete-guide-to-strength-and-conditioning-training-9781399421362)

Technique	Score												Areas for IPP
	0	1	2	3	4	5	6	7	8	9	10	10+	
Basic movement patterns													
Run										x			
Jump – bilateral, unilateral, multiplanar					x								
Land – bilateral, unilateral, multiplanar							x						
Skip								x					
Hop									x				
Roll		x											Develop roll technique
Rotate							x						
Balance (static and dynamic)										x			
Weight transfer											x		
Brace									x				
Fundamental movement patterns													
Animal movements – crawls										x			
Squat and lunge				x									
Hip hinge			x										Develop hip hinge
Push (vertical and horizontal)								x					
Pull (vertical and horizontal)								x					
Brace (rotation and antirotation)							x						
Hang/climb						x							
Jumping and landing mechanics													
Bilateral landing										x			
Unilateral landing					x								
Multiplanar landing					x								
Bilateral jumping										x			
Unilateral jumping						x							
Plyometrics			x										Introduce plyo in training
Acceleration, deceleration, change of direction (COD)													
Running gait								x					
Start variation – forwards, cross/drop step						x							
COD – cutting, swerving, 45 degrees, 90 degrees, 180 degrees						x							

Figure 3.4 Example movement competency development template (for a blank template, please visit: bloomsbury.com/uk/complete-guide-to-strength-and-conditioning-training-9781399421362)

road map aims to provide you with the guidance to do this regardless of the goals of the client.

> **Take-home messages**
>
> - It is important to identify and agree short-, medium- and long-term process and performance goals that lead to outcome goals and ensure that these take account of barriers.
>
> - Create performance targets that are specific, measurable, achievable, realistic and time-bound, and revise performance targets in line with regular review processes.
>
> - Use individual performance plans to further develop the client.

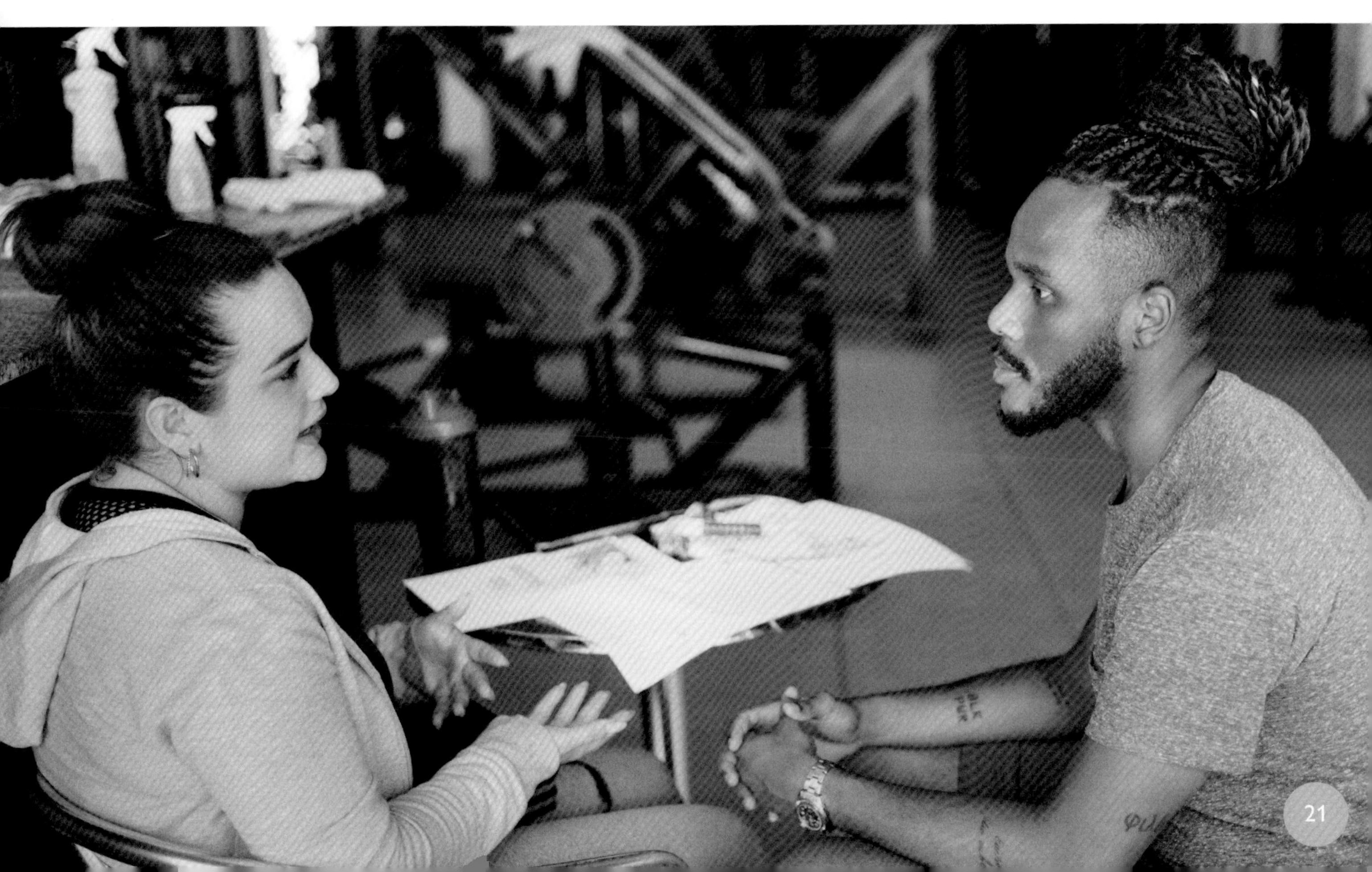

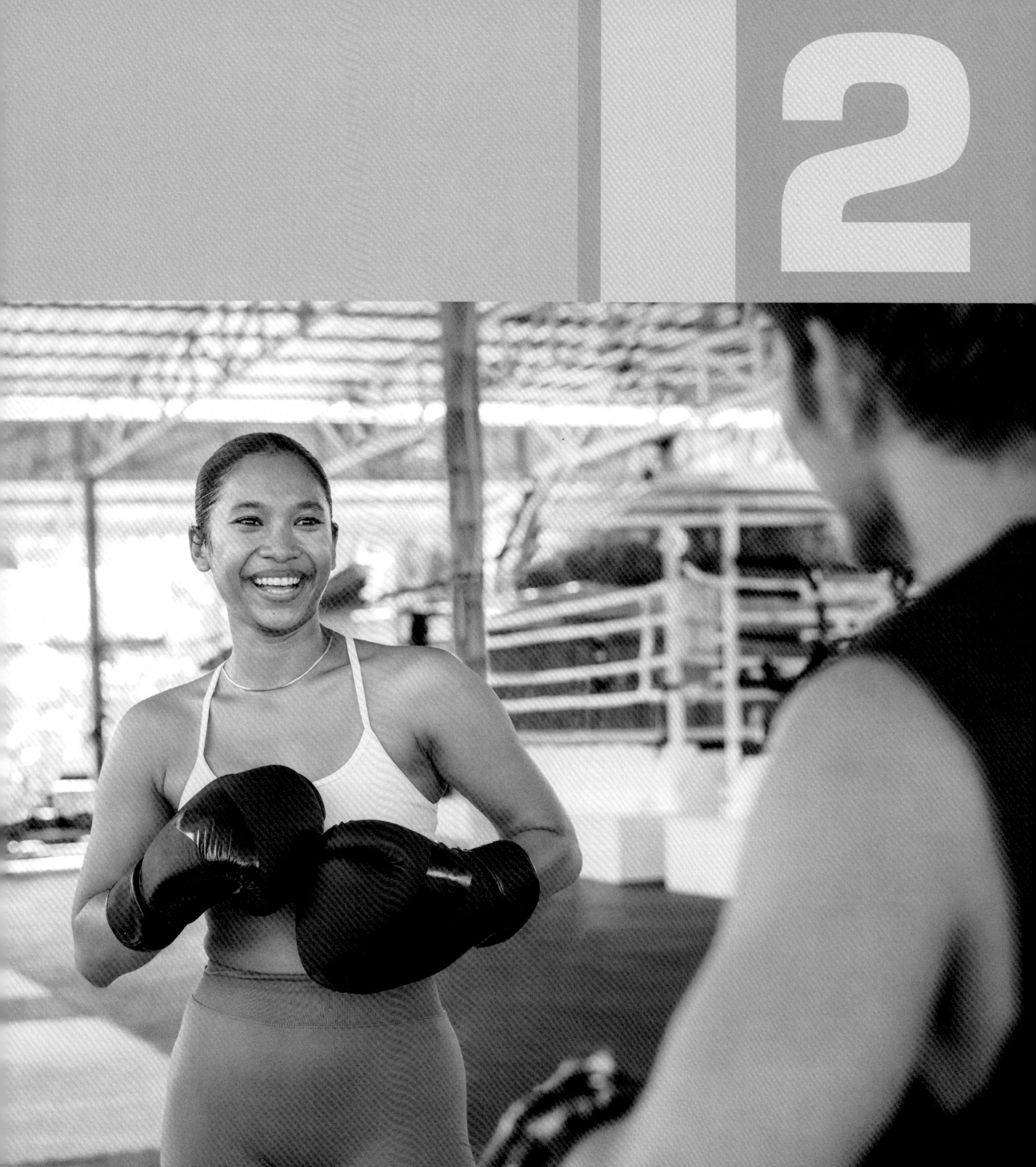

2

PART **TWO**

THE FUNDAMENTALS OF STRENGTH AND CONDITIONING

In part 1, we discussed the initial consultation between the S&C practitioner and the client, in which a needs analysis and goal setting process was undertaken. Once this has been completed, the practitioner can move on to designing an appropriate training programme that considers the information gathered.

This can be a complex process, so in this part we'll begin by talking through the components and principles of fitness that are the fundamentals of any S&C training programme. The rest of the chapters in this part go on to examine these in depth one by one, providing information on how to train them. We then go on to provide sample programmes for each component of fitness. As the range of potential clients is vast in terms of age, sex, ability, goals etc., we have selected a variety of clients from a range of typical scenarios to help you in this process. You will find all of these programmes in Appendix 2.

Part 3 covers how to test each of these components, and then part 4 provides detailed general training strategies. Taken together, these three parts will enable you to create programmes relevant to different components of fitness and suitable for different sports.

CREATING AN S&C PROGRAMME

Creating an S&C programme is a multifaceted process, and an S&C practitioner should consider a wide range of factors that may influence programme design and delivery. For example, the client's age, injury history, sport, S&C experience, competition level, accessibility to training and other commitments such as work and family requirements all must be considered for an S&C programme to be successfully delivered.

Further to this, each client will have different goals and performance areas compared to other clients competing in the same sport. Therefore, a one-size-fits-all guide to creating S&C programmes cannot be justified and would not provide an opportunity for clients to optimally develop. We have provided some example training programmes (see Appendix 2) for each component of fitness. These outline some possible ways that training programmes can be designed to elicit development of those components of fitness. These programmes are designed to provide a more holistic approach to client physical development, particularly if they compete in a sport that relies on the interaction and use of multiple components of fitness.

The components and principles of fitness

4

The areas covered in this chapter are:

- The components of fitness that are typically targeted for development by S&C practitioners

- The general principles of fitness that can help S&C practitioners when designing training programmes

Introduction

One of the most difficult tasks for the practitioner is deciding what to include in an S&C training programme. The easiest way to do this is to consider which components of fitness are relevant to the goals of the client, so that they can be assessed and developed. However, the practitioner should first understand what these components are. Therefore, this chapter will identify and describe components of fitness with examples across a range of sports and events that prioritise the importance of each component.

So, what are the components of fitness? Let's find out.

Components of fitness

Fitness is a multifaceted construct that is made up of health-related components known as components of fitness. Each component can be developed separately or in conjunction with other components.

What these components are can vary depending on the source used and the definition of 'fitness' itself.

The ACSM describes health-related physical fitness as an ability to perform daily activities with vigour and the demonstration of traits and capacities that are associated with a low risk of premature development of hypokinetic diseases.

When designing S&C programmes, it is helpful to consider the range of components of fitness that could be targeted for improvement.

We will examine each of these in more detail in chapters 5 to 13, but below is a brief overview of each component.

AEROBIC OR CARDIOVASCULAR ENDURANCE

Cardiovascular endurance (also known as *aerobic capacity*) can be described as the ability of the heart and lungs to deliver oxygen to the working muscles and for the muscles to use this oxygen to generate work.

ANAEROBIC ENDURANCE

This refers to the ability to maintain high-intensity effort without relying on oxygen as the main *energy*

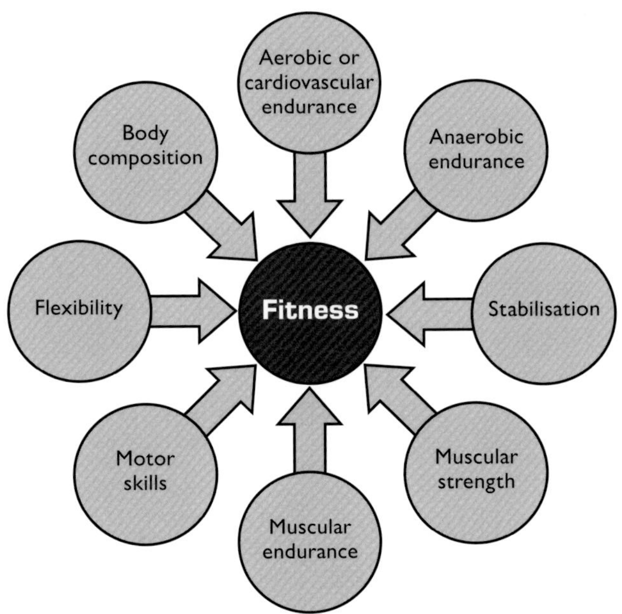

Figure 4.1 Components of fitness

source. The *anaerobic* system contributes to energy production when the aerobic system can no longer supply the required energy for the intensity of activity being performed. This can be for a sustained period or over repeated bouts.

STABILISATION

The term stabilisation is often used interchangeably with core *stability*, which refers to the ability to control the position and motion of the trunk over the pelvis and legs to facilitate force transfer between the upper and lower extremities (i.e. in gross motor tasks). This requires an ability to provide a stable base during a range of movements. Stabilisation is a component of fitness that is required for all clients regardless of their participation in sport or athletic events.

MUSCULAR STRENGTH

The term *muscular strength* can be thought of as the maximum amount of force that a muscle or muscle group can generate and is associated with resistance training that uses relatively high intensity and low repetitions.

MUSCULAR ENDURANCE

This is the ability of a muscle or muscle group to perform repeated *contractions* against a resistance for a period of time and is associated with resistance training that uses relatively low intensity and high repetitions.

MOTOR SKILLS

Motor skills is an umbrella term referring to various components that contribute to performing physical actions. The components of motor skills include:

- **Speed** – The ability to move quickly from one point to another. It can be improved through muscle coordination, efficient body movement, core strength and flexibility.
- **Power** – A combination of strength and speed. It can be developed through plyometric and resistance training.
- **Agility** – The ability to change direction at speed in response to an external stimulus.
- **Balance** – The ability to always maintain equilibrium. The brain receives balance information from various sources: *proprioception*, the *vestibular system* and vision.
- **Coordination** – The ability to move the limbs precisely in a particular direction.

FLEXIBILITY

This can be thought of as the ability to move a joint through a range of motion using forces that act on a joint, such as gravity or assisted stretching. This shouldn't be confused with the term mobility, which is related to the range of motion achievable by active muscle recruitment.

BODY COMPOSITION

This refers to the amount and relative proportions of fat mass and fat-free mass (lean *tissue*) in an individual.

SPORT-SPECIFIC COMPONENTS OF FITNESS

Different sports draw on different components of fitness. For example, a snooker player has very different components of fitness requirements to a high jumper, as shown in figure 4.2.

Once you have gathered all of the client information and determined what the goals of the S&C programme are, you need to identify what you think would be the main components of fitness that are relevant to the client's goals. A client may have goals that link to a particular sport or event, or they may just have general fitness goals. In the latter case, you would need to discuss which components of fitness they would like to develop. To help you do this, figure 4.2 provides an overview of a range of sports and events and what would be considered the main components of fitness related to each one. You will see that some have multiple components that are considered important. We call these hybrid sports or events.

	Cardio	Muscular strength	Muscular endurance	Flex	Balance	Speed	Agility	Power
Snooker				✔	✔			
Rugby	✔	✔	✔	✔	✔	✔	✔	✔
Sprinting		✔		✔	✔	✔		✔
Sprint cycle		✔				✔		✔
Netball	✔	✔	✔	✔		✔	✔	✔
Football	✔	✔	✔	✔	✔	✔	✔	✔
Tennis	✔	✔	✔	✔	✔	✔	✔	✔
High jump		✔			✔		✔	✔
800m swim	✔		✔	✔				✔
Recreational running	✔		✔			✔		
Body toning		✔	✔					

Figure 4.2 Main components of fitness for a range of sports and events

Principles of fitness

When designing an S&C programme, it can be useful to consider fundamental factors that can affect physiological adaptation and therefore the outcome and potentially the success of the programme. These factors are called principles of fitness and include:

SPECIFICITY

This refers to the way in which the body can adapt to the demands of the types of exercise performed. For example, type 1 muscle fibres (*see* p. 45) will adapt to endurance training, while type 2 muscle fibres (*see* p. 45) will adapt to more intense strength or explosive training. Although a somewhat controversial area, adaptation to the type (or specificity) of the training may occur. For example, a client who trains predominantly on a treadmill will become better at using the treadmill even though there will be a transfer of fitness to other forms of cardio-type exercise. This is referred to by the ACSM as the 'specificity principle', which states that the physiological adaptations to exercise are specific to the type of exercise performed.

OVERLOAD

The principle of overload suggests that exercise below a minimum intensity will not result in physiological adaptation. For adaptation to occur, overload must be achieved. Overload can be described as placing a greater stress or load on the body than it is usually accustomed to. If this occurs on a regular basis, the body can undergo physical changes to adapt to the greater workload. There are many ways in which overload can be achieved. For example, lever length, speed, resistance and gravity are examples of variables that can be manipulated to achieve overload.

PROGRESSION

S&C training programmes should progress in terms of workload otherwise adaptation will not occur.

Once the body has adapted to a specific workload, it will not adapt any further. This is often referred to as staleness or plateau. Progressive overload can be described as the systematic increase of a combination of frequency, volume and intensity to elicit adaptation. The rate of progression can be affected by various factors:

- **Fitness level** – Less fit clients generally progress fitness components at a faster rate than fitter clients.
- **Experience** – A client with training experience can often progress their training workload at a faster rate than those with no experience.
- **Injury** – An injury to a specific site can reverse any gains previously made. It is important to remember that the rest of the body may be trained to prevent total body reversibility.
- **Environment** – The environment can affect progression in several ways. For example, exposure to changes in altitude and extreme temperatures can impact the adaptation of the body or system to training.

REGRESSION (REVERSIBILITY)

It is possible for specific fitness components to diminish within 2 weeks of cessation of exercise. This principle is known as regression. For example, although the loss of muscular strength and aerobic endurance is very much dependent on the client, in general, muscular strength can diminish after about 3–4 weeks whereas aerobic endurance can diminish after about 2 weeks.

INDIVIDUALITY

Individuals progress at different rates, so it is important that frequency, volume and intensity are manipulated to suit the client. In any S&C programme, progression should be encouraged when the client can cope with the current workload.

RECOVERY TIME

Recovery time is crucial to the success of any S&C programme. Rest and active recovery periods are typical strategies used. Clients should be monitored frequently for signs of exhaustion and *overtraining*, such as a drop in performance, increase in *resting heart rate* and regular illness. Recovery of the muscular, cardiovascular and *neural* systems depends on many factors, such as the intensity of the training session, client fitness levels, age, gender, psychological factors and dietary interventions. As a general guideline, clients should be given a 24–48-hour recovery period following a bout of strenuous exercise.

Note: Manipulation of training variables and periodisation will be covered in more detail in chapter 24.

Take-home messages

- Practitioners should understand and use the components and principles of fitness as the foundations of strength and conditioning training.

- The manipulation of the principles of fitness within training programmes will determine how each component of fitness is developed.

- It is important to understand which components of fitness are required for different sports and individuals when developing training programmes.

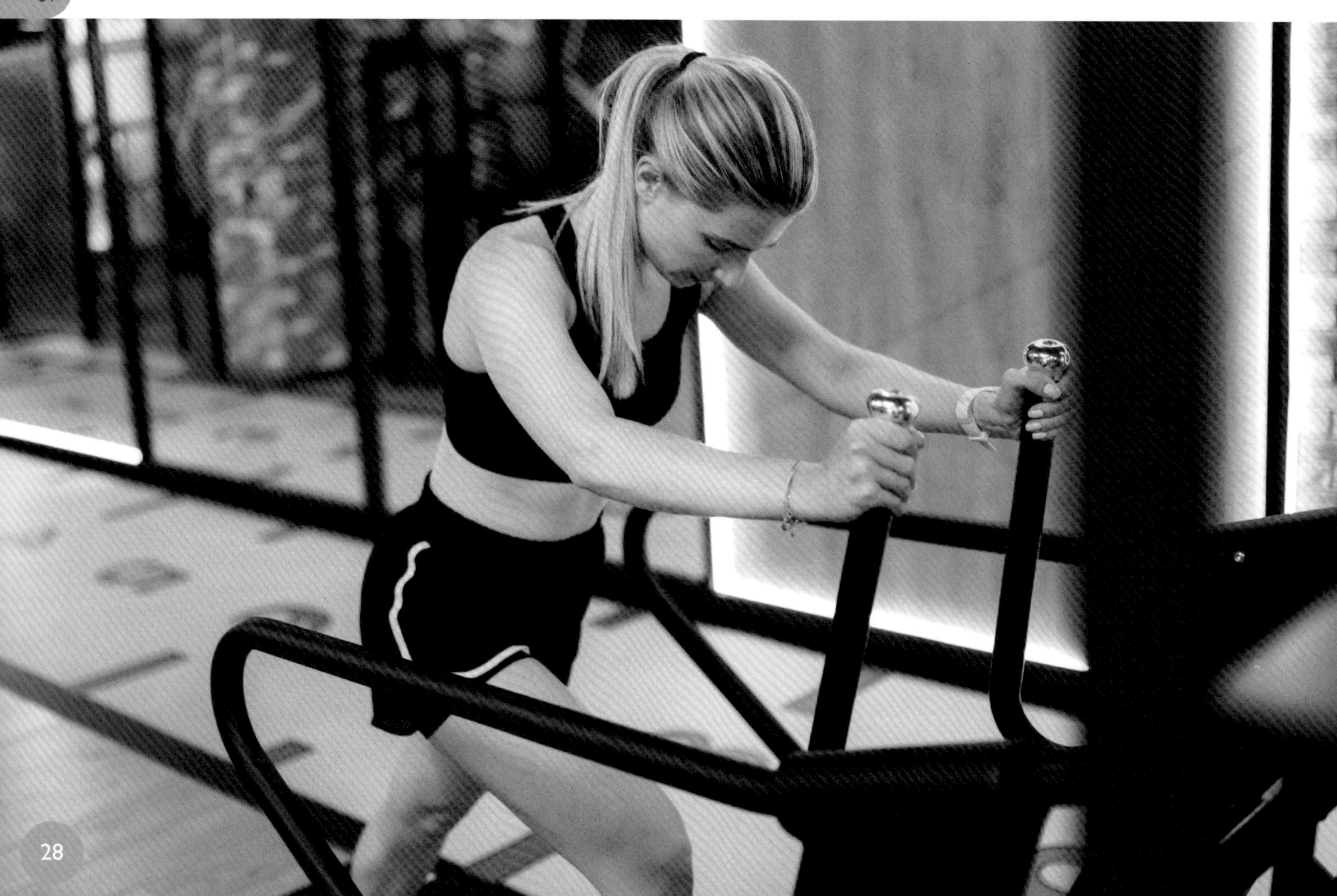

//Aerobic endurance 5

The areas covered in this chapter are:

- What aerobic endurance is and how the body responds and adapts to aerobic training

- What factors can affect adaptations

- Suitable training methods

- The training variables related to the aerobic system

Introduction

Now that we've explored the components and principles of fitness, it's time to move on to investigate different *energy systems* and performance characteristics and how they can be developed and trained through the manipulation of the components and principles of fitness.

What is aerobic endurance?

Aerobic endurance is also known as cardiovascular endurance or aerobic capacity and refers to the ability of the heart, lungs and associated vessels to deliver oxygen to working muscles (and subsequently for the muscles to use this oxygen to generate work output). The aerobic energy system utilises fats and *carbohydrate* (using carbs in the form of glucose is known as aerobic glycolysis) for the purpose of producing *adenosine*

triphosphate (ATP) in the presence of oxygen to supply the demand for energy.

At rest, approximately 70% of ATP is provided by fats and 30% from carbohydrates. As intensity increases, more oxygen must be transported to the working muscles to produce the required energy with a shift in preference to carbohydrate for ATP provision. If the intensity remains at submaximal capability the aerobic system should provide enough energy to cope with the demand. If the intensity increases beyond the maximum capability of the aerobic system, the extra demand for energy must be provided by the anaerobic system (which we explore in chapter 6).

Aerobic (or cardiovascular) fitness can be measured directly by the volume of oxygen taken into the body, transported and utilised every minute by each kilogramme of the body, and is known as VO_2. The maximum amount of oxygen an individual can transport

"

and use in 1 minute at sea level is known as VO_2max. The unit of measurement for VO_2max is $mlO_2.kg^{-1}min^{-1}$ (relative to bodyweight).

The aerobic energy system can be developed by training at ranges from approximately 50 to 70% of VO_2max. Intensity levels below 100% VO_2max can be referred to as aerobic-type training and although related to events that last more than 90 seconds, aerobic training is associated with high-volume sessions. When training at this level, energy (from ATP) comes predominantly from aerobic glycolysis and fat.

Adaptations to aerobic training

There are various adaptations that can occur as a result of regular aerobic training. Typical adaptations include the following:

- **Blood** – Increases in plasma volume and *haemoglobin* (the iron-containing oxygen-transport metalloprotein in the red blood cells) can occur, which may enhance oxygen delivery during exercise.
- **Heart** – Left ventricle cavity size and thickening of the wall can lead to an increase in *stroke volume* and *cardiac output*, which in turn leads to increased oxygen delivery and thermoregulatory ability (these are known as central adaptations).
- **Capillaries** – Peripheral adaptations include increased *capillary* density, which, along with an increased number and size of *mitochondria* and aerobic *enzymes*, can increase the amount of oxygen extracted from the blood.
- **Fibres** – *Slow twitch* type 1 muscle fibres can potentially increase in size and *fast twitch* type 2b muscle fibres can be converted to more fatigue-resistant fast twitch type 2a fibres. The net result of this is increased power of the aerobic system, greater fat breakdown and reduced reliance on anaerobic glycolysis (anaerobic energy source).

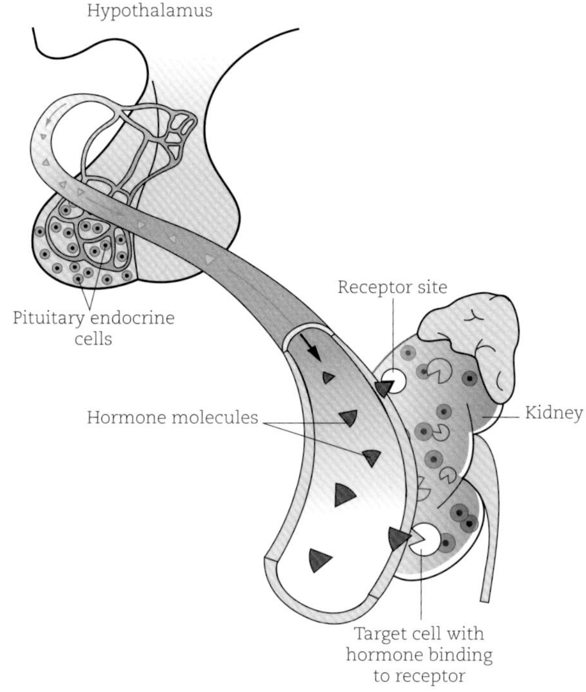

Figure 5.1 Hormone and receptor sites

- **Hormonal factors** – The nervous and the *endocrine system* work in conjunction to regulate functions such as temperature regulation, *blood pressure*, blood glucose and blood calcium levels. The nervous system operates relatively quickly as a network of connecting nerve fibres that transmit electrical signals, whereas the endocrine system operates more slowly using chemical messengers called *hormones* that are secreted into the bloodstream from groups of cells known as *glands* (when hormones are released from nerve endings, they are known as *neurotransmitters*).

As with the nervous system, the endocrine system works on a lock and key basis: hormones act as keys, and receptor cells act as locks, as can be seen in figure 5.1. For example, hormones released from the

Table 5.1	MAIN HORMONAL ADAPTATIONS TO AEROBIC EXERCISE	
Hormone	**Function**	**Training effect**
Insulin	A peptide hormone produced by the pancreas. *Insulin* regulates carbohydrate and fat metabolism and promotes storage of glucose.	Long-term exercise can result in improved insulin sensitivity and an increased rate of *protein* synthesis.
Cortisol	A steroid hormone produced by the adrenal gland in response to exercise (as well as stress). Cortisol is involved in the breakdown of *triglyceride* and protein to produce glucose. Extended exercise can increase cortisol levels resulting in the breakdown (catabolism) of protein for fuel.	Levels decrease progressively with training. This can result in lower heart rate and blood pressure levels during submaximal exercise (lowering the oxygen demand for a given intensity).
Epinephrine and norepinephrine	These hormones are classified as catecholamines and are produced by the adrenal glands. Epinephrine elevates cardiac output, increases blood glucose and supports fat metabolism. Norepinephrine performs similar functions as epinephrine and is also involved in vasoconstriction to parts of the body not involved in exercise.	While exercise initially triggers a surge in these hormones, regular training can result in a blunted response to the same level of exertion over time, resulting in improved mood and reduced stress.

pituitary gland will only bind with specific receptor cells in the kidneys. Information is then passed on to target cells, which will stimulate the kidneys to perform a specific function.

The main endocrine glands include the pineal, pituitary, thyroid, parathyroid and adrenal glands. There are other tissues in the body that secrete hormones, such as the hypothalamus, *pancreas*, thymus, ovaries, testes, kidneys and stomach, but these are not referred to as endocrine glands.

The main hormonal adaptations as a result of aerobic exercise can be seen in table 5.1.

FACTORS AFFECTING ADAPTATION

There are many factors that can limit the improvement of VO_2max. These include:

- **Initial level of endurance** – In general, the higher the initial level of fitness, the smaller the potential improvement. Improvements in VO_2max generally occur in the first two months of training, which is why pre-season conditioning is considered important in relation to performance for some sports.

- **Age** – Improvements in endurance tend to decrease with age, but regular training can slow the rate of decrease. VO_2max drops by approximately 1% per year after the age of 25–30 years, but endurance training can reduce this to nearer 0.5% per year up until the age of about 50 years, However, factors such as perimenopause and menopause have been suggested to accelerate the rate of decline for women.

- **Hereditary factors** – The initial level of endurance and relative improvement of an individual is genetically determined. The response to aerobic training is specific to the individual and can be dependent on hereditary factors by as much as 80%.

Training methods for aerobic endurance

There is a wide variety of approaches to aerobic training, including easy recovery and long steady state training, and threshold training.

EASY RECOVERY AND LONG STEADY STATE TRAINING

This type of training is often used to facilitate recovery (physiologically and psychologically). Sometimes called long slow distance (LSD) training, this typically lasts between 1 and 2 hours at intensities below 60–70% VO_2max. In many sports and athletic events, easy recovery sessions are an important, yet overlooked, part of an overall training programme.

THRESHOLD TRAINING

This type of training is very subjective and can often differ in description but is usually performed at an intensity between 80% and 90% VO_2max. This is normally at an exercise intensity at which the body can only just tolerate levels of blood lactate (a by-product of energy production through anaerobic glycolysis). If too much blood lactate is produced it can affect muscle contraction, meaning that exercise intensity has to be reduced.

The inclusion of threshold training in addition to submaximal exercise has been shown to be effective as it can lead to a decrease in lactate production and/or an increase in lactate removal, which can subsequently improve performance. Tempo running is a term that is often used to describe running at a pace slightly slower than threshold. This type of running can be sustained for significantly longer intervals than faster running.

Training variables for aerobic endurance

There are several key variables that must be considered when designing training programmes. The interaction between volume, intensity and frequency of training is referred to as *training load*. It is important for the practitioner to balance training load with appropriate rest and recovery in order to elicit the required training response.

VOLUME

Volume refers to the amount and quality of training performed in a specific time. In other words, a combination of frequency and duration. For example, a client might perform three 5km (3.1 mile) runs in a week, which would equate to a training volume of 15km/week (9.3 miles/week).

INTENSITY

The term intensity refers to how hard an activity is, so for cardiovascular endurance, how hard would it be to cycle or run at a particular pace? As intensity increases, the amount of oxygen required to cope with the demand also increases, so heart rate increases proportionately to deliver more oxygen. The increase

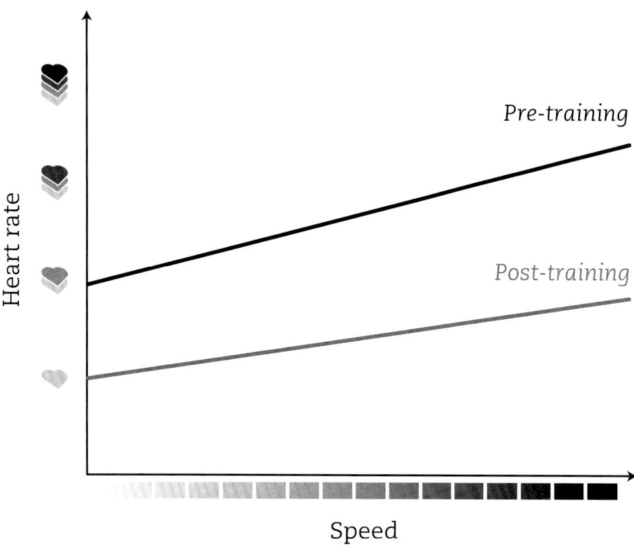

Figure 5.2 Graph showing heart rate against speed

in heart rate due to an increase in exercise intensity has a linear relationship, which can be explained as follows. If intensity (in this case speed, as in figure 5.2) was increased at regular intervals and heart rate measured after each increase, the points on the graph would follow a straight line. Regular training would result in a lower heart rate for the same intensity, as can be seen.

FREQUENCY

The term frequency refers to how often training takes place. For example, a client might have three training sessions per week but only do cardiovascular training in two of them and resistance training in the other. In this case, the frequency of training is three times per week, but the frequency of cardiovascular training is two times per week.

REST

This refers to the rest period between bouts of training activities. For example, a training programme might mimic the demands of a sport where there is a 1-minute burst of activity followed by a 20-second rest period, which is then repeated several times. This can also be referred to as a work-to-rest ratio.

RECOVERY

This is just the amount of time between sessions when no training takes place. Inadequate recovery can affect adaptation and lead to overtraining and possible injury. Too much recovery time might negatively impact client development. During recovery periods, low-intensity cardio training can be performed, which is known as active recovery. This has been shown to be an efficient method of alleviating the effects of ***delayed onset muscle soreness (DOMS)***.

Take-home messages

- When training at VO_2 levels associated with aerobic endurance, energy (from ATP) comes predominantly from aerobic glycolysis and fat.

- There are many adaptations to aerobic training, which include the adaptation of hormonal factors.

- A range of training methods can be used to develop aerobic endurance, including steady state and threshold training.

- Training variables (volume, intensity, frequency, rest and recovery) can be manipulated to develop and maintain aerobic endurance.

Anaerobic endurance

The areas covered in this chapter are:

- What anaerobic endurance is and how the body responds and adapts to anaerobic training

- An overview of training methods

Introduction

This chapter will investigate anaerobic endurance, its role within exercise and how it can be developed through the manipulation of the principles and components of fitness. The aerobic and anaerobic energy systems operate as different entities but often in conjunction during varying intensity bouts of exercise. Therefore, it is important to understand how they work and how they can be developed within training to optimise performance.

What is anaerobic endurance?

Anaerobic means 'without oxygen', so anaerobic endurance refers to the ability of the body to maintain exercise at a level that requires energy from sources other than oxygen.

There are several related thresholds that can be used to set training intensities. The term *anaerobic threshold* (AT) can be thought of as the point at which the energy demand of exercise can no longer be met by the aerobic system, meaning that the anaerobic system would need to contribute. At all exercise intensities, the by-product *lactic acid* (LA) is produced. At low intensity, LA can be broken down to produce ATP (mainly by type 1 muscle fibres). At higher intensity, the rate of production of LA can exceed the rate of its removal. This is referred to as lactate threshold (LT) or onset of blood lactate accumulation (OBLA), which results in the feeling of pain and fatigue. At this point, the rate of ventilation (the flow of air into and out of the *alveoli* in the lungs) surpasses normal rate and is known as *ventilatory threshold* (VT).

Adaptations to exercise

Adaptations to anaerobic training mainly occur in the muscle groups used during the training. Typical long-term adaptations include the following:

- **ATP-PC** – There may be an increase in the resting levels of ATP and *phosphocreatine* (PC), which is a

high-energy *molecule* that is stored in muscles and mainly used for rapid ATP production.

- **Glycogen** – The long-term effect of interval-type training can result in an increase in the storage of glycogen, which is the form of glucose stored in the muscles and liver.
- **Enzymes** – There is also an increase in the enzymatic activity involved in the process of anaerobic glycolysis. An example of this is the enzyme myokinase, which plays a role in intracellular energy *homeostasis*.
- **Recovery** – There can also be an improvement in recovery from high-intensity exercise, especially with a well-developed aerobic system.

These combined adaptations can lead to an increase in performance as a result of a more efficient anaerobic system.

Anaerobic training can also result in some training effect of the aerobic system if the exercise durations or repetitions are long enough. Indeed, to increase AT, aerobic training is considered essential. If the aerobic system is trained to its maximum potential, then this would delay the point at which the anaerobic system would be required to help provide the energy for the higher-intensity exercise.

Anaerobic speed reserve is the difference between maximal aerobic speed (MAS) and maximal sprint speed (MSS). The greater the aerobic capacity of a client, the greater the MAS, which in turn reduces the anaerobic speed reserve and means the client can train at greater intensities while maintaining aerobic respiration.

Training methods

Exercise at intensity levels approaching 100% VO_2max or above can be referred to as anaerobic-type training. At this level the supply of energy comes predominantly from ATP-PC and anaerobic glycolysis. Typically, anaerobic endurance can be divided into short-term or long-term categories depending on the energy systems targeted (ATP-PC or anaerobic glycolysis). Short-term anaerobic endurance training is designed to increase the ability to perform maximal work for a short period of time and long-term anaerobic endurance training is designed to improve the ability to maintain exercise at a relatively high intensity for a longer period.

SHORT-TERM ANAEROBIC ENDURANCE TRAINING

The main goal of short-term anaerobic endurance training is the development of the capacity of the ATP-PC system. Typically, training bouts of less than 15 seconds should be performed at anaerobic levels. This often looks like 1:10 work-to-rest ratios (meaning the rest between repetitions should be 10 times the duration of the work period) with recovery durations of 3–5 minutes to allow PC resynthesis if sets are to be repeated. Low-intensity exercise during recovery is recommended as it can help to increase blood flow and aid PC resynthesis. Table 6.1 shows typical short-term anaerobic endurance training in relation to repetitions, work time and recovery time. The number of sets would be specific to each client; therefore, it is advised that in the first training session with a client you would try and estimate the number of sets the client can cope with by judging the point at which you feel the client has reached fatigue.

LONG-TERM ANAEROBIC ENDURANCE TRAINING

The primary goal of long-term anaerobic endurance training is the development of the anaerobic glycolysis system and the ability to buffer the hydrogen ions that are produced by this energy system (in other words, to help prevent acidosis, which is when pH levels in the blood fall). This production of hydrogen ions occurs mainly during intense bouts of exercise of between 30 and 180 seconds' duration and is believed to interfere

Table 6.1	**TYPICAL TRAINING FOR SHORT-TERM ANAEROBIC ENDURANCE**		
	Repetitions	**Distance/time**	**Recovery**
Running	10	100m	3–5 mins
Cycling	10	10 secs	3–5 mins
Typical adaptations	• Increase in ATP, creatine and PC stores. • Increase in concentration and activity of enzymes involved in the phosphagen system (creatine kinase and myokinase).		

Table 6.2	**TYPICAL TRAINING FOR LONG-TERM ANAEROBIC ENDURANCE**		
	Repetitions	**Distance/time**	**Recovery**
Running	10–12	100m	10–60 secs
Running	8	400m	3–5 mins
Cycling	10–12	30–180 secs	2–5 mins
Typical adaptations	• Increase in concentration and activity of enzymes involved in the anaerobic glycolysis system (phosphofructokinase). • Increased capacity to buffer acid production within the muscle and the blood.		

with muscle contraction. To replenish PC levels and return pH levels towards normal, a long recovery with a work-to-rest ratio of between 1:4 and 1:5 is recommended. Alternatively, shorter bouts of exercise (20–120 seconds) with shorter rest periods and 1:1 work-to-rest ratios (termed lactate tolerance training) can be used. Table 6.2 shows typical long-term anaerobic endurance training in relation to repetitions, work time and recovery time.

HIGH-INTENSITY INTERVAL TRAINING (HIIT)

Intermittent (interval) exercise or training at relatively high intensity has increased in popularity. This is in part because it reflects the conditions of many sports or events, which involve bursts of intense activity followed by less intense periods. Interval training typically involves repeated bouts of high-intensity exercise (above threshold) interspersed with periods of rest or active recovery. The work-to-rest ratio is dependent on many factors, including the experience of the client and the goal of the training programme. Typical work-to-rest ratios can be seen in table 6.3.

High-intensity interval training is quite demanding, so it is recommended that these general guidelines should be followed:

• The client should undertake a period of continuous training before starting interval training, to establish a good cardio fitness level.

Table 6.3 — TYPICAL WORK-TO-REST RATIOS FOR HIIT ZONES

Intensity (HIIT zone)	Work-to-rest ratio	Work duration	Rest duration
95–100%	1:3	Up to 10 secs	15–30 secs
85–90%	1:2	10–45 secs	30–90 secs
75–85%	1:1	45–120 secs	90–120 secs

- The pace should be a gradual increase that raises the heart rate to the required % of maximal heart rate (MHR).
- The number of repetitions should reflect the condition and age of the performer.
- The rest interval should enable the performer to reduce the heart rate to a baseline level.
- Only manipulate one variable at a time.

Those new to this type of training should begin with the maximum recommended rest period and should gradually reduce this as they become accustomed to the training. It should also be noted that medium and long work-to-rest ratio training sessions have been shown to be physiologically more demanding (and show a greater utilisation of carbohydrates) than short work-to-rest ratio sessions. This should be considered when planning training sessions, as interval training can have a negative effect on performance at a later time due to increased glycogen depletion.

Take-home messages

- It is important to understand the concept of anaerobic threshold and the link between lactate and ventilatory threshold.
- When training at VO_2 levels associated with anaerobic endurance, energy (from ATP) comes predominantly from anaerobic glycolysis and ATP-PC.
- A range of training methods can be used to develop anaerobic endurance, including short-term, long-term and HIIT.

//Stabilisation

The areas covered in this chapter are:

- An understanding of the systems and mechanisms associated with stabilisation

- An overview of training methods

Introduction

This chapter will focus on the stabilisation of the lumbopelvic-hip complex and how the ability to generate and withstand force through this region is vital for sports performance. A variety of methods to train core stabilisation and mobilisation will be covered in this chapter.

What is stabilisation?

The core is also referred to as the lumbopelvic-hip complex. Even though an accepted definition is lacking, core stability can be thought of as the ability to control the position and motion of the trunk over the pelvis and legs to facilitate force transfer between upper and lower extremities (i.e. in gross motor tasks). In simple terms, core stability relates to the ability to maintain neutral spine (optimal trunk alignment) during the transfer of load through the body to the extremities. To do this, the central nervous system must recruit the relevant muscles for both stability and mobility.

One proposed model is that of Panjabi, who suggests that the mechanisms of stabilisation include three systems that are interdependent, as shown in figure 7.1. Continuous interaction from all three systems is required to maintain stability.

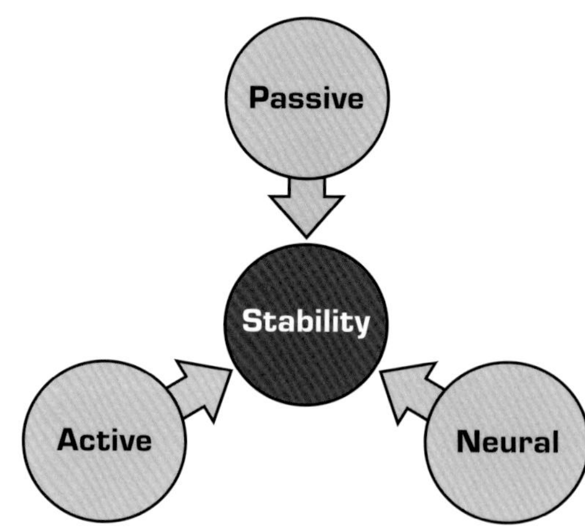

Figure 7.1 Core stabilisation subsystems (adapted from Panjabi, 1992)

The three systems are:

1. **Passive system** – This comprises static tissues such as vertebrae, intervertebral discs, *ligaments* and passive muscle properties. Stabilisation contribution from this system is only achieved around the end range of motion.
2. **Active system** – This mainly comprises core musculature. This system provides dynamic stabilisation to the spine and the proximal appendicular skeleton. Movement information from this system is also relayed to the neural control system.
3. **Neural control system** – This system is the control centre for incoming and outgoing signals relating to movement and stabilisation control.

Core stabilisation exercises are often included in exercise programmes under the premise that there is a link between reduced function of the core musculature and musculoskeletal injury. Despite the lack of clear evidence to support a direct link, the authors strongly advise the inclusion of core stabilisation exercises as there is a large body of evidence that suggests a relationship between core stability and reduced risk of injury as well as the many other published benefits.

LOCAL STABILISERS AND GLOBAL MOBILISERS

There is a widely accepted classification system that classifies muscles that are predominantly responsible for stabilisation as 'local'. These muscles are deep, with attachments on or near vertebrae, and typically perform eccentric endurance tasks rather than short-term or explosive concentric tasks.

Muscles classified as 'global' tend to be superficial and connect the trunk to the extremities. They mainly

Table 7.1	MUSCLES TYPICALLY ASSOCIATED WITH STABILISATION AND MOBILISATION
Area of stabilisation	**Main stabiliser muscles**
Core or trunk area	**Stabiliser muscles with little mobilisation ability:** *Transversus abdominis*, multifidus, pelvic floor, *diaphragm*, internal obliques, quadratus lumborum **Muscles with a greater mobilisation ability:** Rectus abdominis, external oblique, erector spinae
Hip	**Stabiliser muscles with little mobilisation ability:** Gluteus medius and minimus, piriformis, gemellus (inferior and superior), obturator (internus and externus), quadratus femoris **Muscles with a greater mobilisation ability:** Gluteus maximus, iliopsoas, tensor fasciae latae, hamstrings, adductors, rectus femoris
Shoulder	**Provides stabilisation mainly of the scapula:** Rhomboid, trapezius, serratus anterior, subscapularis **Provides stabilisation mainly of the humeral head:** Infraspinatus, teres minor/major, supraspinatus

function concentrically to produce large torques for movement and power. Table 7.1 represents a list of muscles that are commonly associated with either stabilisation or mobilisation at the core, hip and shoulder. They are taken from various sources of muscle categorisation for the purpose of exercise programming.

MECHANISMS OF STABILISATION

The mechanisms of stabilisation are not fully understood, but it is thought that several may contribute. For instance, intra-abdominal pressure, thoraco-lumbar *fascia* gain and the hydraulic amplifier effect are thought to contribute to stabilisation. These are covered below:

- **Intra-abdominal pressure** – The contents of the trunk area, including the stomach, intestines and various organs and fluid, are collectively termed the abdominal ball or fluid ball, which is cylinder-like in shape. It is suggested that when the core muscles contract, the walls of the abdominal ball are tightened and compressed. This creates an increase in pressure known as intra-abdominal pressure. This pushes against the spine and prevents it from making any excessive movements, helping to keep it in the correct posture.

- **Thoraco-lumbar fascia gain** – The thoraco-lumbar fascia is a sheet of connective tissue, almost *tendon*-like, that covers most of the muscles in the back and attaches to the spine, pelvis and sacrum. When the muscles of the inner unit are activated, tension is produced in the thoraco-lumbar fascia. It has been suggested that this tension creates an *extension* force on the spine (in other words, causes it to stiffen) and thus provides a degree of stabilisation that contributes to the overall stabilisation of the spine. The exact mechanism of thoraco-lumbar fascia gain is still under investigation and a topic of much debate.

- **Hydraulic amplifier effect** – When the erector spinae muscles contract, the thoraco-lumbar fascia that surrounds these muscles resists their expansion. This resistance increases the strength of the erector spinae muscles and it has been suggested that this contributes to the stabilisation of the spine.

Training methods

Stabilisation training should focus on maintenance of neutral spine, optimal posture and the transfer of loads from the core to extremities. As core stability provides a stable base for the transfer of loads, it is thought to be a key factor of fundamental movement patterns.

For this reason, core stability and movement mechanics are often integrated in training (*see* table 24.3 on p. 150). Assessment of movement (movement screening) considers various functions, such as neuromuscular control, proprioception, joint stability, mobility, strength and balance, however it is not typically performed by S&C practitioners unless specific knowledge is gained through continued professional development (CPD) or through experience.

Unfortunately, in relation to this type of training, several terms appear in the literature, which can be confusing. For the purpose of this book, the term 'motor control stabilisation exercise' (MCE) will be used. MCEs focus on the activation of the deep local trunk muscles, with progression towards more dynamic and complex tasks that involve the activation of local and global trunk muscles. The rate of progression should be dictated by the ability of the client to perform the exercises. A starting point that is often advocated is awareness of neutral spine position followed by stabiliser contraction and the use of abdominal bracing. So, what are these, and how are they assessed?

NEUTRAL SPINE POSITION OR ZONE

When the spine is in a neutral position (also known as neutral spine), which is midway between lumbar *flexion* and extension, it is considered the optimum position of power and balance for dynamic movements. Neutral spine can be found by using repositioning exercises such as pelvic tilts. These involve a client tilting the pelvis forwards and backwards several times, then returning to the neutral position as described below.

Client:

1. Stand in an upright position with the feet shoulder-width apart.
2. Attempt to flatten the lower spine by pulling the crotch area up towards the chest.
3. Attempt to increase the hollow in the lower back by extending the buttocks backwards.
4. Repeat this movement several times at a slow, controlled pace.
5. Try to find the neutral position midway between the two extremes.

Practitioner:

1. Make sure that any movement occurs only in the lumbar spine; do not allow any movement at the shoulders or in the legs.
2. Watch for the full range of motion between the full anterior and the full posterior tilt.
3. Inform the client when the pelvis is midway between these two points.

ABDOMINAL BRACING

Contraction of the stabilising muscles can be very difficult to perform consciously, which is where abdominal bracing comes in. Abdominal bracing is a method that is often used to improve the neuromuscular control of local stabilisers. It requires contraction of the transversus abdominis (TA), which is considered to be one of the most important local muscles in core stabilisation.

The following method can be used to instruct clients to practise abdominal bracing:

1. Lie with your back on the floor, knees bent and feet flat on the floor. Relax and try not to flatten the spine against the floor; instead, maintain a normal lumbar curve.
2. Find a position 5cm (2in) below the navel and 5cm (2in) to either side of that position. Press in lightly on each side using the first two fingers of each hand. This should be the location of the TA. Slide one hand under the natural curve of the lower spine so that you can feel any pressure changes from the body through the hand.
3. Cough! As the TA is one of the muscles responsible for the forced expiration of air during coughing, you should feel the contraction under your fingers. The pressure on the hand under the lumbar spine should not change: try to maintain constant pressure throughout the contraction.
4. Aim to replicate the contraction felt when coughing, without coughing. Aim to contract at about 30% of maximum contraction capability.
5. Once you can contract the TA, perform the same action making sure that you are not holding your breath or activating the rectus abdominis. You can place a hand just below the diaphragm to check for contraction of the rectus abdominis.

Note: Once clients are capable of TA contraction without holding their breath or contracting the rectus abdominis, use the same method in a standing position.

FUNDAMENTAL MCES FOR S&C PROGRAMMING

When clients are able to consciously contract local stabilisers, they can progress to more complex and dynamic MCEs. There is an enormous range

Table 7.2	**EXAMPLE OF PROGRESSIVE MCE EXERCISES**			
	Recruitment	**Stabilisation**	**Dynamic stability**	**Performance**
Method	Mostly bilateral (BL) to develop motor control and coordination	Mostly BL to develop eccentric/motor control BL offset, asymmetrical and symmetrical	BL and unilateral (UL) to develop power and deceleration BL offset, asymmetrical and symmetrical UL (linear)	BL and UL to develop *acceleration* and explosive sport-specific performance BL offset, asymmetrical and symmetrical UL (multiplane)
Pre-requisite	Novices For beginners to S&C	Competent bodyweight BL squat technique <20% asymmetry in loaded squat	Competent BL landing control Competent bodyweight UL squat technique Squat >1.25 × body mass (8RM) or 1.5 × body mass (1RM)	Competent BL drop jump mechanics Competent UL landing control Squat strength >1.5 × body mass (8RM) or 2 × body mass (1RM) Competent UL deceleration and change of direction
MCE dynamic	Squat patterns Lunge patterns Hip hinge Crawls/animal movements Hang Press-up Push Pull Neutral spine Abdominal brace Brace and resist Weight transfer	Skips in place BL squat jump (SJ) (in place, forwards) BL countermovement jump (CMJ) (in place, forwards) Split jump (same leg land) Step and land (forwards, lateral, standing and from running on the spot) Hop in place (forward/lateral/angle) Ladder and hurdle varied linear and lateral running *Supine* and *prone* bridge Supine foot slides Superman (contralateral) Donkey kicks	Step-land-push back (forwards, lateral, standing and from running on spot) SJ and CMJ to box Step-up jump (same and alternating leg) BL drop jump (30cm/12in box) Rotational jump and land Tuck jump UL bounding Plyo press-ups Pull-ups (assisted) Push press (UL) Single-arm rows (bear stance) Side bridge Dead bugs, bear crawls, bicycle crunches Superman (ipsilateral) Superman donkey kicks	Continuous UL SJ/CMJ to BL landing UL SJ/CMJ to box Continuous CMJ (hurdles) SJ/CMJ weighted Lateral hop (band/rope/med ball) COD sport-specific drills with perturbation Plyo offset press-ups Pull-ups Push press Bent-over rows Single-leg bridges Jack-knife and V-sits

of exercises available to the practitioner, but table 7.2 provides a progressive list of MCEs that can be incorporated into an overall programme. It should be noted that other components of fitness such as strength, speed and power can also be developed using these exercises.

Training benefits

Core stability exercises have often been associated with improved client performance and/or decreased incidence of injuries. Training programmes incorporating general and sport-specific core stability exercises have been shown to improve balance, back muscle strength and endurance. However, it is unclear whether the improvement is translated into athletic performance. Some research has found that postural stability plays an important role in functional movements and/or performance in sports such as shooting, gymnastics and team sports, such as football. Dynamic balance, which is suggested to be one of the most important motor skills (the ability to maintain or regain balance on an unstable surface with minimal extraneous motion) has also been shown to develop with core stability training along with trunk endurance.

Take-home messages

- It is important to understand core stabilisation subsystems and the definitions and identification of stabiliser (local) and mobiliser (global) in relation to muscle roles.

- Methods of spinal stabilisation include intra-abdominal pressure, thoraco-lumbar fascia gain and hydraulic amplifier effect.

- Neutral zone is important in relation to posture along with contraction of the transversus abdominis.

- Physiological and neural factors can contribute to stability.

Muscular strength and endurance

The areas covered in this chapter are:

- An explanation of what muscular strength and endurance are

- The terminology associated with resistance training

- Physiological adaptations to resistance training and the factors that can affect adaptation

- The effects of ageing on muscle mass

- The pros and cons of free weights versus resistance machines

- The training variables related to the muscular system

- The importance of exercise order when planning and designing training programmes involving weights

Introduction

This chapter will explore the development of muscular strength and endurance. The sport-specific development of the neuromuscular system for clients and teams enables the muscles to generate adequate force and power outputs to cope with the demands of their sport or activity while minimising the risk of injury. It is also important for the wider population, especially as we age. A variety of training methods designed to develop muscular strength and endurance are also included.

What is muscular strength and endurance?

Muscular strength can be thought of as the maximum amount of force that a muscle or muscle group can generate and is associated with resistance training using relatively high intensity and low repetitions.

Muscular endurance is the ability of a muscle or muscle group to perform repeated contractions against a resistance over a period and is associated with resistance training using relatively low intensity and high repetitions.

Resistance training

Resistance training, which is also known as weight training, is essentially exercise that uses muscular contraction against a resistance. It can be used to develop components such as muscular strength, muscular power (*see* chapter 10) or muscular endurance as well as building a robustness to, and reducing, injury risks.

Resistance training activities are varied and can include the use of free weights (such as barbells, dumbbells and kettlebells), bodyweight, resistance bands, medicine balls, weighted vests and resistance machines. Regardless of the method used, muscular contraction takes place. This can be classified according to the length of the muscle during the contraction. Let's take a look at these different types of contraction now:

ISOTONIC CONTRACTION

Isotonic contraction refers to a muscle contraction while lifting and lowering a resistance against gravity. It can be divided into two types:

1. *Concentric contractions* – These occur when the *agonist* shortens in length when contracting against a resistance. An example would be a biceps curl when the weight is being lifted upwards (the *origin* and *insertion* move towards each other). When using free weights, the muscle doing the main work is always contracting concentrically when the weight is moving upwards, against gravity.
2. *Eccentric contractions* – These occur when the agonist lengthens when contracting against a resistance – for example, when the weight is being lowered during a biceps curl. Here, the origin and insertion are moving away from each other.

ISOMETRIC CONTRACTION

This is when there is no change in muscle length when contracting against a resistance. This type of resistance training is associated with good strength gains, but it

is important to be aware that isometric contractions can raise blood pressure.

ISOKINETIC CONTRACTION

This is a type of muscle contraction where the muscle is changing length, but the speed of contraction remains constant. This type of contraction requires specialist equipment such as an isokinetic dynamometer, which is expensive and not readily available.

Adaptations to exercise

Essentially, there are two main groups of muscle fibres:

1. Slow twitch (type 1) fibres (otherwise known as slow oxidative, SO) are used typically for endurance-type activities and posture control. Oxygen and fat are the main fuel sources for contraction, as they have many mitochondria to help produce the energy. The number and size of mitochondria can be increased by endurance training. They also have many capillaries to supply oxygen via gaseous exchange.
2. Fast twitch (type 2) fibres are typically used for short, powerful activities and are generally broken down into the categories type 2a and type 2b. Type 2a fibres use both aerobic and anaerobic energy pathways whereas type 2b uses only anaerobic path-

ways. Fast resistance training can influence strength and power output and therefore influence sport performance.

Changes in neurological, physiological and hormonal factors can all play an important role in adaptations made by the body, including the development of strength and power. Let's look at each in turn:

NEUROLOGICAL FACTORS

Improvements in neural function can contribute to gains in muscular strength. These improvements usually occur in the early stages of resistance training, since gains in strength have been reported without concomitant increases in muscle mass. Neural factors thought to assist in the development of strength include the improvement of recruitment patterns during muscular contraction, and increased rate of muscle unit firing (rate coding). It has also been suggested that resistance training can lead to a reduction in the sensitivity of **Golgi tendon organs** (a proprioceptor located in muscle/tendon that inhibits excessive muscle force production), which are believed to impair the force capability of muscle. This decreased sensitivity can result in the disinhibition of the target muscle, which in turn leads to greater force production.

PHYSIOLOGICAL FACTORS

Typical physiological adaptations to resistance training include hypertrophy, increase in muscle mass, muscle fibre adaptation and improved bone density. Hypertrophy (enlargement of muscle fibres) in humans occurs due to an increase in the *size* of individual muscle fibres and not due to an increase in the *number* of muscle fibres, which is known as **hyperplasia**. As can be seen in figure 8.1, during the first few weeks of a strength training programme there will be little hypertrophic gain, as strength gains are normally attributed to metabolic and neural factors such as increased

enzyme activity and improved muscle fibre recruitment. After the first few weeks of training, increases in the cross-sectional area of muscle fibres can lead to greater muscle force production. Increases in muscle size can be assessed by measurements of girth, ultrasound, computed tomography (CT) or magnetic resonance imaging (MRI).

In general, greater increases in hypertrophy are seen in males compared to females. Typical increases in muscle fibre size of between 27% and 33% in slow twitch type 1 and fast twitch type 2 fibre types have been observed in untrained individuals following several months of strength training. Fast twitch type 2 fibres tend to increase in size more than slow twitch type 1 fibres, so those with a relatively low percentage of fast twitch fibres will have a limited potential for hypertrophy. Slow twitch type 1 fibres tend to hypertrophy due to a reduction in protein breakdown and fast twitch type 2 fibres enlarge due to an increase in protein (from the Greek *prota* meaning 'prime importance') synthesis.

Adaptations, neural or physiological, can be attributed to or associated with training at specific repetition maximum intensities. Table 8.1 shows typical

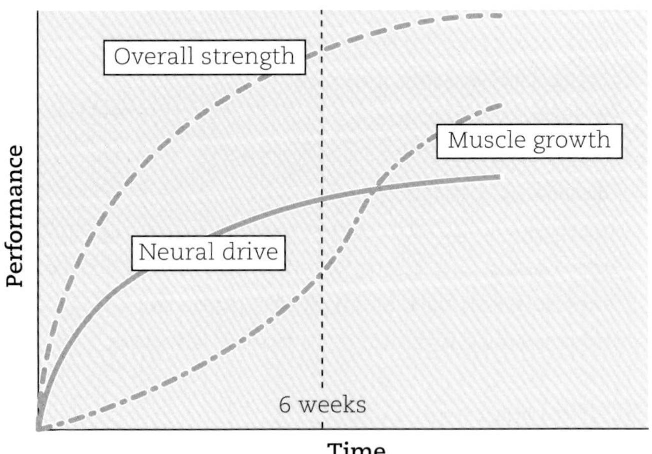

Figure 8.1 Neural and hypertrophic adaptations

adaptations in relation to number of maximum repetitions (or percentage of repetition maximum).

Note: The main fibre type adaptation is the conversion from fast twitch type 2b to fast twitch type 2a fibres. This is usually only observed when the training intensity is over 40% of 1RM. It is thought that when heavy resistance training is performed over a long period, fast twitch type 2b fibres that are regularly recruited can adapt to become fast twitch type 2a fibres, which are more fatigue-resistant than fast twitch type 2b. This change is mediated through changes in myosin heavy chain (MHC) isoforms from type 2b to type 2a.

HORMONAL FACTORS

There are several hormones related to physiological function that can be affected by regular exercise, such as those described in table 8.2.

Adaptive responses in the endocrine system have been shown to take place in relation to the intensity and duration of resistance training. Acute hormonal responses to resistance training include increases in anabolic hormones such as testosterone, growth hormone (GH) family, insulin, insulin-like-growth-factor-1 (IGF-1) and decreases in catabolic (to break down) hormones such as cortisol. Strength training can increase testosterone levels in both young and older males, but not always in females. It appears that the greater the volume of muscle recruited, the greater the anabolic response.

Resistance training with moderate intensities, high volume and relatively short recovery periods (hypertrophy training) tend to produce the greatest increase in testosterone, GH and IGF-1. This type of training also produces the greatest catabolic response through an increase in cortisol, though the overall balance is towards anabolism. Training using greater loads and longer recoveries (1–3RM and 5–8 minutes' recovery) can result in lesser increases in anabolic hormones than observed from hypertrophy training. This can explain

Effects of ageing

Loss of muscle mass is known as sarcopenia. It is one of the main causes of weakness and lack of mobility as we age and has been recognised as a disease by the World Health Organization (WHO). Maximal strength capacity is normally reached around the age of 30 years for both men and women. It declines a decade or so later and appears to diminish severely after the age of 65. This loss occurs predominantly in those who are sedentary, as it has been shown that regular strength training at any age can increase muscular strength. It has also been shown that those who are active in early life and remain active can delay loss of muscle mass.

Age-related loss of muscle mass is thought to be due to the decline of muscle protein synthesis. Physical inactivity can increase the rate of muscle mass loss and the associated decrease in physical function is linked to increased morbidity and mortality. Physical activity including resistance exercise should continue into old age for the prevention, and in some cases the treatment, of decline in muscle function.

why those training to increase muscle mass would be advised to use moderate loads, several sets, and short recovery rather than maximal strength training.

Free weights versus resistance machines

There is an ongoing debate in the industry around the use of free weight exercises, resistance machine exercises or both in relation to training and testing. There are advantages and disadvantages to both, so the choice must take into account the individual needs of the

Table 8.1	TYPICAL ADAPTATION AS A RESULT OF RESISTANCE TRAINING AT SPECIFIC REPETITIONS	
Reps	**% RM**	**Adaptation**
1	100	Increased strength as a result of neural factors.
2–3	95	Increase in contractile proteins.
4–5	90	Improved use of ATP and PC.
6–7	85	
8–9	80	Increased strength and hypertrophy effects.
10–11	75	
12–13	70	Main hypertrophic effects. Improved glycolysis.
14–15	65	Increased endurance, slight strength and hypertrophic gain.
15–20	60	Increase in aerobic enzymes. Improved fat metabolism.

Table 8.2	EXERCISE-RELATED HORMONES AND THE EFFECTS OF TRAINING	
Hormone	**Function**	**Training effect**
Human growth hormone (HGH)	A peptide hormone secreted by the anterior pituitary gland that stimulates cellular growth. HGH can increase muscle protein synthesis, increase bone mineralisation, and promote fat metabolism. It is thought to be stimulated by high-intensity exercise, such as heavy strength training, explosive power training or high-intensity cardio exercise.	Most research involves response to single resistance or anaerobic training sessions. Resting values are increased but less so in trained people.
Insulin-like growth factor (IGF)	IGF is a peptide hormone produced in the liver that supports the function of HGH to repair protein damaged during exercise.	There's some evidence to support increases in IGF as a result of resistance training.
Testosterone	A steroid hormone produced mainly by the testes in males and the ovaries in females. **Testosterone** is responsible for muscle protein resynthesis (which plays a significant role in skeletal muscle growth).	Most research involves response to single resistance training sessions. Resting values are increased but less so in trained people. Most studies used male subjects. No changes found yet in women.

Table 8.3	ADVANTAGES AND DISADVANTAGES OF FREE WEIGHTS AND RESISTANCE MACHINES	
	Advantages	**Disadvantages**
Free weights	• Many exercises can be performed with limited equipment. • Uses synergists and stabilisers in a functional way. • Full range of motion is available. • Can mimic the movements of many sports or events. • Relatively portable.	• More instruction is required for safety and correct technique. • Often require a training partner for safety purposes. • Do not always appeal to a broad range of users.
Resistance machines	• Relatively easy to learn and therefore to instruct. • Can be used to isolate muscle groups for rehab purposes. • The weight setting can be changed easily.	• The plane of motion is set by the machine, which is not functional. • Can sometimes limit range of motion. • Seated positions do not replicate most functional movements. • Seat supports negate the use of core stabilisers. • Relatively expensive compared to free weights. • They are not portable.

client. Table 8.3 outlines some of the advantages and disadvantages relating to the choice of exercise modality.

Training variables

As with aerobic training there are a range of variables that can be manipulated in resistance training: volume, intensity, frequency, rest and recovery.

VOLUME

The volume in relation to resistance training can be measured in two ways:

1. Sets × repetitions
2. Sets × repetitions × load

The load refers to the amount of weight lifted, and repetitions refers to the number of times the weight is lifted. Sets just refers to how many times this is repeated. For example, for a client who performs 3 sets of 10 repetitions of 80kg, the volume can be calculated as 30 reps at 80kg = 2400kg.

There is no optimal number of repetitions and sets for muscular development. Strength gains have been observed in programmes that range from a single set to multiple sets across the range of *repetition maximum (RM)*. Repetitions and sets can be influenced by the phase of training (such as *hypertrophy*, strength, endurance etc.), therefore programme design should be informed by guidelines relating to specific phases, which are shown in table 8.4.

Table 8.4	GENERAL RESISTANCE TRAINING GUIDELINES		
	Strength	**Hypertrophy**	**Endurance**
Intensity (% 1RM)	≥85	67–85	<67
Sets	2–6	3–6	2–3
Reps	1–6	6–12	12+
Frequency (sessions/week)	1–2 (per muscle group)	1–2 (per muscle group)	2–3 (per muscle group)
Rest (minutes)	2–5	1.5	Approx. 0.5

INTENSITY

Training intensity (otherwise known as the load) refers to the amount of weight to be lifted. This can be expressed as RM. This is the maximum weight that can be lifted for a specific number of repetitions. For example, 10RM is the maximum weight that can be lifted for 10 repetitions. Intensity can also be expressed as a percentage of the maximum weight that a client can lift. For example, 80% of 1RM. This just means 80% of the maximum a performer can lift.

FREQUENCY

This is the same as it is for aerobic endurance. However, in this case it refers to muscles being trained and not just the training session. For example, a client might do three training sessions a week but only train a particular muscle (the chest, for instance) once, so the training frequency for the chest is once per week.

The optimum number of training sessions per week depends on factors such as the type of session, training status and ability to recover. For untrained clients two to three days' training per week has been found to be effective in the initial stages of training and one to two days per week has been found to be sufficient to maintain strength in novice trainers. Competitive or experienced strength-trained clients typically train five to seven days per week.

REST

In relation to resistance training, rest is the period between sets of exercises. The main aim of rest intervals between sets is to replenish intramuscular stores of ATP and PC following depletion. A rest interval of 3–5 minutes will generally allow replenishment of ATP/PC stores. In general terms, the higher the intensity of the repetitions performed during each set, the longer the rest interval required between the sets. However, the interval chosen should reflect the training goals. Typical rest intervals for different goals are:

- Power – 5–8 minutes
- Strength – 3–5 minutes
- Hypertrophy – 1–2 minutes
- Muscular endurance – 30–60 seconds

RECOVERY

The recovery period refers to the time in between training sessions when no exercise takes place. This is important, as following a period of strenuous exercise it is common for skeletal muscles to become sore. This soreness, associated with post-exercise self-perception, has been termed delayed onset muscle soreness (DOMS). Even though the exact mechanism of this soreness is not fully understood, it has been suggested that it is caused by damage at a microscopic level. During high-intensity strength training the ATP-PC energy system is primarily used. Training daily is possible, since ATP-PC can be fully restored within 24 hours.

Exercise order

Within a training session, large muscle mass exercises should precede small muscle mass exercises to avoid fatigue affecting the larger muscle groups. For example, if triceps were exercised to fatigue prior to performing a chest exercise, the triceps would not be able to fully assist the pectorals (chest muscles), so reducing the performance of the chest muscles. It is also important to provide symmetry by alternating upper-body and lower-body exercises as well as front (anterior) and back (posterior) exercises.

Muscle symmetry

Creating muscle symmetry can be an important factor, as a strength imbalance between opposing muscle

Table 8.5	TYPICAL STRENGTH RATIOS FOR AGONIST AND ANTAGONIST MUSCLE GROUPS	
Joint	**Movement**	**Ratio**
Ankle	*Plantarflexion/dorsiflexion*	3:1
Ankle	*Inversion/eversion*	1:1
Knee	Extension/flexion	3:2
Hip	Extension/flexion	1:1
Shoulder	Flexion/extension	2:3
Elbow	Flexion/extension	1:1
Lumbar	Flexion/extension	1:1

Table 8.6	DESCRIPTIONS OF COMMONLY USED RESISTANCE TRAINING METHODS
Training method	**Description**
Single sets	Performing one set of each exercise.
Multiple sets	Performing more than one set of each exercise.
Circuit sets	A series of resistance exercises with a rest period between each exercise.
Super sets	Performing several exercises for the same body part or pairing exercises for agonist and antagonist.
Pyramids	Increasing the resistance and decreasing the repetitions over several sets.
DeLorme-Watkins	This system involves increasing the intensity based on 10RM. For example, if a client has a 10RM of 40kg for the shoulder press, they will perform: set 1 – 10 reps of 50% of 10RM = 20kg; set 2 – 10 reps of 75% of 10RM = 30kg; set 3 – 10 reps of 100% of 10RM = 40kg.
7s, 14s and 21s	Sets that include multiples of 7.
Drop sets (stripping)	Continuous lowering of the resistance with fatigue at each set.
Complex training	Combination of resistance training and plyometrics.
Pre-exhaustive	Isolation exercise followed by a compound exercise, e.g. leg extension then squat.
Post-exhaustive	Compound exercise followed by an isolation exercise, e.g. bench press then pec fly.

groups may be a limiting factor in the development of strength or speed and can also be a factor in increasing the risk of injury to joints or muscles surrounding joints. Muscle balance testing to compare the strength of opposing muscle groups can be used to identify asymmetry. For example, the strength ratio of the quadriceps to hamstrings should be approximately 3:2 to reduce the risk of injury. Table 8.5 shows reported values for joint agonist-*antagonist* strength ratios.

When developing a programme that includes muscular strength and endurance it is useful to know the terms associated with training as shown in table 8.6

Take-home messages

- A range of general resistance training activities can be used in an isometric, eccentric, concentric and isokinetic way to develop muscular strength and endurance.

- The magnitude and rate of adaptation from training is dependent on multiple factors including the training age/experience of the client, training frequency and programme adherence.

- Progressive overload is the optimal method to use to incur adaptations while minimising risks of under- or overtraining.

- Muscular strength is especially important as we age.

- There are advantages and disadvantages of strength training using free weights versus machine weights.

- There are a wide range of ways to adapt and manipulate training variables to achieve different outcomes.

- Exercise order is an important consideration. Large muscle mass exercises should precede small muscle mass exercises.

- One of the aims of S&C is to create muscle symmetry and correct imbalances.

//Speed

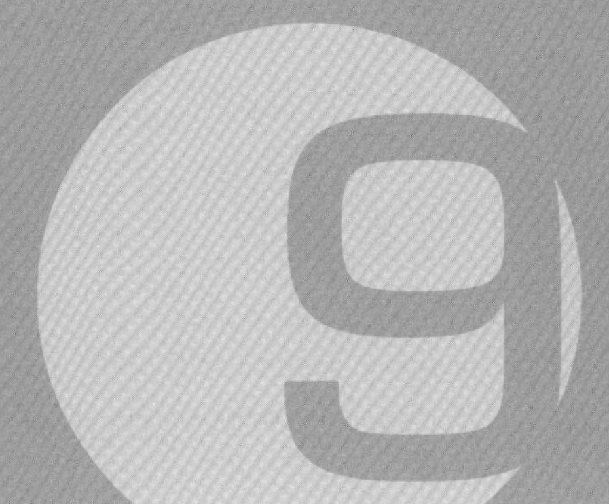

The areas covered in this chapter are:

- An explanation of what speed is

- The different phases of a sprint

- The training variables that are associated with speed training

- An overview of training methods

Introduction

Speed is a component of performance that is closely linked with muscular strength, endurance and power. To move at speed (e.g. to sprint) or to move something at speed (e.g. an arm swing during a tennis serve) is a complex process that requires the neuromuscular capacity to generate force quickly (power) and the technical ability to conduct the action with the precision required for the activity. This chapter will explore the factors that contribute to speed and how they can be developed.

What is speed?

Speed can be described as the ability to move quickly from one point to another. This can be in relation to speed over the ground or to limb speed. The latter is important for sports such as martial arts.

Speed over the ground is often measured in relation to sprinting. Sprint speed has several phases depending on the distance of the sprint, as shown in figure 9.1.

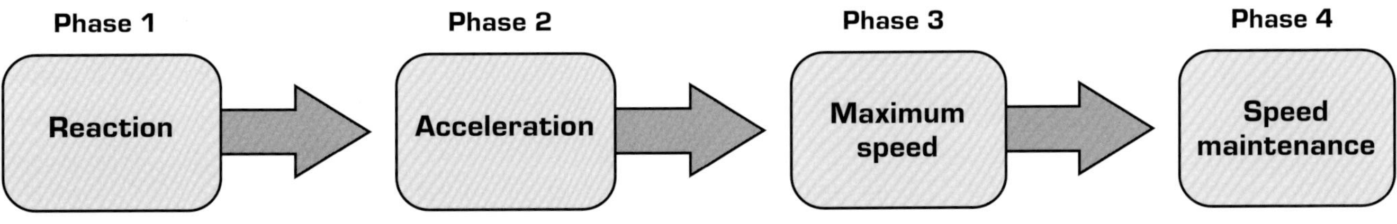

Figure 9.1 Phases of a sprint

SPRINT PHASES

Most sprint distances have a reaction (to a stimulus) phase, an acceleration phase, a maximum speed phase and a speed maintenance (also known as deceleration) phase. However, in most team sports, typical sprint distances covered during a game are generally only 10–20m (33–66ft), which means that maximum speed is often not achieved. In these cases, the reaction and acceleration phases can be considered more important than the maximum speed phase.

Reaction phase

Before any movement occurs a performer often has to identify and react to a particular stimulus. This is known as reaction time. Depending on the sport or event, the stimulus could be the movement of a ball or reacting to an opponent or opportunity in a game situation, or it could be as simple as the gun going off at the start of a track race. Reaction times can be improved by regular training and are typically measured to be in the region of approximately 100–200 milliseconds (ms) (0.1–0.2s).

Acceleration phase

In this phase, the term acceleration describes an increase or a change in the speed of a performer. During this phase there tends to be a rapid increase in the number of steps taken (this is known as the stride frequency) and a steadier increase in the length of the stride that is taken. Stride length and stride frequency can be described as follows:

$$\text{Stride length} = \frac{\text{distance covered}}{\text{number of strides}}$$

$$\text{Stride frequency} = \frac{\text{number of strides}}{\text{time taken}}$$

Maximal speed phase (30–80m/33–88 yards)

Highly trained or elite-level performers usually reach their individual maximal speed at approximately 50–60m (55–66 yards), whereas in less trained individuals, maximal speed is normally reached at approximately 30m (33 yards). This phase is associated with a more upright running position as opposed to a lean forwards in the acceleration phase. The hamstrings are considered important during the maximal speed phase due to the cycle-like motion in which they play a major role.

Speed maintenance/deceleration phase

Many sports require the performer to repeat maximal (or close to maximal) sprints with varying recovery intervals. This ability is known as speed maintenance or speed endurance. Maintaining maximum speed beyond 80m (88 yards) is difficult for most performers. Once at maximum speed, a performer needs to be strong, as fatigue and tiredness can cause deceleration. Interval-type training is a strategy often used to improve speed maintenance.

Training methods

There are a number of training methods used to improve the different phases of speed. Methods include: resisted sled training, uphill-downhill training, weighted-vest training and assisted or overspeed training. Let's look at each in turn now.

RESISTED SLED TRAINING (RST)

Resisted sled training is commonly used as a means to develop sprint performance and in particular the early acceleration phase, although research is limited in relation to the long-term effects.

The towing load selected should reflect the sport and the physical status of the client but is usually limited to less than 20% of body mass, as loads in excess of this could alter the running biomechanics of the client and limit the development of the *stretch-shortening cycle* (the muscle contraction response to a rapid stretch). In

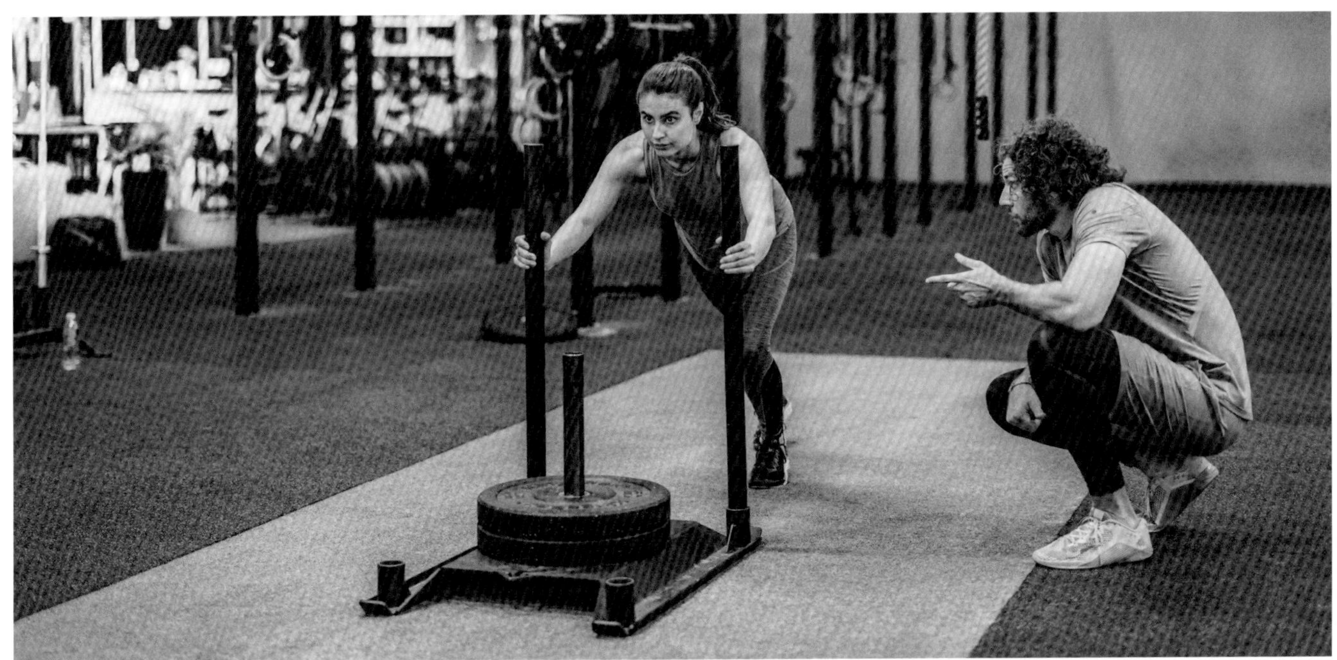

Figure 9.2 Resisted sled

addition, the effect of the surface must be considered, since towing a load on grass will produce a different load than towing on a running track due to the variance in friction.

UPHILL-DOWNHILL TRAINING

This type of speed training involves short sprints that start with a slight incline followed by a horizontal section then a slight decline. Though there is a lack of conclusive evidence in relation to the optimum gradient and sprint distances, it has been suggested that training with uphill and downhill gradients of approximately 3 degrees and an overall distance of 30–50m (33–55 yards) can positively impact on maximum running speed.

WEIGHTED-VEST TRAINING

The use of wearable resistance is a popular training method to help sprint performance, even though

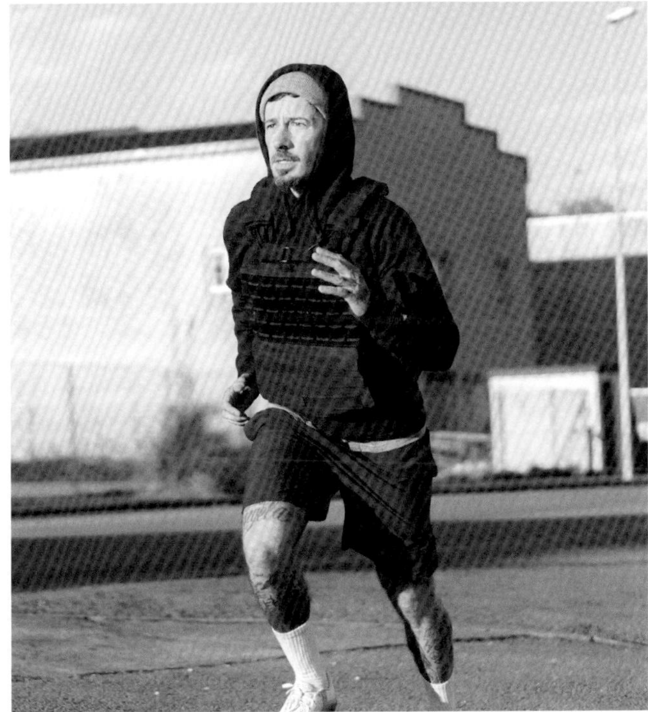

Figure 9.3 Weighted-vest training

longitudinal evidence to support its use is limited. The use of weighted vests loaded with up to 15–20% of body mass could increase vertical force at foot contact, thereby increasing the load on the extensor muscles and hence enhancing the stretch-shortening cycle (similar to an increase in vertical jump resulting from a box drop jump).

ASSISTED OR OVERSPEED TRAINING

Assisted training has been in use for many years. Its objective is to achieve supramaximal speed using methods such as downhill running or towing. However, its effectiveness has not been determined conclusively. Although some research has reported an increase in maximum running speed as a result of this type of training, speeds above 110% of maximum speed are not recommended as the greater stride lengths that are incurred can lead to a braking effect, which could result in major changes in sprinting biomechanics and eccentric muscle damage.

Take-home messages

- Speed is the ability to move quickly from one point to another, whether that's over the ground or limb speed.

- There are four phases to a sprint: a reaction (to a stimulus) phase, an acceleration phase, a maximum speed phase and a speed maintenance phase. For many sports, since there is insufficient time to reach maximum speed, the training focus is the reaction and acceleration phases.

- Various training methods can be used to increase speed and improve speed endurance, including resisted sled training, uphill-downhill training, weighted-vest training and assisted or overspeed training.

- The components of sprint speed are important and can be addressed using stride length and stride rate.

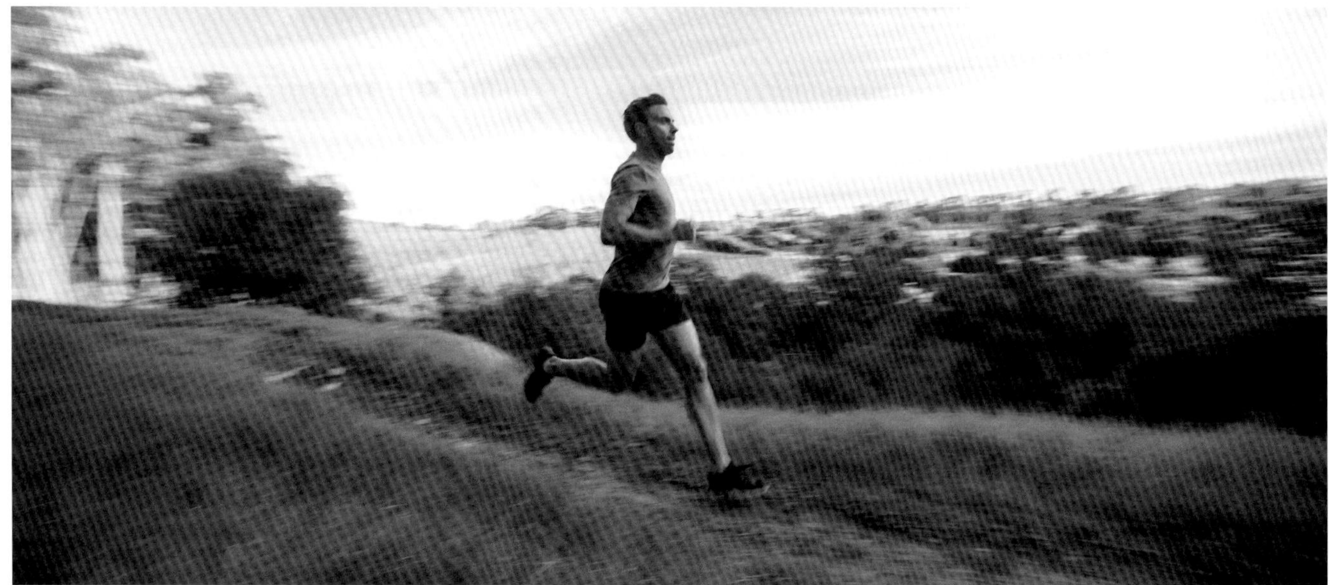

Figure 9.4 Overspeed training

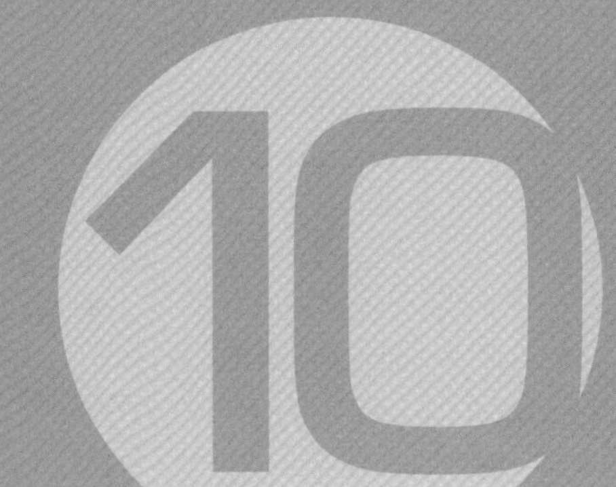

The areas covered in this chapter are:

- An explanation of what power is and how it can be measured and calculated

- A discussion of optimal training methods

- The relevant intensities associated with those methods and how they can be monitored and programmed

Introduction

A large variety of sports involve performing specific actions that require an object to be moved with force at speed. This may include the body acting to propel itself (e.g. sprinting) or components of the body acting to move an external object (e.g. striking a football or hitting a hockey puck using a stick). Therefore, power as a component is closely related to muscular strength and endurance and speed, as both of these components are required to generate power. This chapter will look at how the components combine to generate power and how they can be developed.

What is muscular power?

It is often stated that muscular power is an important characteristic of many sports, especially those involving sprints, jumps and changes of direction. In order to understand the training requirements, power can be thought of as the rate of doing work and is measured in *Watts* (W). Therefore, power can be expressed as:

> **power = work ÷ time**

Work done (such as moving an amount of weight) is measured by the force needed over a certain distance. Therefore, power can also be expressed as:

> **power = force × velocity**

This equation shows that the ability to generate power is influenced by the force a muscle can generate and the speed of contraction.

Training methods

The production of power and training for that production can be looked at separately. Maximum power output is affected by the load, as can be seen in figure 10.1, which shows the relationship between force and velocity.

For example, if using loads close to 1RM then the force will be near maximum (peak force), but the speed of contraction will be slow, and the resulting power will be minimal. Conversely, if the load is very light, the force will be minimal and the speed of contraction near to maximum (peak velocity), again resulting in low power output.

As far as training for power is concerned there is no current consensus as to the optimal training load, since research has shown that training with loads below 50% of 1RM is effective for power development whereas others have shown that loads above 50% are just as effective. For this reason, a mixed methods approach using a variety of training loads is often advocated, as low load can impact the high velocity area of the force-velocity relationship (*see* fig. 10.1) and high load can impact the high force area.

Even though the literature can be somewhat confusing with regards to optimal training methods, the authors recommend that strength is developed prior to more specific training that emphasises power and speed as advocated by Harris *et al.* (2000). Table 10.1 shows an example of high velocity, high force and mixed methods training for an agonist-antagonist muscle pair in relation to repetitions and percentage of 1RM.

VELOCITY-BASED TRAINING

Micro-electro-mechanical systems (MEMS) that obtain sport performance measures during training or competition are now in widespread use by coaches in many sports and events. Devices with built-in transducers and accelerometers, which are inexpensive and non-invasive, can be used to measure the intensity, directionality and magnitude of a client's movements. Devices can be attached to the client or a barbell to provide instant feedback in relation to acceleration performance. As well as being used for testing variables such as power (peak, average, set average) and velocity (peak, average, set average), devices such as these enable the coach to implement velocity-based training (VBT), which is essentially a method of resistance training based on velocity to inform or enhance practice.

It is widely known that the number of completed repetitions of a given percentage of 1RM differs between clients with the intention often cited as the cause of the difference. This simply means that some will try harder than others and therefore achieve different results! For this reason, VBT has been suggested as an alternative training method that can produce instant objective data. Contemporary research has suggested that there are three main applications for using VBT:

1. **Estimating 1RM** – Some researchers have used the relationship between velocity and %1RM to estimate 1RM.
2. **Prescribing load** – Volume and relative intensity can be manipulated depending on the magnitude of velocity loss.

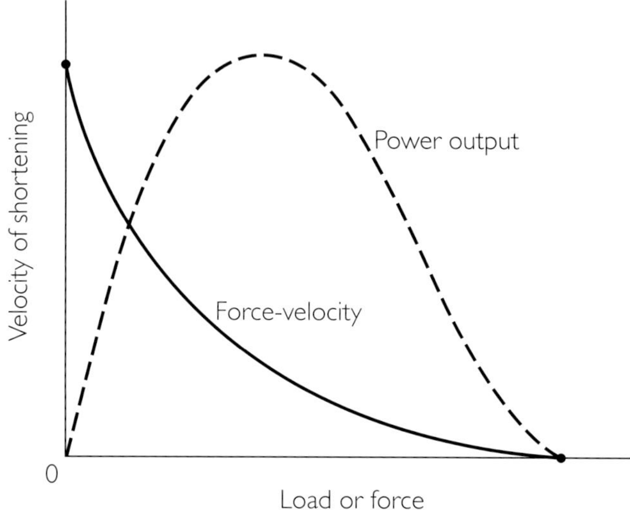

Figure 10.1 Force-velocity relationship

<table>
<tr><td>Table 10.1</td><td colspan="3">EXAMPLE OF HIGH VELOCITY, HIGH FORCE AND MIXED METHODS POWER TRAINING</td></tr>
<tr><td></td><td>High velocity</td><td>High force</td><td>Mixed methods</td></tr>
<tr><td>Squat
Bench press</td><td>Monday & Thursday:
5 reps @ 80% 1RM
5 reps @ 80% 1RM</td><td>Monday & Thursday:
15 reps @ 30% 1RM
15 reps @ 30% 1RM</td><td>Monday:
5 reps @ 80% 1RM
Wednesday:
8 reps @ 60% 1RM
Friday:
15 reps @ 30% 1RM</td></tr>
<tr><td>Dead lift
Bent-over row</td><td>Tuesday & Friday:
5 reps @ 80% 1RM
5 reps @ 80% 1RM</td><td>Tuesday & Friday:
15 reps @ 30% 1RM
15 reps @ 30% 1RM</td><td>Monday:
5 reps @ 80% 1RM
Wednesday:
8 reps @ 60% 1RM
Friday:
15 reps @ 30% 1RM</td></tr>
</table>

Note: The number of sets and rest periods will be dependent on the experience of the client.

3. **Velocity feedback** – It has been demonstrated that real-time velocity feedback can increase motivation and competitiveness.

Load-velocity profiling

Like any training variable it is important to establish a baseline so that programmes can be manipulated based on relevant information. One method of using VBT is to create a load-velocity profile that monitors velocity of the movement against %1RM over time so that future training sessions can be monitored (squat, deadlift and bench press are typical exercises that are used to create load-velocity profiles). Table 10.2 provides a protocol for developing a load-velocity profile assuming the 1RM is known.

Once data has been collected, velocity against %1RM can be plotted on a graph and a line of best fit applied. Table 10.3 shows an example of data recorded from three separate profiles of a specific lift, first at baseline, then follow-up 1 at 4 weeks and follow-up

Table 10.2	PROTOCOL FOR DEVELOPING A LOAD-VELOCITY PROFILE
Step	**Description**
1	Client completes a standardised warm-up.
2	Client completes 3 reps at 20, 40 and 60% of 1RM after being instructed to perform at their maximum capacity. Record the repetition with the fastest mean velocity (MV) for each set.
3	Client completes 1 rep at 80 and 90% of 1RM. Record the MV for each set.

2 at 8 weeks. The time between follow-up profiles is dependent on many factors, such as training status, periodisation phase and recovery, but is often used to provide information across training sessions.

Table 10.3	EXAMPLE DATA (BASELINE, 4 WEEKS AND 8 WEEKS)		
	Mean velocity (m/s)		
%1RM	**Baseline**	**Follow-up 1**	**Follow-up 2**
20	1.4	1.3	1.5
40	1.15	1.05	1.25
60	0.85	0.75	0.95
80	0.53	0.45	0.63
90	0.4	0.32	0.5

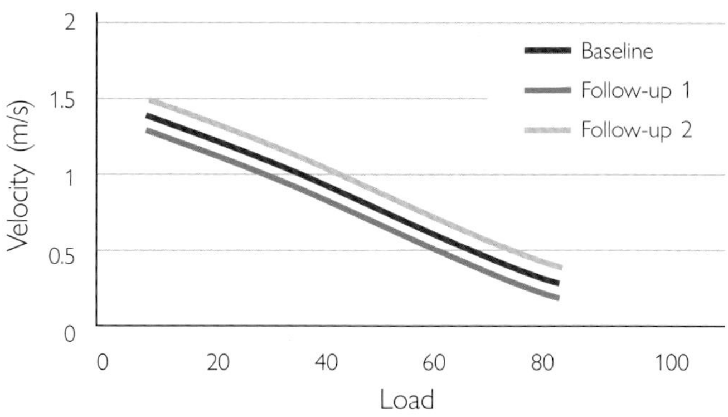

Figure 10.2 Load-velocity profile for example lifts

Data can then be plotted as in figure 10.2, which shows the load-velocity profile for all three sets of lifts. It can be seen that the profile in follow-up 1 is faster than the baseline, which indicates an improvement, potentially in neuromuscular capacity. The profile in follow-up 2, however, is slower than baseline, which could indicate fatigue or overtraining.

Velocity loss threshold

There are many ways in which the profile can be used to inform training. One method that is used to provide information during training sessions is velocity loss threshold (VLT). This is where the practitioner develops a load profile for a client performing a lift at a specific percentage of 1RM. The velocity is then tracked in real time during training and if it falls below a particular threshold (20% for example) then the set is terminated. This type of training is used by practitioners to manage fatigue. For example, during off-season periods, a greater VLT can be implemented (20–40% is common) whereas during in-season sessions the VLT may be smaller (less than 20%).

Note: The practitioner must exercise caution with this type of training: clients often sacrifice technique for speed of execution, so it is important to maintain the intended stability and range of motion.

PLYOMETRIC TRAINING

This type of training is generally used to improve performance in areas such as jump height, sprint speed and peak power output. Derived from Greek and meaning 'changing length', the term plyometric (first used by track coach Fred Wilt in 1975) can be described as rapid eccentric loading (the muscle stretching quickly) followed by a brief isometric phase and an explosive rebound (the muscle shortening quickly) using fast twitch fibres to increase the efficiency of force production or performance.

Essentially, there are two mechanisms involved during plyometric movements:

1. **Stretch-shortening cycle** – When muscle fibres are stretched rapidly there is a response known as the stretch-shortening cycle. This response has the effect of stimulating a contraction of the muscle fibres that are being stretched, which results in a greater muscular force than would be elicited normally. However, plyometric exercises must be performed rapidly, as the response will only occur if the ground contact time is less than 0.2 seconds.
2. **Elastic potential energy** – The elastic potential energy of connective tissue (muscle and tendon) is thought to contribute to power development.

Table 10.4	PLYOMETRIC FOOT CONTACT GUIDELINES			
	Low intensity	**Moderate intensity**	**High intensity**	**Total per session**
Beginner	60–100	60	40	100–120
Intermediate	100–150	60–100	40–80	150–200
Advanced	150–200	100–150	60–100	180–220

For those with no history of this type of training, it is advised to follow general guidelines before undertaking any form of plyometric exercises. These are outlined below:

- **Strength base** – Ensure a good strength base. Strength ratios of 2 × bodyweight for 1RM squats (lower-body plyometrics) and 1.0 to 1.5 × bodyweight for bench press (upper-body plyometrics) are recommended for both male and female performers (note that this is only a recommendation and this type of training can still be undertaken by those who do not meet this strength requirement if the practitioner thinks it is appropriate).
- **Age** – Although there are no specific age guidelines, younger performers should be closely supervised. The training history should be considered, and progression should be slow.
- **Jump height** – For box jumps or reactive jumps, the height is typically 75–110cm (30–43in), as jumps above this might not elicit the stretch-shortening cycle.
- **Rest periods** – Plyometric exercises can cause depletion of energy stores and fatigue of the central nervous system (CNS). A work-to-rest ratio of 1:5 is generally used for adequate recovery. Although there is no consensus regarding the optimum rest periods between high-intensity plyometric sessions, the authors recommend a period of between 48 and 72 hours.

- **Volume dosage (reps, sets, load etc.)** – Foot contacts performed during a training session can be used to as a measure of work done. General guidance for number of foot contacts per session can be seen in table 10.4.

Take-home messages

- Various training activities can be used in the development of power.

- The authors advise developing strength before moving on to develop speed and power.

- Practitioners must be aware of the relationship between power, force and velocity in skeletal muscle and understand the stretch-shortening cycle utilised in jumping.

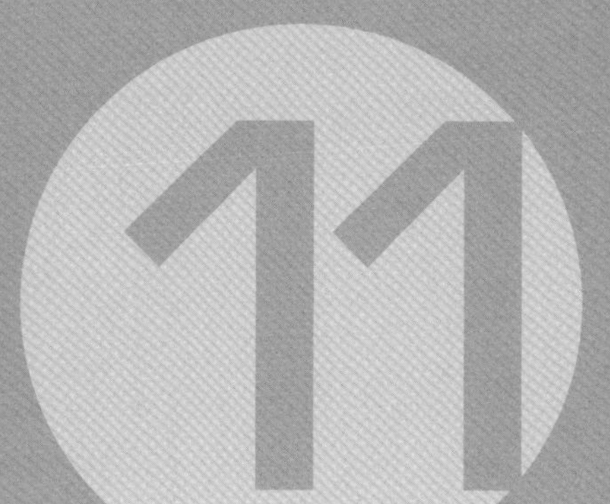

//Agility

> **The areas covered in this chapter are:**
>
> - What *agility* is and why it is important
>
> - Typical training methods and the relevant intensities associated with those methods

Introduction

So far, each of the components of fitness that have been covered in this part of the book have had clear definitions and methods of development. However, agility is a component that can have a different definition depending on the sport and physical action required. The general consensus is that agility is the ability to respond to a stimulus within a sport-specific manner. This chapter will therefore look at the unique ways in which the different components of agility can be developed.

What is agility?

Although it is widely recognised that agility plays a crucial role in many sports, there is no current consensus on the definition of the term. Sheppard and Young (2006) have defined agility as a rapid whole-body movement with a change of velocity or direction in response to a stimulus. In other words, deceleration, change of direction, and acceleration, and this is the framework we will use.

Agility is generally considered to be made up of several components, such as balance, coordination, strength and power, which should be addressed when designing training programmes. It should be mentioned, though, that straight line speed does not appear to be linked with agility performance. Speed and agility can be considered as distinct qualities that can be trained separately. Training for agility, therefore, should recognise the specific demands of the sport, such as movement patterns and pace changes and the relationship with decision making. Key to all of this is balance, which we'll take a look at now.

BALANCE

Balance is a fundamental component of agility and can be described as the process by which individuals maintain equilibrium and move their bodies in a specific relationship to the environment. Muscular strength contributes to balance, as does information from proprioception (feedback in neural awareness of joint position), the vestibular system (inner ear) and vision.

When the body is at rest it is known as being in static balance and when the body is in motion it is known as being in dynamic balance. Balance can be measured in both static and dynamic situations. Balance is not only required for effective movement in sport: it's important in older age, when falls represent the most frequent and serious type of accident. The Royal Society of Prevention of Accidents (2025) estimates that approximately 3,500 older adults die each year due to falls.

Training methods

When designing training programmes, agility can be thought of in two ways: programmed and random.

PROGRAMMED AGILITY

If a movement is considered agile but does not involve the reaction to a stimulus then this can be classified as programmed agility. Take the example of a high jumper who needs to be agile enough to take off at a different angle to the approach run. The individual has calculated the direction of the movement and has no need to change this in response to any external stimulus. Movements such as these are sometimes referred to as closed skills.

RANDOM AGILITY

If a movement is considered agile and does involve a reaction to a stimulus then this can be classified as random agility. When a goalkeeper reacts to a well-struck volley by heading for the far corner but the ball takes a deflection, the goalkeeper is agile enough to change body position quickly in order to make the save. These movements are referred to as open skills.

Agility is not considered a main component of fitness for all sports or events. The practitioner needs to use their knowledge and experience to decide if agility is an important component to include in a client training programme. Table 11.1 shows the importance of agility across a range of sports and events.

Table 11.1	AGILITY IMPORTANCE ACROSS A RANGE OF SPORTS AND EVENTS		
	Low	**Medium**	**High**
Football			✔
100m sprint	✔		
Netball			✔
Hammer throw		✔	
Darts	✔		
Snooker	✔		
Cycling	✔		
Badminton			✔
Tennis			✔
Archery	✔		
Karate			✔
Judo			✔
Recreational running	✔		

Take-home messages

- There is no single definition of agility, but in general, agility is the ability to respond to a stimulus within a sport-specific manner.

- Agility, which can be programmed and random, is often confused with change of direction.

- Different sports have different agility requirements.

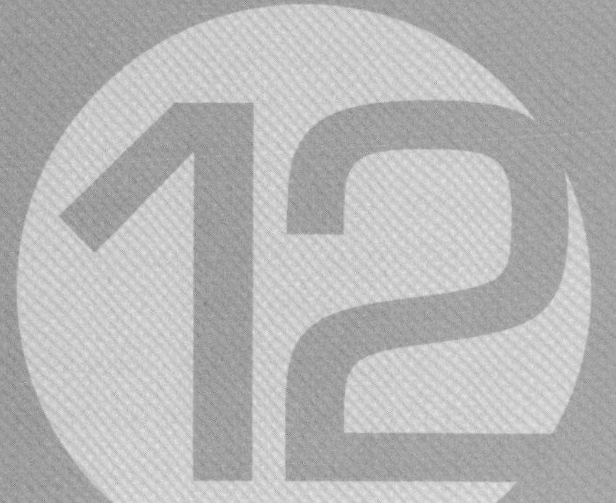

//Flexibility

Introduction

Flexibility is a component of performance that links closely with the previous chapters in this section. Flexibility can be a limiting factor that controls the range at which the neuromuscular system can generate force, speed and power at each individual joint. This chapter will explore what flexibility is and how it can be developed.

What is flexibility?

Flexibility can be thought of as the available range of motion at a joint. Flexibility is joint specific in that an individual can be flexible at one joint but not necessarily at others.

Types of stretching

There are many types of stretching exercises that are used to maintain or increase joint range of motion.

These include static, dynamic and ballistic stretching and PNF (proprioceptive neuromuscular facilitation). The most effective stretching occurs when muscles are warm, as this reduces tissue stiffness, so an appropriate warm-up is always recommended prior to stretching.

STATIC STRETCHING

A static stretch is held for a period of time at a point of mild tension. If the stretch is held long enough, the tension usually subsides and the stretch can be increased, if required. If a partner or another group of muscles assists in the stretching process, it is known as an active stretch. If there is no assistance, it is known as a passive stretch. It is important to note that static stretching should be performed slowly to reduce the effect of the stretch reflex, which is a reflex action that causes a muscle to contract when it's being stretched. In simple terms, the faster the stretch, the more powerful the contraction.

The acute effects of static stretching on strength and power performance have been a heavily debated topic for many years. In an attempt to provide clarification about whether or not short-duration static stretching (StS) should be included as a warm-up component, Chaabene and colleagues concluded that StS should be included before the uptake of recreational sports activities due to its potential positive effect on flexibility and musculotendinous injury prevention. However, they also suggested that in high-performance individuals StS must be used with caution due to its negligible but still prevalent negative effects on subsequent strength and power performances, which could have an impact on performance during competition. ACSM guidelines relating to static stretching are shown in table 12.1.

DYNAMIC STRETCHING

A dynamic stretch refers to stretching in motion, where an agonist muscle is contracted to elicit a stretch in an antagonist muscle. When this occurs, it is known as *reciprocal inhibition*. This type of stretching is usually carried out in a slow and controlled manner in order to minimise the risk of injury and to mimic the types of movement that may be used in the exercises to follow.

BALLISTIC STRETCHING

Ballistic stretches are where bouncing movements caused by momentum or gravity are performed near the end range of motion. This type of stretching is usually carried out only by those who are familiar with it, as there is little control of the movement and therefore a greater risk of injury than with other types of stretching.

PNF

Proprioceptive neuromuscular facilitation (PNF) is a type of partner-assisted stretching that is normally used when flexibility is limited. Originally used as a rehabil-

Table 12.1	ACSM FITT GUIDELINES FOR STATIC STRETCHING
Frequency	Minimum 2–3 sessions per week; ideally 5–7 sessions per week
Intensity	To the end range of motion at a point of tightness, without pain
Time	10–30 secs, 2–4 times per stretch
Type	Static, preceded by a warm-up

itation method for *cerebral palsy*, tension is built up in a muscle prior to it being stretched. When tension in a muscle reaches a certain level, the Golgi tendon organ (GTO) – a collection of specialist cells – located at the musculotendinous junction initiates a reflexive relaxation of the muscle during the subsequent stretch.

Although the mechanisms of PNF are not fully understood, autogenic inhibition (also known as the inverse myotatic reflex) and reciprocal inhibition are commonly cited as two of the main mechanisms involved. It is the GTO that responds to tension in the muscle. If tension becomes too great, the GTO inhibits muscle contraction, causing the muscle to relax. It is thought that through regular PNF stretching, there is an alteration to the output from the muscle spindles and the GTOs to the central nervous system, which results in increased flexibility.

Note: It is recommended that this type of stretching only be performed by those qualified to do so.

There are various methods of PNF stretching, such as hold-relax, contract-relax and hold-relax-contract, which are explained below:

• **Hold-relax** – During hold-relax PNF, a passive stretch is held for up to 10 seconds, followed by an isometric contraction of up to 6 seconds against resistance. There is then another passive stretch of up to 10 seconds, during which the stretch is subsequently increased.

- **Contract-relax** – The contract-relax technique is very similar to the hold-relax technique but instead of an isometric contraction, the muscle undergoes an isotonic contraction, as it is contracted while moving into the stretch. A passive stretch is then carried out to finish, as with the hold-relax technique.

- **Hold-relax-contract** – The hold-relax-contract method is very similar to the contract-relax technique apart from that the second passive stretch is replaced with an active contraction and the client 'pushes' into the stretch.

Training benefits

Performing stretching exercises has been shown to result in many benefits, such as improving range of motion. One of the main benefits of maintaining range of motion is that it allows clients to carry out daily activities as long as possible throughout their lives. It is also believed that being flexible can improve coordinated movements that would decrease the risk of injury caused by awkward movement. However, the degree to which flexibility directly impacts on reducing injury risk is a debate in current research.

It is recommended that people with tight muscles would probably benefit most from static stretching whereas those who are naturally supple should engage in no more than light stretching. The most effective stretching occurs when the muscles are warm, so it is prudent to incorporate static stretching into cooldown routines.

As with agility, flexibility might not be considered to be a main component of fitness that is needed by a client. Table 12.2 provides an overview of the importance of flexibility across a range of sports and events.

Table 12.2	FLEXIBILITY IMPORTANCE ACROSS A RANGE OF SPORTS AND EVENTS		
	Low	**Medium**	**High**
Football		✔	
Rugby		✔	
Netball		✔	
Basketball		✔	
Darts	✔		
Snooker	✔		
Cycling		✔	
Badminton		✔	
Tennis			✔
Archery	✔		
Karate			✔
Judo			✔
Show jumping	✔		
Recreational running		✔	

How to put together a programme to improve flexibility

As outlined above, flexibility is a component of fitness that links closely to mobility and range of motion. If an athlete can actively utilise wider ranges of motion and elicit neuromuscular control within muscle group end ranges, then this may benefit performance within their sport and reduce injury risks. However, it is unlikely that a practitioner will design a training programme that aims to solely develop a client's flexibility. Rather, it is a component of fitness that may be incorporated into training programmes or be built into a warm-up or cool-down. It is also a component that needs to be regularly trained within programmes to maintain flexibility. A range of different techniques (static, dynamic and PNF stretching etc.) that can be used to improve flexibility have been detailed in this chapter and are regularly incorporated into hybrid training programmes that aim to develop multiple components of fitness through a multifaceted approach. Many of the sample programmes provided within this book (*see* Appendix 2) contain aspects of flexibility training within them and can be used as a practical application reference for this chapter.

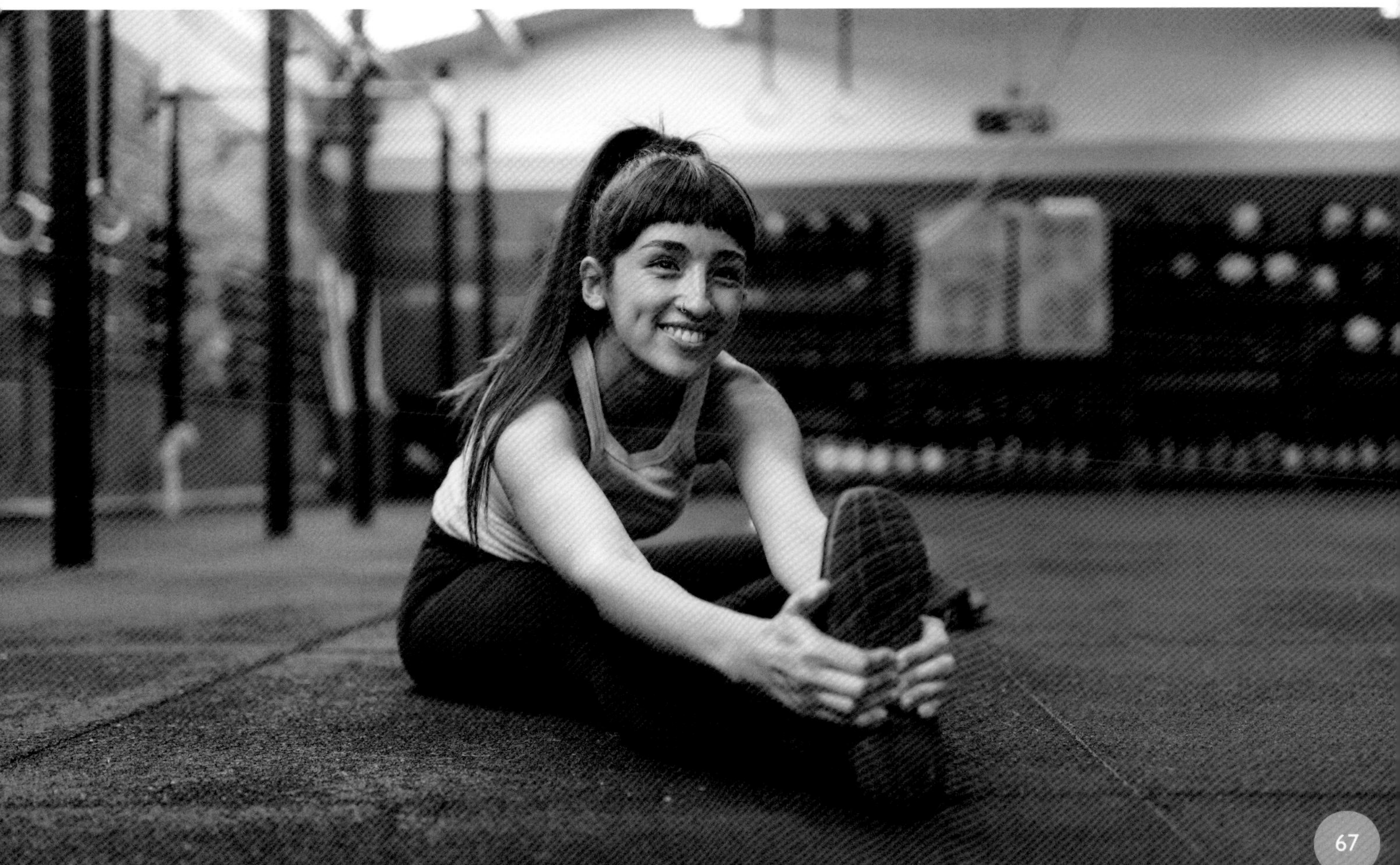

13

The areas covered in this chapter are:

- What body composition is and why it is important

- The difference between subcutaneous and visceral fat

- Health risks associated with increased body fat percentage

- Benefits associated with reduction in body fat percentage

- Training methods used for obese and deconditioned clients

Introduction

Understanding body composition and how it can impact performance is an important tool for an S&C practitioner to possess. Having a high percentage of fat or a low lean muscle mass can have ramifications on overall health and well-being as well as physical performance. This chapter discusses what body composition is. Chapter 23 delves into how it can be measured and monitored.

What is body composition?

The term body composition can be thought of as the amount of fat mass (FM) and the amount of fat-free mass (FFM) (which is everything that is not fat). An increase in fat-free mass (by way of muscle tissue) or a decrease in fat mass can be goals for athletes and the general public alike. So let's discuss what fat is and training methods that can be used to reduce it!

We can start by exploring the meaning of the terms *obesity* and overweight, which have been defined by the ACSM as:

- **Overweight** – Bodyweight that exceeds the normal or standard weight for a particular person based on height and frame size.
- **Obesity** – The percentage of body fat at which an individual's risk of disease increases.

Fat can be stored under the skin (known as subcutaneous fat) or in the abdominal cavity, and surrounds organs such as the liver, pancreas and intestines (known as visceral fat). As we age, the amount of visceral fat tends to increase. This can be a health issue as it produces damaging molecules such as free radicals that may contribute to the development of insulin resistance, type 2 diabetes, high blood pressure, *atherosclerosis* and cancers. Fortunately, visceral fat can be easier to use as fuel for exercise, which makes it vitally important to keep exercising as we age.

Current figures show that currently in the UK about two-thirds of the adult population are overweight or obese and that more than one-third of adults are classed as inactive. However, physical activity levels are rising, which may lead to an increased uptake in those wanting to access strength and conditioning.

There are many factors that can affect body composition, such as hypothalamic, endocrine and genetic disorders, diet and physical inactivity. In terms of the cause of obesity, there are specific genes associated with the condition with suggestions that genetic factors may be linked to excess weight gain from the first few months of life. In fact, children of obese parents have a much higher risk of becoming obese than if their parents were of normal weight. Food intake is also a major contributing factor to weight gain. It is only in relatively recent times that energy-dense, low-cost food has been readily available, leading to overindulgence and hence weight gain. There is a common misconception that obese people have slower *metabolic rates* than non-obese people. Unfortunately, many studies suggest the opposite to be true in that energy usage at rest (known as resting metabolic rate) increases with bodyweight.

Training benefits

Regular training that targets a change in body composition can have many benefits. Those that are because of increased muscle mass include improved insulin sensitivity and increased resting metabolism. Benefits of increased fat loss are linked to a reduction in chronic illness such as coronary heart disease (CHD), diabetes, *hypertension* and several cancers. It should also be noted that regular physical activity such as aerobic endurance and resistance training can reduce the risk of becoming obese by up to 50% compared to people with sedentary lifestyles.

Training methods

This is where body composition differs from other components of fitness in that all other components have specific training methods associated with them, whereas there are several ways in which to target body composition. Methods of training for an increase in muscle tissue is covered in chapter 8; therefore, this chapter will focus on reduction of fat mass as a way of changing body composition.

There is a consensus that a combination of increasing *calorie* expenditure (physical activity) and decreasing calorie intake (eating food) is the most effective method for fat loss in the long term. In relation to physical activity, aerobic-type activity combined with light resistance training is considered the most effective method. Daily routines such as parking at the furthest end of car parks, using stairs rather than lifts and getting up to change the TV channel should be encouraged for those clients who are deconditioned and new to strength and conditioning. For clients who are classed as obese, there are exercise guidelines published by the ACSM that you could use, as shown in table 13.1.

How to put together a programme to improve body composition

You may have clients with a weight loss goal and little history of physical activity whom we can assume will be deconditioned. For this type of client, we can combine aerobic endurance and resistance training into

Table 13.1	ACSM PHYSICAL ACTIVITY GUIDELINES FOR OBESITY	
	Aerobic training	**Strength training**
Mode	Because of the stress on the joints, low-impact activities should be chosen (i.e. walking and swimming).	In the initial stages, this may involve calisthenics to provide overload, but the client may then move on to resistance equipment.
Intensity	Low to moderate intensity: 40–85%HRmax; 6–15 RPE.	Use loads within the client's capability. Overload by increasing intensity gradually.
Duration	20–60 mins per session. Increase intensity with slow progression.	Perform 1–3 sets of 12–15RM. 1–2 mins' rest between exercises.
Frequency	At least 5 days per week.	2–3 sessions per week.
Precautions	Avoid impact activities. Use non-weight bearing alternatives. The expenditure should be approximately 150–400Kcal per day.	Avoid impact or jarring exercises.

General precautions:
- It is recommended that a dual approach be adopted: increase caloric expenditure and decrease caloric intake (no less than 1200Kcal/day).
- Negative energy balance (calories in minus calories out) of 500–1000Kcal/day.
- Aim for a maximum weight loss of 1kg/week.
- Obese people have an increased risk of hyperthermia so watch out for overheating.

an overall programme. Table 13.2 shows how a general aerobic training programme can be progressed over several weeks and table 13.3 shows how a resistance training programme can be progressed.

The programme assumes that during the initial stage of the programme (the first 4 weeks) clients will be unfit. For this reason, the intensity level is kept low, and the duration short.

Take-home messages

- The body is made up of fat mass (FM) and fat-free mass (FFM).

- Obesity is a condition that is linked to many chronic health concerns.

- Guidelines suggest that a combination of aerobic exercise, resistance training and dietary advice is the optimal way to improve body composition.

Table 13.2	AEROBIC ENDURANCE TRAINING PROGRESSIONS FOR DECONDITIONED CLIENTS WITH A GOAL OF WEIGHT LOSS			
Programme stage	**Week**	**Sessions per week**	**Activity intensity (% HRM)**	**Activity duration (min)**
Initial stage	1	3	40–50	15–20
	2	3–4	40–50	20–25
	3	3–4	50–60	20–25
	4	3–4	50–60	25–30
Improvement stage	5–7	3–4	60–70	25–30
	8–10	3–4	60–70	30–35
	11–13	3–4	65–75	30–35
	14–16	3–5	65–75	30–35
	17–20	3–5	70–85	35–40
	21–24	3–5	70–85	35–40
Maintenance stage	24+	3–5	70–85	20–60

Table 13.3	RESISTANCE TRAINING PROGRESSIONS FOR DECONDITIONED CLIENTS WITH A GOAL OF WEIGHT LOSS			
Programme stage	**Week**	**Sessions per week**	**Activity intensity (% 1RM)**	**Rest duration (seconds)**
Initial stage	1	1	50–60	30–45
	2	1–2	50–60	30–45
	3	1–2	50–60	30–45
	4	1–2	50–60	30–45
Improvement stage	5–7	2–3	60–65	45–60
	8–10	2–3	60–65	45–60
	11–13	2–3	60–65	45–60
	14–16	3–4	65–70	60–90
	17–20	3–4	70–70	60–90
	21–24	3–4	70–70	60–90
Maintenance stage	24+	3–4	70	60–90

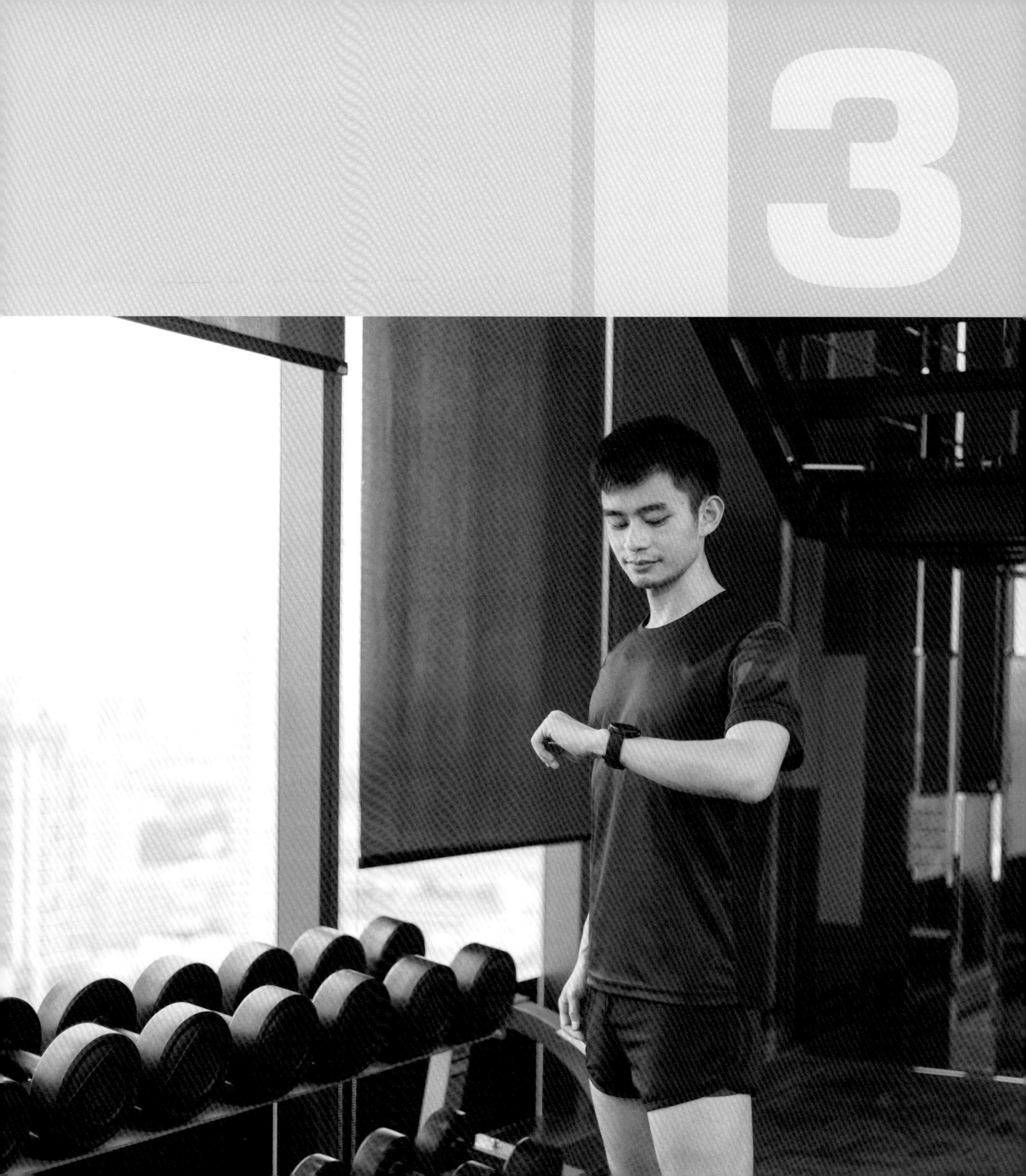
3

PART **THREE**

TESTING THE COMPONENTS OF FITNESS

In part 1 of the S&C road map we discussed the process of client consultation that is used to gather information required to develop a tailored S&C programme. In part 2 we looked at components of fitness and how to develop programmes related to them. In part 3 we describe a range of tests that can be used to measure each component. Testing of components can be done at the same time as the practitioner is developing the S&C programme, as it is useful to know at what level the client is before training starts.

Once the training programme starts you will then need to re-test your client at certain intervals as this can indicate if specific gains are being made. There is no specific time interval for re-testing that suits all clients. A minimum period of 6 weeks is usually recommended, as this allows time for the client to adapt to the training programme. Many sports teams use a period of 13 weeks, as this accommodates 4 testing sessions per year. It is not recommended to re-test after periods longer than 13 weeks since this is thought to reduce motivation.

Some of your clients' goals might be specific and measurable in relation to a specific component of fitness. For example, your client might want to reduce body fat by a certain percentage. If the goal is not achieved following the re-test, then you might consider changes to the programme, such as an increase in intensity of aerobic training.

The first chapter in part 3 deals with the considerations and the knowledge that a practitioner should have in relation to client testing. The rest of the section will describe how to perform a range of tests used to assess components of fitness.

Performance //assessment

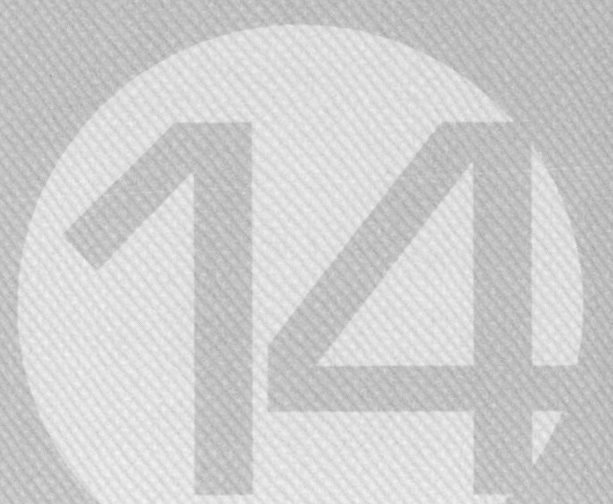

The areas covered in this chapter are:

- The range of benefits that regular performance assessment brings

- Where testing can take place

- The different types of health and fitness tests

- Testing-related terminology

- Test methodology

- Data protection, data collection, data analysis and data feedback, including interpreting client data in order to understand the different types of client and their needs

- Understanding the importance of validity and reliability with regards to testing and how an awareness of procedures can impact on this

- Programming training and future testing, including building in reassessments/reviews to support client progress, motivation and adherence

Introduction

Regular testing of clients is vital for tracking performance in relation to specific goals. This is known as performance assessment and is used to inform training *adaptations* and minimise risk of injury. Practitioners should be aware that there are a multitude of available physiological and psychological tests. There are many factors to consider when selecting which of these tests to use, such as the environment where testing takes place, and whether to use direct or indirect, maximal or submaximal, and static or dynamic testing.

Practitioners should also be aware of the importance of collecting, analysing and interpreting data and having the ability to present this in a suitable format for other professionals. This can inform how training is programmed as well as future testing.

Testing

Testing can have many benefits, including those outlined in table 14.1.

There are various different types of testing, which we will explore in detail now:

LABORATORY AND FIELD TESTS

Testing can take place in a laboratory or in a field environment (in an applied setting). Laboratory tests tend to be more accurate, though in recent years some field tests have become increasingly more accurate compared to their laboratory versions. Laboratory tests normally have more control over and are impacted less by external factors that may affect results. For example, field-based tests may be impacted by weather conditions (temperature, humidity, differing playing surfaces) whereas these factors can be accounted for and controlled within a laboratory. However, field-based testing methods may be more sport-specific or functional, which means that the outcomes of these tests may better translate to the performance of the specific sport compared to laboratory-based tests.

DIRECT AND INDIRECT TESTING

When a test measures directly what it is investigating this is known as direct testing. An example is a laboratory-based VO_2max test where measurements of the maximal volume of oxygen consumed are taken via the collection of expired gases. Alternatively, an example of an indirect test of VO_2max would be the multistage fitness test or the Cooper 12-minute run test in which the stage number and distance run is used to estimate or predict VO_2max. Smartwatches are also a useful and relatively inexpensive tool that can measure VO_2. However, they give estimates that can have a degree of error. Even though the estimate might not be entirely accurate, they can be useful to track the progress of your client.

Table 14.1	BENEFITS OF FITNESS TESTING
Benefit of testing	**Description of benefit**
Identify strengths and weaknesses	This can help to establish an overall picture of the client's physical condition. It also provides baseline data for client training programmes and can help to assess the health status of the client, which can act as a potential monitor for overtraining.
Monitor progress	By repeating tests at specific intervals, the effectiveness of the training programme can be monitored. Results can also be used as a motivational tool.
Grouping	This can provide information that allows grouping of clients according to ability.
Education	This can help provide a better understanding of the demands of a particular sport or event.
Recovery guide	This can be used as a tool to assess recovery from injury and readiness for training.
Motivation	Testing can be used to set standards and motivate clients.
Goal setting	Short- and long-term objectives can be established.

MAXIMAL AND SUBMAXIMAL TESTING

The decision to use maximal or submaximal tests depends largely on the requirements for the data, the client being tested and the aims or reasons for the test being carried out. Maximal testing requires clients to exercise to volitional fatigue (this is the point at which the client chooses to stop based on their perception that they cannot continue rather than the point of failure). Even though adverse cardiovascular events (such as heart attack) during maximal testing are rare, practitioners should ensure that adequate screening has taken place beforehand. This should be done to ensure the client has no health issues and has current experience of exercising to high intensity. Submaximal testing refers to tests that do not require the client to go to maximal fatigue. Other factors such as proximity to competition and possibly fatiguing effects of the test should also be considered.

STATIC AND DYNAMIC TESTS

Tests can be broadly categorised as static or dynamic. With static tests there is no form of exertion required by the client whereas with dynamic tests there is a requirement. Table 14.2 shows a range of typical static and dynamic tests.

Table 14.2	TYPICAL STATIC AND DYNAMIC TESTS
	Typical tests
Static tests	Heart rate, blood pressure, body mass index, lung function (peak expiratory flow, forced vital capacity), anthropometric measurements (height, weight, waist circumference), sit and reach
Dynamic tests	Muscular strength, muscular endurance, power, speed, VO_2max, lactate threshold

Testing-related terminology

For those involved in regular testing activities it is useful to understand the following terms:

VALIDITY

Validity can be thought of as the degree to which a test or instrument measures what it purports to measure and can be determined by comparing the results of the test with those of a gold-standard test (for what is being measured), also known as the *criterion measure*.

OBJECTIVITY

This is the degree to which multiple testers agree on the magnitude and outcome of the measurement. A clearly defined scoring or measurement system can enhance the test objectivity, as can the experience of the tester.

RELIABILITY/REPRODUCIBILITY

The reliability (also known as reproducibility) of a test refers to its consistency. For example, if the same test is repeated (without a change in client status) and similar results are obtained, then the test is deemed reliable. Reliability also refers to the amount of variation that occurs in the test results between repeated trials. The main source of variation that can affect the reliability of the test is known as *experimental error*.

Experimental error

Error can be influenced by factors such as the tester's experience and complexity of the test, such as in the use of *skinfold* calipers, which involves identifying the correct anatomical sites, lifting the correct thickness of skinfold, and reading the dial at the correct angle. There can also be errors associated with equipment, especially when calibration is required. Standardising test procedures can help to reduce test errors. The steps below explain how to do this:

Table 14.3	PRE-, DURING- AND POST-TEST GUIDELINES
Procedure	**Guidelines**
Pre-test	• Clients should be screened and familiar with procedures/equipment to be used. • Assistants should be fully briefed in advance of the test. • Obtain the client's informed consent and ensure that medical clearance has been given (where appropriate) prior to any testing. • Ensure all clients are fully screened. • Standardise the pre-test conditions. • Ensure a normal diet in the days leading up to testing and do not eat 2 hours prior to the test (water is allowed unless the test specifies not).
During-test	• Encouragement and motivation should be standardised during the test. • On a test day, avoid smoking, alcohol, tea or coffee and any similar substances. • All clients should wear appropriate clothing (let them know in advance). • Explain the test procedure and objectives to all involved in the testing. • All clients should be free from illness or injury on the day of the testing.
Post-test	• Check the test in terms of compliance. • Check data collection for accuracy. • Organise client feedback.

- Standardise the test environment, temperature (between 18°C and 23°C/64.4°F and 73.4°F) and humidity (less than 70%) of an indoor testing environment. Ensure there is good ventilation.
- Take repeat measures at the same time of day as the original test.
- Follow a consistent procedure, i.e. the number of clients tested at a time, the presence or absence of observers, the amount of motivation given by observers, the sequence of the tests and the amount of rest time between tests.
- Standardise the amount and content of the warm-up and practice allowed by all clients.
- Record precise details of the test protocol (method) and measuring techniques used, for future repeatability.

Pre-test, during-test and post-test procedures such as those in table 14.3 should also be addressed, as these can help to reduce the risk of experimental errors.

NORMATIVE- AND CRITERION-REFERENCED STANDARDS

When evaluating test results, it is useful to compare against standards known as normative-referenced standards or criterion-referenced standards. Standards can be related to age, gender and fitness levels. These can also be referred to as norm tables.

Test methodology

There are many factors that the practitioner should consider when designing a test methodology. The following are just a few areas:

EVIDENCE-BASED PRACTICE

For practitioners, it is important that there is a rationale for using specific training exercises or programmes. One way to do this is to ensure that any practices used are supported by peer-reviewed (essentially an academic term for quality control), scientifically robust research. Using the findings of published research to influence practice will help to create safe programmes that, if carried out correctly, will provide the means to reach training goals and targets. It is important to be inquisitive and think critically as a practitioner in order to make calculated conclusions about things that may be observed within the industry.

The rise of personal trainer, sport science, strength & conditioning and physical trainer-related accounts on various social media platforms has resulted in infinite training resources that are readily available. However, these posts should be treated with the same level of critical thinking as a scientific research article. If evidence and a rationale are not provided, they should be treated with caution and independent research should take place to explore any claims made by the posts. If the social media post sounds too good to be true, then that is probably the case. For example, it is important that any social media post that claims 'this is the only exercise you will ever need' or 'one exercise to get rid of muscle pain' is treated with a critical eye, as it is unlikely that they are supported by scientific evidence and there is no truth to the claims being made.

Note: It is the duty of all practitioners to evidence and provide a rationale for any programmes or training methods prior to use.

SCIENTIFIC SEARCH ENGINES

There are an enormous number of accessible research papers and articles so it can be difficult to find appropriate ones that are related to a field of interest. However, there are various ways in which specific research studies can be found. Scientific search engines are a very useful and pragmatic way to locate articles of specific topics. Popular search engines include Google Scholar, PubMed, Medline and Scopus, among others. Within each of these search engines there are advanced search options that allow users to use keywords to search for all related articles in a field.

STRENGTH OF SCIENTIFIC EVIDENCE

Not all research is considered to be of the same value and strength of findings. Citing peer-reviewed research is vital when using scientific evidence for practice. This research (commonly referred to as papers) has gone through a review process before being accepted for publication in journals, which ensures it is scientifically robust and accurate in its findings. However, not all journals carry the same value, and some have a more stringent review process than others. Each journal has an impact factor, and this alludes to the reputation the journal has and how impactful the research published in the journal is. A higher impact factor normally suggests a better, more impactful journal, which infers it only accepts research of high standards for publication.

When reviewing a research paper, practitioners should consider areas such as the number of participants, the type of participants, the methodology and the statistical tests used for the research. This will help to see if the claimed findings can be replicated and are suitable for the population a practitioner may be working with. For example, the findings and practical applications from a paper performing research with professional participants may not be suitable to use with recreational clients. When using research to support better practice, context should always be considered to ensure its suitability for the population it may be used with.

Figure 14.1 provides more information regarding the strength and quality of different types of peer-reviewed research. Generally, research that amalgamates the

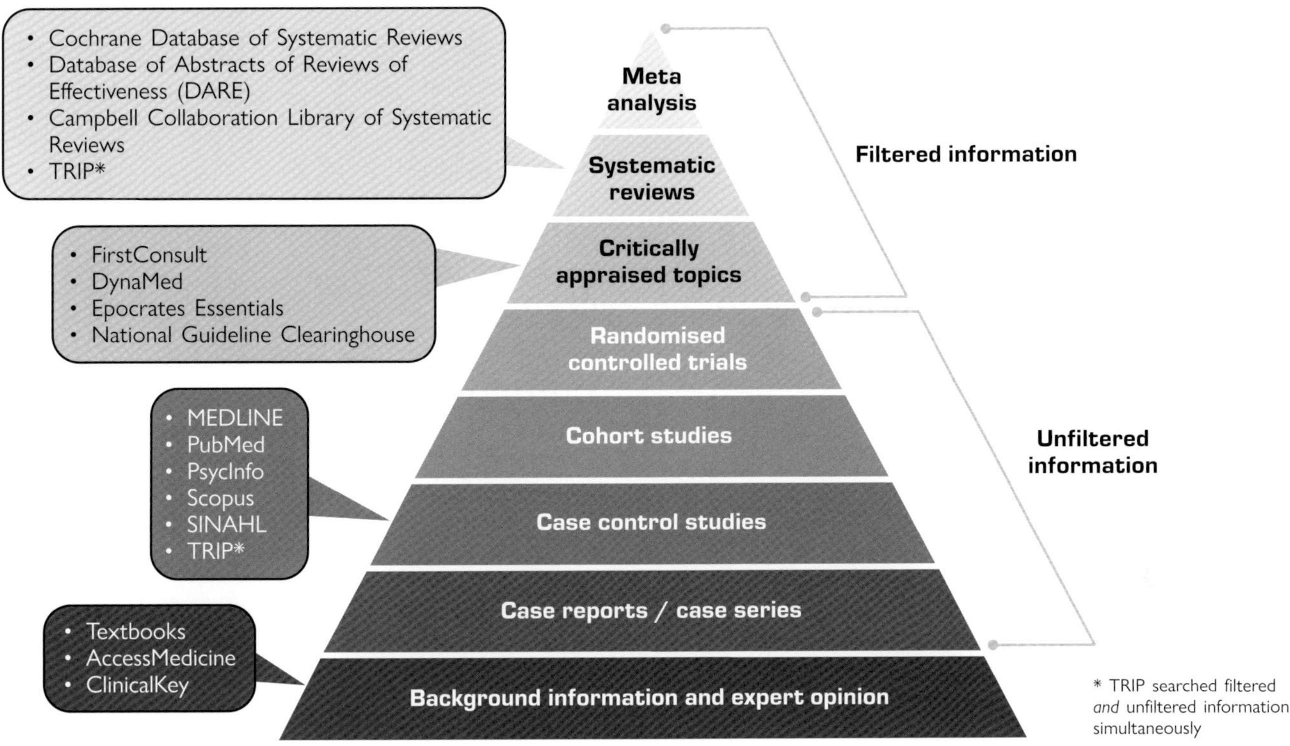

Figure 14.1 The scientific research pyramid

findings of a range of studies written on the same topic, known as a meta-analysis or review paper, carries the greatest level of strength and quality of findings. This is because this type of paper reviews the findings of previous research and draws in-depth collective conclusions on the research area. There are different types of reviews, but they are all considered to be high in quality (top of the research pyramid). Studies that involve a group of individuals are found below reviews on the pyramid (lower in quality) and are broadly split into randomised controlled trials, cohort studies and case control studies. Generally speaking, the more individuals these studies use, the more likely that the findings will be representative of the population they are testing for. For example, a study performed using a group of 50 hockey players will likely provide more representative findings than a study that uses five hockey players, therefore the research will carry greater influence and strength.

Research considered to have the lowest level of quality are case studies (research that analyses the effects of an experiment on one individual) or opinion pieces that do not include any experimentation but instead call on an industry expert to provide their opinions on a particular topic.

Data protection

When collecting any personal client information there is a responsibility of the practitioner to ensure that all information is dealt with in a confidential way. Essentially, the Data Protection Act 2018

Component	Test	Units	Target range	Score	Class
Body (anthropometric) data	Height	cm	See BMI		
	Weight	kg	See BMI		
	Heart rate	bpm			
Body composition	BMI	Index	<25		
	Skinfold	Fat %	M: <25% F: <30%		
	Electrical imp	Fat %	M: <25% F: <30%		
Blood pressure	Blood pressure	mmHg	120/80<140/90		
Lung function	FVC	L	Age-related scores		
	FEV1	L	Age-related scores		
	EIB	% drop	<10% drop		
Flexibility	Sit and reach	cm	M: ≥22cm F: ≥22cm		
	Modified sit and reach	cm	M: ≥14.4cm F: ≥14.8cm		
Cardio endurance	Multi-stage fitness test	Level	M: level ≥7 F: level ≥6		
	Cooper 12-minute test	m	Age-related scores		
	Rockport walk test	bpm s	Set baseline		
Balance	Stork test	s	≥25s		
Power	Vertical jump	cm	M: ≥41cm F: ≥ 31cm		
Speed	30m sprint	s	M: ≤4.4s F: ≤4.7s		
Client name:		Date:	Environment:		
Time:	Conditions:				

Figure 14.2 Test result sheet (for a blank template, please visit: bloomsbury.com/uk/complete-guide-to-strength-and-conditioning-training-9781399421362)

(legislation.gov.uk/ukpga/2018/12/contents) determines responsibilities when collecting and storing information. The main areas of the act advise the following:

- Personal data should only be collected for lawful purposes.
- Personal data should only be used for the purposes for which it has been collected.
- Personal data should not be kept for longer than is necessary.
- Measures should be taken to ensure that personal data is kept confidential and stored appropriately.

Before any testing is carried out, consent from a client must be obtained in writing, having fully explained the nature of the chosen tests. This can be done using a health and fitness assessment consent form (*see* Appendix 3).

Data collection

Test results should be recorded in a standardised manner, such as that shown in figure 14.2. Once results have been recorded, they can be compared with normative data and classified.

Data analysis terms

When interpreting any test data there are common terms that are useful to know. Let's explore some of them now:

PRECISION

This is related to the accuracy of the measurement taken. For example, a 30m (33-yard) sprint should be measured to the nearest hundredth of a second (0.01s) and *not* to the nearest second, whereas heart rate monitors only record to the nearest beat per minute so an averaged heart rate of 167.5bpm should be correctly

recorded as 168bpm. The following terms are related to precision:

- **Mean** – The mean or arithmetic average is the sum of the scores divided by the number of scores.
- **Median** – The middle score or 50th percentile. Order the numbers from low to high; the middle one is the median.
- **Mode** – This is the most frequently observed score. It is not typically a useful indicator of the average value for a measurement.
- **Range** – The range is the maximum score minus the minimum score. It gives a measure of the variability of the data.

ANALYSING DATA

One of the first steps in the analysis of data is to verify if the data set is normally distributed, as this can inform the type of analysis that is performed. Normal distribution of data indicates that most of the data points are close to the average, while relatively few points tend to one extreme or the other. For example, a normally distributed data set plotted on a graph would have a bell-shaped appearance, such as that in figure 14.3.

When plotting data, the x axis (horizontal) represents the value of the measurement, and the y axis (vertical) is

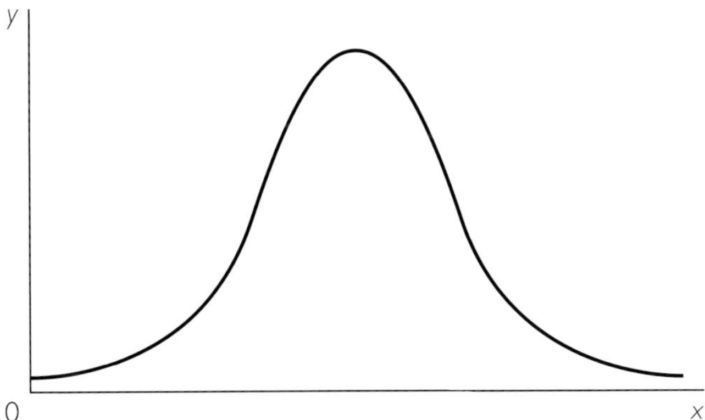

Figure 14.3 Normal distribution of data

the number of data points for each value on the x axis. The **standard deviation** shows how the data points are clustered around the mean. When data points are bunched together and the bell-shaped curve is steep, the standard deviation is considered small. When the data points are spread apart, it represents a larger standard deviation. As can be seen in figure 14.4, one standard deviation away from the mean in either direction on the horizontal axis accounts for approximately 68% of the data in the group. Two standard deviations can account for approximately 95% and three standard deviations can account for about 99%.

Once the distribution of data has been established there are various analyses that can be carried out depending on the required outcome. Common outcomes include **correlation** and differences.

CORRELATION

The term correlation (denoted as 'r') describes the relationship between two sets of data and can be a positive relationship or a negative relationship. For example, figure 14.5 shows the relationship between 1RM squat strength and 30m (33-yard) sprint times. The values of 'r' can range between minus one (-1), known as a negative relationship, and plus one (+1), known as a positive relationship. The closer 'r' is to either +1 or -1, the stronger the association or relationship. Typically, the value of 'r' is then squared (R^2). In figure 14.5, R^2 is 0.9221, which indicates that 92% of the variation in 30m (33-yard) sprint time can be explained by the 1RM squat.

The most common correlations in fitness testing are the Pearson product-moment correlation and the Spearman's rank correlation. A correlation can only indicate a possible relationship between variables or groups of measurements but does not confirm or establish a causal relationship. In other words, it cannot state exactly that one of the groups of measurements has a direct effect on the other group of measurements.

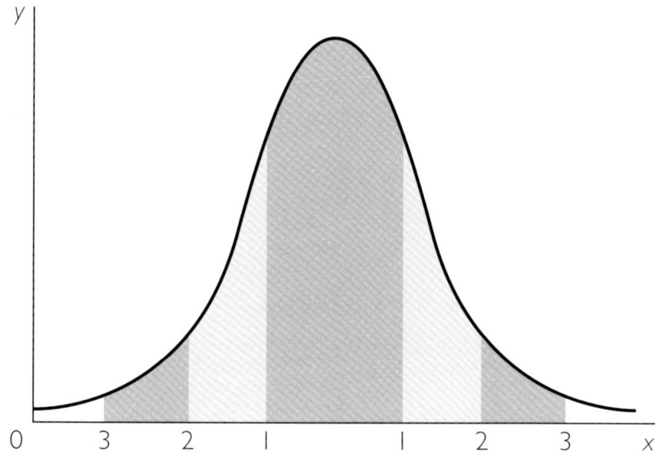

Figure 14.4 Standard deviation away from the mean

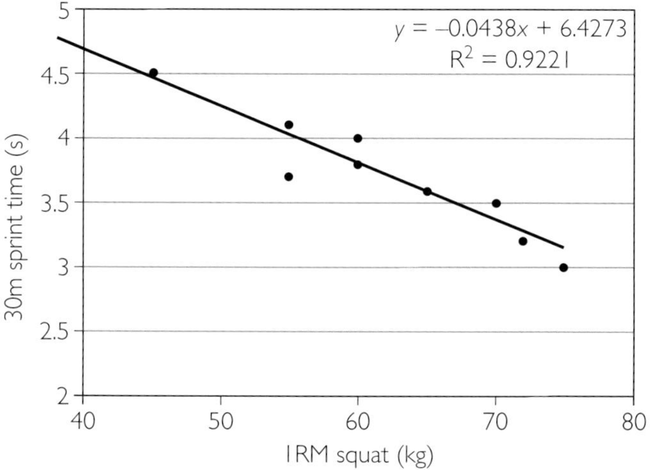

Figure 14.5 Sprint times related to squat strength

DIFFERENCES

Improvement in performance is one of the most common outcomes required from testing. The *t* test is most frequently used to test for differences between sets of data (i.e. test for differences in performance). The data in table 14.4 can illustrate the use of a *t* test.

Table 14.4	SQUAT PERFORMANCE FOR FEMALE VOLLEYBALL TEAMS A AND B		
	Team A year 1	**Team A year 2**	**Team B year 1**
Mean	59kg	62kg	58kg
Standard deviation	11kg	12kg	11kg
P value (relative to Team A, year 1)		0.006 (<0.05)**	0.34 (>0.05)

** indicates a significant P value (<0.05)

To compare squat performance of team A between year 1 and year 2 a paired t test is used (paired = when data sets are from the same group). The result of the paired t test shows that the 'P' value obtained is 0.006. As this is less than 0.05 (the usual threshold chosen for statistical significance), it shows that the squat performance for team A was significantly greater in the second year than the first year (if the 'P' value was above 0.05 this would show that team A's squat performance was not significantly greater).

When comparing team A in season 1 to team B, an unpaired t test would be used (unpaired = data sets from two different groups). Results of the unpaired t test show that the 'P' value obtained is 0.34. As this is greater than 0.05, it shows there is no significant difference in performance between the two teams.

While t tests provide an understanding of how significant differences between two sets of data are, it is also possible to calculate the magnitude or size of the observed differences using effect sizes. Cohen's d effect sizes are the most commonly used measure to calculate the size of a difference between two groups. The equation to calculate Cohen's d effect sizes is as follows:

$$\frac{\text{Group A mean} - \text{Group B mean}}{\text{pooled standard deviation}}$$

Table 14.5	COHEN'S d EFFECT SIZES	
	Cohen's d	**Effect size**
	0.2	Small
	0.5	Medium
	0.8	Large

The pooled standard deviation refers to the average standard deviation of both groups. Table 14.5 shows how Cohen's d values can be interpreted in terms of the size of the difference between two groups.

Using the same example, we can input the mean and standard deviation to calculate the effect size for the differences between year 1 and year 2 for team A:

$$\frac{\text{Year 1 mean} - \text{Year 2 mean}}{\text{Mean Year 1 and Year 2 standard deviation}}$$

$$\frac{59 - 62}{11.5}$$

$$= 0.26$$

Therefore, according to the effect size, there is a small difference in squat performance between year

1 and year 2 for team A. By using t tests (p values) and effect sizes in conjunction with one another, it is possible to identify if differences between data sets are significant and also the size of the differences that have been observed.

NORMATIVE/BASELINE DATA – ANALYSING CHANGES IN PERFORMANCE

When analysing performance test data, it is important to compare this with baseline values or normative data values. Baseline test values are the values that were recorded from the first or previous tests that were carried out by the same client. Repeat test results can be compared to baseline levels to track changes in performance. Normative data can be taken from published research from equivalent populations of individuals using similar testing equipment to calculate test scores.

SMALLEST WORTHWHILE CHANGE (SWC)

It is important to remember that measured changes in performance may not be meaningful changes and will depend on how they are measured and what technology is used to measure them. For a change to be practically meaningful, it must be greater than the SWC, which is a measure that will account for variation in performance that may be caused by error rates of testing equipment, environmental factors or varying performance states of individuals (e.g. varying individual fatigue levels). The SWC can be calculated using this equation:

SWC = 0.2 * between subject standard deviation

Data feedback

Once testing has taken place, practitioners (sport scientists, strength and conditioning coaches, personal train-ers etc.) need to extract and analyse data and then communicate the findings back to the client or group being tested. This can be in the form of written reports or verbally, depending on the situation. Findings may also have to be communicated to other individuals who are associated with those being tested. Analysis of the data can then be used to inform the planning process and subsequent testing.

EXTRACTING KEY DATA

Identifying key measures to track changes in performance

The first step in extracting key data is to establish which metrics (a specific category of data that can be used to answer performance-based questions) and measurements can be used to inform/track changes in performance. For example, research has shown that using jump height is not a good indicator of maximal power output during the countermovement jump test; a power-related metric measured on a force plate is a more suitable metric to use to track performance changes.

Each monitoring tool or testing equipment will produce a range of metrics and it is the role of the practitioner to highlight key metrics from these ranges that can be used to inform key stakeholders (a person with an interest in the specific area being discussed) about performance outcomes without providing too many data points and unnecessary information. Modern technology used to monitor performance (e.g. force plates, accelerometers, motion capture cameras etc.) can provide tens if not hundreds of different metrics, so it can be difficult to streamline these outputs and identify the key metrics required to make informed performance-based decisions.

Artificial intelligence (AI) and machine learning are becoming increasingly commonplace within the sports industry, particularly as the volume of data available to practitioners, obtained from the testing and monitoring of athletes, has exponentially increased. While the use of AI may assist with the cleaning, wrangling and processing of large data sets, its use requires a specialised skill set often associated with data scientists. The ability to use coding languages such as Python or R is also becoming more commonplace within the sports science and S&C industry, thus some practitioners may possess the skill set to use AI to process the data they collect. However, an S&C practitioner still needs the necessary skills to be able to interpret results and make meaningful inferences from the data to inform training programmes.

Identifying key measures for different stakeholders

While having the resources and ability to collect objective data points to measure performance outcomes is important, possessing soft skills and an understanding of the target audience that the results will be shown to is equally as important. Key stakeholders who support clients (technical coaches, medical staff, family members and the clients themselves) may have experience from a variety of backgrounds and therefore may have ranging abilities in interpreting data. Equally, they may have interest in different aspects of the test and the data being collected. Using the countermovement jump test as an example again, if the test is being used in the rehabilitation process for a client returning from injury, there may be results from the test that are used differently by various people. A technical coach may look at the maximal power output and compare the results to a baseline pre-injury level of performance as an indicator of how the client is progressing through the rehabilitation process. However, a sport scientist or physiotherapist may be more interested in observing the power output differences between the injured and healthy limb to minimise asymmetries that may be indicative of a higher risk of re-injury.

CREATING WORKING RELATIONSHIPS WITH KEY STAKEHOLDERS

Collaboration between key stakeholders (clients, coaches, physios)

In sport, the acronym MDT stands for multi-disciplinary team, which consists of everyone who supports clients to achieve optimal performance levels. This includes the technical, performance, medical and management teams, who must all collaborate and work towards a collective goal to provide a client/team with the support required to succeed in their sport. Everyone within the MDT has specific areas of expertise and responsibilities that they must use to perform their role effectively while also working with the others to achieve overarching objectives. An MDT that is successful in working in their individual parts in conjunction with the wider group will provide clients with the tools to succeed in their development.

Data feedback

As touched on above, various stakeholders may be interested in different metrics, depending on their role. Similarly, they may also have differing levels of competency and understanding of data and how it can be used to inform practice and performance. Therefore, it is vital that practitioners develop working relationships with the coaching, medical and performance teams. This will help to determine the level of understanding of each staff member regarding data analysis. Furthermore, it is helpful if performance practitioners understand the others' areas of interest and how they like to visualise data so that they know how to best deliver information to their wider team. For example, some technical coaches may not necessarily be interested in data but would like the practitioner to explain if the results are good or bad and how best to proceed. On the other hand, some staff may want to analyse the data in depth to inform their decision-making process.

It is therefore important to be adaptable to working with a wide range of staff and understand their working processes.

VISUALISING DATA – CREATING FEEDBACK REPORTS

Data visualisation

There are many different ways in which data can be displayed and analysed. Therefore, the ability to effectively display data in ways that the reader will be able to easily interpret is an important skill to develop. When designing reports to display data, practitioners should consider who will be viewing them and the way in which they can analyse data. This understanding comes from forming working relationships with colleagues and understanding how they would like to have information fed back to them.

Often, simplicity is key for developing reports. Graphs, tables and other data feedback methods should be easy for stakeholders to interpret without the need for an explanation from the designer. In terms of report design, it is important to be consistent and concise, so the following guidelines should be used:

- Each graph should only display one or two metrics.
- The axes should be scaled appropriately so that the data is clear to see.
- Text and numbers should be a neutral colour and a size that is readable.
- Coloured bars or data points can be effective in highlighting data but only one or two colours should be used, as the use of many colours can make it difficult to interpret the data.
- Informative, concise graph and axes titles that include the units of the measure they are showing should be used so that an explanation of the graph is not required to understand what it is displaying.
- The type of graph or table used affects how easy it will be for others to interpret the data. Commonly, a simple bar, column, line or scatter graph or a combination of these (e.g. a column graph with a line graph showing another metric and displayed on an additional axis within the same graph) are adequate to display the data and can be easily interpreted by the reader.
- Radar plots and pie charts are effective visually in displaying higher-level data and general trends of data but may be less suitable than tables or scatter/ bar graphs in providing precise values.

Table 14.6 is an example of a table that has an appropriate layout and adequate information included within the column titles, including an explanation of the metric and the units of measurement. As all numbers have metres or number of occurrences as units, decimal places have been removed to make the table easy to read. MD = match day.

Figure 14.6 shows an example of a well-designed graph (left) and a poorly designed graph (right). The well-designed graph includes a title, values representing the size of each bar, appropriately scaled axes and an axis title including units of measurement.

Modification of data visualisation for different stakeholders

To reinforce previous points, reports displaying data may look different depending on who is viewing them and what metrics they may be interested in. For example, a team manager may like the data to be displayed in rank order so that they can see how their clients are performing compared to other team members of competitors. On the other hand, medical staff may prefer detailed reports on one client with specific metrics included that can help to identify risks of injury or progress within rehabilitation programmes.

Table 14.6	AN EXAMPLE OF A TABLE DISPLAYING LOCOMOTOR DATA OF A FOOTBALL PLAYER ACROSS A TRAINING WEEK INCLUDING FOUR TRAINING SESSIONS (MD-5, MD-4, MD-2, MD-1), ONE MATCH (MD) AND TWO REST DAYS (MD-3, MD+1) MEASURED USING A BACK-MOUNTED GPS DEVICE					
Day	Training day	Total distance (m)	High-speed running [19.8km/h](m)	Sprint running [>25.2km/h] (m)	Accelerations (#)	Decelerations (#)
Mon	MD-5	3420	100	0	22	12
Tues	MD-4	8670	850	122	50	28
Wed	MD-3	0	0	0	0	0
Thur	MD-2	6730	340	54	58	30
Fri	MD-1	3980	130	0	25	15
Sat	MD	10,510	960	156	65	32
Sun	MD+1	0	0	0	0	0

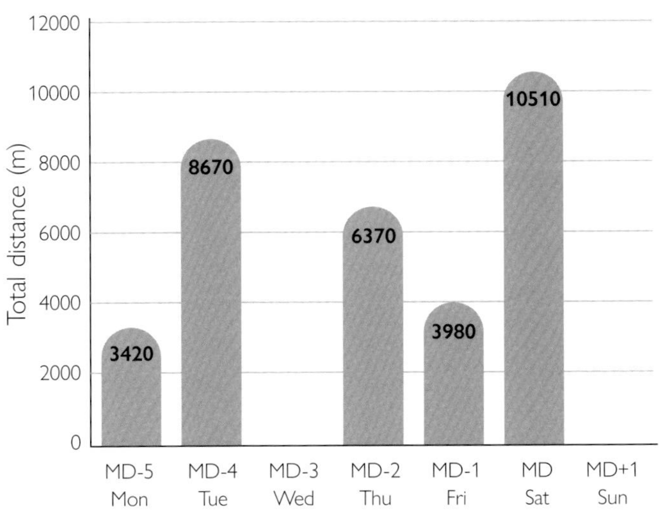

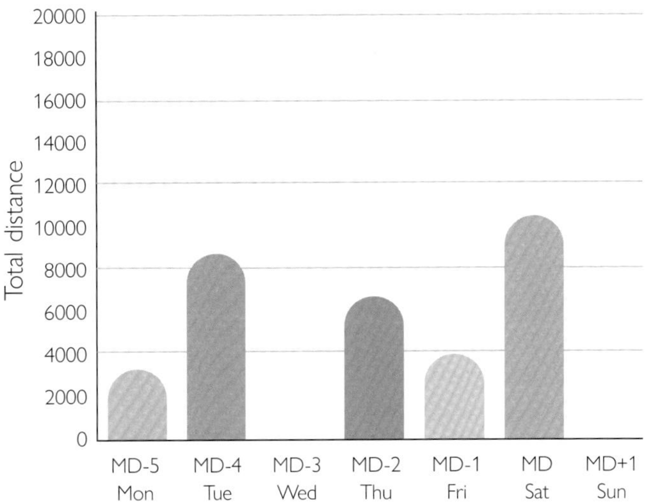

Figure 14.6 Graphs showing the total distance covered by a football player during each day of a training week including four training sessions (MD-5, MD-4, MD-2, MD-1), one match (MD) and two rest days (MD-3, MD+1) measured using a back-mounted GPS device

Programming training and future testing

DATA ANALYSIS AND VISUALISATION FOLLOW-UP

The most important aspect of data analysis is the ability to plan and understand the next steps required to progress depending on the outcome of testing. Training programme design, content and delivery should consider the current performance status of a client based on testing and assessments. Using objective and subjective data to make informed decisions on how best to train clients provides practitioners with a rationale when designing training programmes. For example, if a sprinter is found to have low eccentric hamstring strength during Nordic hamstring testing, then one aim of their programme should be to address this, as it is commonly known that high eccentric hamstring strength is a factor that reduces hamstring injury risks.

Following the analysis of testing results and delivery of feedback, programme planning should never be an isolated event carried out by one practitioner. The programme should be designed collectively by members of the MDT so that everyone is aligned on the programme's rationale, aims, goals/outcomes and timescale. It is also vitally important that this process is completely transparent, and the client is aligned with and in agreement with their training programme before continuing. Only once all relevant parties are content and in agreement with the programme design should it be undertaken.

PLANNING RE-TESTING

An important aspect of training programme design is the time frame of when re-testing will occur. Re-testing a client should be done strategically and periodically to identify if a training programme is helping the client to succeed in the aims that were highlighted at the beginning of the programme. For example, if a training programme is 12 weeks long then it may be useful to conduct tests at the midpoint after 6 weeks to provide an insight into the efficacy of the training programme. This then provides an opportunity for the training programme to be modified to realign with the aims that it was originally created under. Furthermore, testing batteries should be planned at periods when clients are not fatigued (i.e. not following competition) and at points so that any fatigue induced by tests does not impact competition performance.

Take-home messages

- Data analysis, visualisation and feedback are vital skills to learn and develop.

- They allow practitioners to translate their findings from training, competition and testing data into manageable reports that are designed so that they can be correctly interpreted by relevant stakeholders that are involved in the client's development and performance.

- The correct interpretation of data can allow practitioners to better understand and plan further training programmes and testing sessions to allow clients an optimum environment where they can develop and perform in their sport.

Aerobic endurance testing 15

Introduction

Aerobic endurance is a component of fitness that is important not just for athletic performance but for general health as well, as having a good level can reduce the risk of chronic diseases such as heart disease and diabetes. Aerobic endurance tends to be one of the most common client goals. The general public often use the term 'wanting to get a bit fitter' rather than 'wanting to improve aerobic endurance'. This chapter looks at how to measure the progress of aerobic endurance using scientifically robust tests and investigates how they can be used for the development of aerobic endurance.

Testing

Cardiovascular endurance can be measured as volume of oxygen (VO_2). As exercise intensity increases, the volume of oxygen consumed increases directly until it reaches a plateau, as shown in figure 15.1. This plateau is termed VO_2 max and is also known as aerobic capacity, aerobic power or maximal oxygen uptake. When bodyweight is not taken into account it is called absolute VO_2 and is measured in litres per minute. When bodyweight is taken into account it is

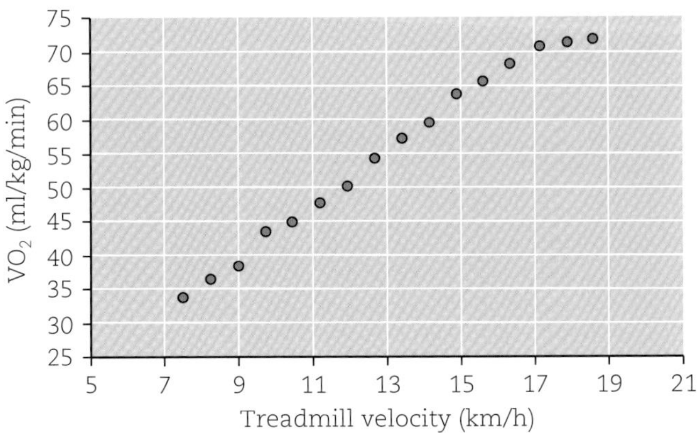

Figure 15.1 Relationship between exercise intensity and volume of oxygen

known as relative VO_2 and the units of measurement are millilitres of oxygen per kilogram bodyweight per minute ($mlO_2.kg^{-1}.min^{-1}$).

Cardiovascular endurance testing can be done either at submaximal level or at maximum depending on the client being tested, the experience of the tester and the goal of the test. Testing to maximum level is referred to as a VO_2max test.

The direct method of testing involves the collection and analysis of breath-by-breath *expired air*, which is known as respiratory gas analysis. This can be done in either a lab or field-based environment, as equipment such as portable gas analysers and smartwatches are commonly available.

Some of the more common indirect field-based methods of testing for VO_2 include the multi-stage fitness test (also known as the beep or bleep test), the 30–15 intermittent fitness test, the Harvard step test, the Cooper 12-minute run, the Rockport walking test and heart rate variability. They are referred to as indirect tests because they do not measure the amount of oxygen consumed. Let's take a look at some now:

Multi-stage fitness test

The multi-stage fitness test (MSFT) was first developed by Leger in 1984. It is a suitable test of maximal oxygen uptake (VO_2max) for teams, as the acceleration and deceleration required in the test reflects the needs of many sports.

Equipment required:

A flat, non-slippery surface at least 20m (66ft) in length, 30m (98ft) tape measure, marking cones, pre-recorded audio file

Test protocol:

There are 23 exercise levels, where each exercise level lasts approximately 1 minute and comprises of a series of 20m (66ft) shuttle runs. The starting speed is 8.5km/hr-1 and this increases by 0.5km/hr-1 at each level. A single beep indicates the end of a shuttle, and three beeps indicate the start of the next level. The test is conducted as follows:

1. Measure out a 20m (66ft) section on a flat surface with a marker cone or line at each end.
2. Give clients clear instructions for how to do the test and then perform a warm-up.
3. Start the test. During the test, clients must place one foot on or beyond the 20m (66ft) marker at the end of each shuttle.
4. If a client arrives at the end of a shuttle before the beep, they must wait for the beep and then resume running.
5. Clients are to keep running for as long as possible until they can no longer keep up with the speed set by the beeps.
6. Issue a warning if a client fails to reach the end of the shuttle before the beep. They should be allowed two further shuttles to attempt to regain

Table 15.1 — MULTI-STAGE FITNESS TEST LEVELS

Level	Shuttle	VO$_2$max	Level	Shuttle	VO$_2$max	Level	Shuttle	VO$_2$max	Level	Shuttle	VO$_2$max
4	2	26.8	5	2	30.2	14	2	61.1	15	2	64.6
4	4	27.6	5	4	31.0	14	4	61.7	15	4	65.1
4	6	28.3	5	6	31.8	14	6	62.2	15	6	65.6
4	9	29.5	5	9	32.9	14	8	62.7	15	8	66.2
						14	10	63.2	15	10	66.7
6	2	33.6	7	2	37.1	14	13	64.0	15	13	67.5
6	4	34.3	7	4	37.8						
6	6	35.0	7	6	38.5	16	2	68.0	17	2	71.4
6	8	35.7	7	8	39.2	16	4	68.5	17	4	71.9
6	10	36.4	7	10	39.9	16	6	69.0	17	6	72.4
						16	8	69.5	17	8	72.9
8	2	40.5	9	2	43.9	16	10	69.9	17	10	73.4
8	4	41.1	9	4	44.5	16	12	70.5	17	12	73.9
8	6	41.8	9	6	45.2	16	14	70.9	17	14	74.4
8	8	42.4	9	8	45.8						
8	11	43.3	9	11	46.8	18	2	74.8	19	2	78.3
						18	4	75.3	19	4	78.8
						18	6	75.8	19	6	79.2
10	2	47.4	11	2	50.8	18	8	76.2	19	8	79.7
10	4	48.0	11	4	51.4	18	10	76.7	19	10	80.2
10	6	48.7	11	6	51.9	18	12	77.2	19	12	80.6
10	8	49.3	11	8	52.5	18	15	77.9	19	15	81.3
10	11	50.2	11	10	53.1						
						20	2	81.8	21	2	85.2
12	2	54.3	13	2	57.6	20	4	82.2	21	4	85.6
12	4	54.8	13	4	58.2	20	6	82.6	21	6	86.1
12	6	55.4	13	6	58.7	20	8	83.0	21	8	86.5
12	8	56.0	13	8	59.3	20	10	83.5	21	10	86.9
12	10	56.5	13	10	59.8	20	12	83.9	21	12	87.4
12	12	57.1	13	13	60.6	20	14	84.3	21	14	87.8
						20	16	84.8	21	16	88.2

the required pace before being withdrawn. Record the level attained (*see* table 15.1).

Test results:

Table 15.1 can be used to estimate the VO_2max score from the highest test level completed.

Sources of error:

As with all fitness tests there are associated errors. An awareness of how to minimise errors is important in order to achieve consistent and reliable results for comparison purposes.

Table 15.2	SOURCES OF ERROR FOR MSFT
Error source	**Minimising strategy**
Timing	Scorers need to be consistent in judging if clients reach the line in time. Use the same scorer to minimise error.
Population	Suitable for conditioned clients, as it is a maximal test. Do not use for those who are deconditioned.
Environment	Make sure the floor is suitable and there is enough space for all clients.

30–15 intermittent fitness test

The **30–15 intermittent fitness test (30–15 IFT) has become popular in sport because it is a test of the main intermittent sport-specific physiological determinants (not just aerobic endurance) and is therefore useful for tracking clients' overall fitness levels.**

Equipment required:

A flat, non-slippery surface at least 40m (44 yards) in length, 40m (44-yard) tape measure, marking cones, pre-recorded audio file, 30–15 app

Test protocol:

The test was developed by Bucheit in 2000 and requires clients to perform shuttles between two lines 40m (44 yards) apart. There are four versions of the test. This version commences at 8.5km/hr-1 with the client running for 30 seconds before an active recovery period of 15 seconds as they move towards the next starting marker cones. The velocity of each stage increases by 0.5km/hr-1 until volitional exhaustion is reached. The velocity at the last completed stage is recorded as peak velocity. The test is conducted as follows:

1. Measure out a 40m (44-yard) section on a flat surface with a marker cone or line at each end, as shown in figure 15.2.
2. Give clients clear instructions for how to do the test and then perform a warm-up.
3. Start the test. Clients start at line A, run to line C crossing line B, and then return towards line A.
4. After crossing line B again, they stop after 8.5m (28ft) and walk to line A during the 15-second recovery to be ready for the next stage.
5. Clients are to keep running for as long as possible until they can no longer keep up with the speed set by the beeps.

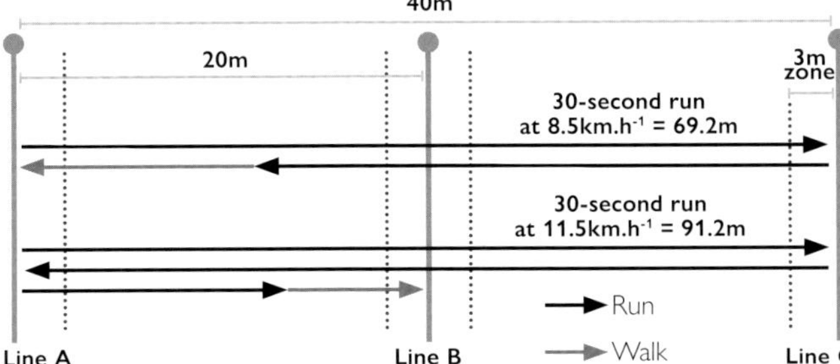

Figure 15.2 The 30–15 intermittent fitness test

6. The test ends when the client cannot reach the next 3m (10ft) zone at the beep on three successive occasions. Record the last completed stage.

Test results:

Client VO_2max can be calculated using the following equation, where G is the gender (1 = male; 2 = female), A is the age (in years), W is the body mass (kg), and V_{IFT} is the peak velocity achieved.

$$VO_2max\ (mlO_2.kg^{-1}\cdot min^{-1}) = 28.3 - (2.15 \times G) - (0.741 \times A) - (0.0357 \times W) + (0.0586 \times A \times V_{IFT}) + (1.03 \times V_{IFT})$$

Sources of error:

Table 15.3	SOURCES OF ERROR FOR 30–15 IFT
Error source	**Minimising strategy**
Timing	Scorers need to be consistent in judging if clients reach the line in time. Brief all scorers prior to the start of the test.
Population	Suitable for conditioned clients, as it is a maximal test. Do not use for those who are deconditioned.
Environment	Make sure the floor is suitable and there is enough space for all clients.

Harvard step test

The Harvard step test is sometimes referred to as the Brouha test because it was developed at Harvard University in 1942 by Brouha and his colleagues to assess aerobic capacity of individuals. This test is simple to conduct and is one of several step tests (such as the Queens College step test and the Chester step test) that can be used to predict aerobic fitness. The test predicts VO_2 based on *heart rate recovery*.

Equipment required:

Step bench of appropriate height, metronome, heart rate measuring device (such as a sport watch or heart rate monitor belt)

Test protocol:

1. With the heart rate measuring device fitted, the client steps on to a bench of height 41.3cm (16¼in) with one leg, then the other and then steps down in the same manner. Fully extend the legs at the top of the step.
2. The step rate is set at 22 full steps (up, up, down, down) per minute for women and 24 steps per minute for men.
3. Clients must maintain the stepping rate for 3 minutes.
4. After 3 minutes the client remains standing.
5. The heart rate is then measured and recorded in bpm.

Test results:

Client VO_2max can be calculated using the appropriate equation:

Men: $VO_2max\ (mlO_2.kg^{-1}min^{-1})$
$= 111.33 - (0.42 \times bpm)$

Women: $VO_2max\ (mlO_2.kg^{-1}min^{-1})$
$= 65.81 - (0.1847 \times bpm)$

Sources of error:

Table 15.4	SOURCES OF ERROR FOR THE HARVARD STEP TEST
Error source	**Minimising strategy**
Timing	Clients not stepping up and down to the rate of the metronome. Allow clients to practise before undergoing the test.
Heart rate	If heart rate is taken manually errors can occur, as the heart rate slows while it is being taken. Use telemetry to avoid this.
Environment	Make sure there is enough space for all clients.
Biomechanical	Taller clients will expend less energy when stepping. Bodyweight can also be a factor. If testing a group with extreme height or weight difference, select an alternative test.

Cooper 12-minute run

This test was designed by Dr Kenneth Cooper in 1968 for US military use. The test involves measuring the distance a client can walk or run in 12 minutes. This test is widely used due to its simplicity and reliability.

Equipment required:

400m (437-yard) track – marked every 100m (110 yards) – or a treadmill, stopwatch

Test protocol:

1. Instruct the client to walk or run as far as possible in 12 minutes.
2. The client should perform a standardised warm-up.
3. The client should start walking or running on the command of the tester, who starts the stopwatch at the same time.
4. The tester should call out the time at regular intervals.
5. After 11 minutes the tester should count down the last minute for the client.
6. After 12 minutes the tester should measure the total distance covered by the client.

Test results:

Client VO_2max can be calculated using the following equation where *d12* represents the distance (measured in metres) covered in 12 minutes:

$$VO_2max = (d12 - 505) / 45$$

The classification table (table 15.5) can then be used to categorise the results based on the distance the client achieves.

Table 15.5	NORMATIVE TABLE FOR ADULTS (VALUES IN METRES)				
Age	Excellent	Above Average	Average	Below Average	Poor
Males 20–29	>2800	2400–2800	2200–2399	1600–2199	<1600
Females 20–29	>2700	2200–2700	1800–2199	1500–1799	<1500
Males 30–39	>2700	2300–2700	1900–2299	1500–1999	<1500
Females 30–39	>2500	2000–2500	1700–1999	1400–1699	<1400
Males 40–49	>2500	2100–2500	1700–2099	1400–1699	<1400
Females 40–49	>2300	1900–2300	1500–1899	1200–1499	<1200
Males >50	>2400	2000–2400	1600–1999	1300–1599	<1300
Females >50	>2200	1700–2200	1400–1699	1100–1399	<1100

Sources of error:

Table 15.6	SOURCES OF ERROR FOR THE COOPER 12-MINUTE RUN
Error source	Minimising strategy
Pacing	Clients need to learn how to pace correctly, so discount the first two or three test results.
Population	The test does not represent team sports that involve changes of direction. Choose a test such as the Yo-Yo test for these populations.
Training status	This is not a reliable test for deconditioned clients. Use for conditioned clients only.

Rockport walking test

The Rockport walking test was developed in 1986 at the University of Massachusetts as a submaximal test to be used predominantly for deconditioned clients. It is based on the time taken to complete a 1-mile (1.6km) walk by using finishing heart rate, weight, age and gender to predict VO_2max.

Equipment required:

400m (437-yard) track (or 1-mile route), stopwatch, measuring device (such as a sport watch or heart rate monitor belt)

Test protocol:

1. Record the weight of the client, then attach the heart rate monitoring device.
2. The client lines up on the starting line of a pre-planned route.

3. The client starts walking on the command of the tester, who starts the stopwatch at the same time.
4. The client walks 1 mile (1.6km) as fast as possible.
5. Immediately on finishing, record the client's heart rate (beats per minute) and the time taken to complete the route.

Test results:

Client VO$_2$max can be calculated using the following equation where Gender = 0 (female) or 1 (male); Time = walk time to the nearest hundredth of a minute, measured in minutes; HR = heart rate (bpm) at the end of the test; BW = bodyweight in kg:

$$VO_2max = 132.853 - (0.0769 \times BW(kg)) - (0.3877 \times age\ (yrs)) + (6.3150 \times gender) - (3.2649 \times time) - (0.1565 \times HR)$$

Table 15.7 can then be used to identify the classification of clients based on gender and age.

Table 15.7	MALE AND FEMALE NORMATIVE VALUES FOR VO$_2$MAX					
Female (values in mlO$_2$.kg^{-1}min^{-1})						
Age	V. poor	Poor	Fair	Good	Excellent	Superior
13–19	<25.0	25.0–30.9	31.0–34.9	35.0–38.9	39.0–41.9	>41.9
20–29	<23.6	23.6–28.9	29.0–32.9	33.0–36.9	37.0–41.0	>41.0
30–39	<22.8	22.8–26.9	27.0–31.4	31.5–35.6	35.7–40.0	>40.0
40–49	<21.0	21.0–24.4	24.5–28.9	29.0–32.8	32.9–36.9	>36.9
50–59	<20.2	20.2–22.7	22.8–26.9	27.0–31.4	31.5–35.7	>35.7
60+	<17.5	17.5–20.1	20.2–24.4	24.5–30.2	30.3–31.4	>31.4
Male (values in mlO$_2$.kg^{-1}min^{-1})						
Age	V. poor	Poor	Fair	Good	Excellent	Superior
13–19	<35.0	35.0–38.3	38.4–45.1	45.2–50.9	51.0–55.9	>55.9
20–29	<33.0	33.0–36.4	36.5–42.4	42.5–46.4	46.5–52.4	>52.4
30–39	<31.5	31.5–35.4	35.5–40.9	41.0–44.9	45.0–49.4	>49.4
40–49	<30.2	30.2–33.5	33.6–38.9	39.0–43.7	43.8–48.0	>48.0
50–59	<26.1	26.1–30.9	31.0–35.7	35.8–40.9	41.0–45.3	>45.3
60+	<20.5	20.5–26.0	26.1–32.2	32.3–36.4	36.5–44.2	>44.2

Sources of error:

Table 15.8	SOURCES OF ERROR FOR THE ROCKPORT WALKING TEST
Error source	**Minimising strategy**
Pacing	Clients need to learn how to pace correctly, so discount the first two or three test results.
Intensity	Clients often adopt a 'comfortable' walking pace. Reinforce the message that this is a maximal test and clients should try to walk as fast as they can.
Training status	This is not a reliable test for conditioned clients. Use for deconditioned clients only.
Training buddies	Clients will often walk in groups and adopt a pace suitable for the least fit. Set clients off at different times.

Heart rate recovery

The ability of the heart to return to near resting levels following exercise can also be used as a measure of aerobic fitness and is known as heart rate recovery (HRR). A shorter recovery is associated with a decreased mortality risk. A longer recovery can be a sign of potential health issues.

Essentially there are two methods of testing HRR. The general method follows a standard protocol and provides a classification whereas the individual profile method follows a protocol that is unique to each client and therefore provides a baseline for future reference.

Equipment required:
Heart rate measuring device (such as a sport watch or heart rate monitor belt), stopwatch, exercise equipment

Test protocol 1 – general method:
1. Fit a HR measuring device to the client.
2. Select the preferred cardio equipment (treadmill, bike, rower, etc.). Repeat testing should use the same equipment.
3. Complete a standardised warm-up appropriate to the environment.
4. Complete a 10-minute bout of exercise at 80% of MHR (70% if deconditioned).
5. Immediately after the exercise, stop and record the client's heart rate.
6. Record the client's heart rate again 2 minutes later.

Test results:
Subtract the heart rate recorded at 2 minutes post exercise from the heart rate recorded immediately post exercise. The difference between the two numbers indicates the following:

Table 15.9	BIOLOGICAL VERSUS CALENDAR AGE SCORE RANGES
Score range	**Biological age versus calendar age**
less than 22	Your biological age is slightly older than your calendar age.
22–52	Your biological age is about the same as your calendar age.
53–58	Your biological age is slightly younger than your calendar age.
59–65	Your biological age is moderately younger than your calendar age.
66+	Your biological age is a lot younger than your calendar age.

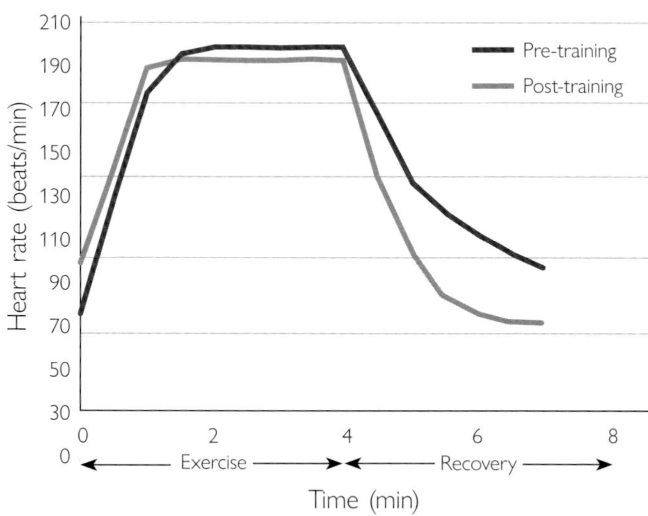

Figure 15.3 Pre- and post-exercise programme recovery profiles

The heart rate recovery test can also be adapted to provide an individual profile, which can then be repeated to monitor progression.

Test protocol 2 – individual profile method:

1. Fit a HR measuring device to the client and record the baseline heart rate.
2. Select the preferred cardio equipment.
3. Carry out the cardio exercise (warm-up, main cardio, cool-down) that has been designed for the client's programme.
4. Record the client's heart rate at regular intervals (30 seconds or 1 minute).

Test results:

A graph such as that in figure 15.3 can be created to show the heart rate profile of the client. Follow-up test results can be plotted on the same graph, which will indicate if the client has improved in aerobic fitness. For example, the post-training line in figure 15.3 shows that the client's heart rate has returned to normal levels quicker than the previous test, which indicates a potential improvement in aerobic fitness.

HEART RATE VARIABILITY

Another method of assessing cardiovascular condition (more specifically the function of the *autonomic nervous system*) is to monitor heart rate variability (HRV). HRV is a measure of the variation in time between heart beats. For example, if resting heart rate is 70 beats per minute, the time between heart beats may vary between 0.9 seconds and 1.3 seconds rather than having a consistent time between them.

A lower HRV is associated with an increased risk of *cardiovascular disease*. A higher HRV is considered healthier as it indicates the ability of the heart to respond rapidly to changes within the body to maintain homeostasis. There are a multitude of factors that can impact HRV including age, genetics, stress, sleep quality, exercise intensity, hormones (especially in females) and diet. Healthy ranges can be seen in table 15.10.

Environmental impacts on field testing

Field-based performance tests may be more sport-specific compared to laboratory-based tests but there are a number of factors that may impact their reliability, validity and repeatability which need to be accounted for. To reduce their impact, the following guidelines should be followed:

- The surface the test is performed on should be consistent for repeated tests. Grass, synthetic outdoor surfaces and indoor surfaces may impact ground reaction forces, which may influence test performance. Even performing a test on a dry grass pitch compared to a saturated one may impact test performance.
- If performed outside, tests should be carried out in a similar climate (e.g. humidity levels) and weather conditions (e.g. no rain/wind) or there should be a method to modify testing scores based on the impact of these factors.

Table 15.10	TYPICAL HEALTHY HRV RANGES
Age group (yrs)	**Average HRV (ms)**
18–25	62–85
26–35	55–75
36–45	50–70
46–55	45–65
56–65	42–62
66+	40–60

- Ideally, the same footwear should be used when tests are repeated. The grip, cushion, force absorption and weight of footwear may impact testing performance. For example, carbon-plated running shoes enhance performance, so may impact testing outcomes if they are used in later tests, when previous tests were carried out using other designs of running shoes.

Take-home messages

- A variety of direct and indirect tests are available to measure VO_2max.

- Practitioners should consider the population they are testing and the equipment available before considering which test is most appropriate to use.

Anaerobic //endurance testing 16

The areas covered in this chapter are:

• Typical field tests for anaerobic endurance that are accessible for the S&C practitioner

• Typical sources of error associated with individual tests

• Physiological adaptations to anaerobic exercise and the factors that can affect adaptation

Introduction

Anaerobic endurance is considered important for improving athletic performance. Having a good level of anaerobic endurance allows the body to perform at high intensity and develop power quickly, which is crucial in many sports and events. While this tends to be the focus in many S&C training programmes, anaerobic endurance can also be beneficial for everyone because it is linked to enhanced energy levels, improved mood and reduced risk of chronic diseases. This chapter looks at how to measure the progress of anaerobic endurance using scientifically robust tests and investigates how they can be used for the development of anaerobic endurance.

Testing

Many anaerobic threshold tests predominantly require the use of laboratory settings although access to portable equipment is allowing for field testing on a more common basis. We have not included a protocol for those that require expensive specialist equipment, take place in a laboratory setting, or require a period of training. We do, however, provide a brief outline of what is involved in such tests – i.e. the lactate threshold (LT) test, ventilatory threshold (VT) test and excess post-exercise oxygen consumption (EPOC) test. The field-based tests we provide protocols for are the Wingate anaerobic test (WAnT) and the running-based anaerobic sprint test (RAST).

Lactate threshold test

Due to the obvious health and safety issues regarding the taking of human fluids (blood in this case) practitioners must undergo a period of training before conducting any blood sampling tests. For the purpose of LT testing, it will be assumed that the sampling protocol will be adhered to following the period of training. It should also be noted that although LT is a common test for predicting performance, blood lactate may not always indicate the lactate production of muscles.

Test results:

A baseline profile of an incremental exercise test can be plotted on a graph such as that in figure 16.1 and subsequent testing can then be used to measure performance. It can be seen in the example that following a period of training the accumulation of blood lactate (OBLA) occurs at a greater running speed, known as a right shift in the curve.

Sources of error:

Table 16.1	SOURCES OF ERROR FOR LACTATE TESTING
Error source	**Minimising strategy**
Equipment	Use of equipment often requires a laboratory setting.
Health and safety	Training is required when dealing with human fluids.
Hydration and glycogen status	**Dehydration** and glycogen depletion can affect blood lactate levels.

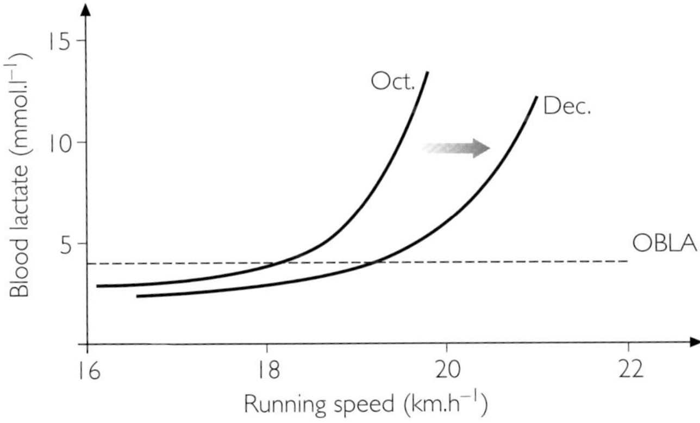

Figure 16.1 Graph showing baseline and follow-up lactate curves

Ventilatory threshold test

This test is typically performed in a laboratory setting by way of a cardiopulmonary exercise test (CPET) in which breath-by-breath oxygen and carbon dioxide levels are recorded. Thresholds known as VT_1 and VT_2 are established during incremental exercise, and these can then be used to set training intensities. The test requires a subjective perception of non-linear increases in ventilation and carbon dioxide production. This type of testing is usually reserved for laboratory conditions by experienced testers although it can be done in a field environment if portable testing equipment is available.

Sources of error:

Table 16.2	SOURCES OF ERROR FOR VENTILATORY THRESHOLD TESTING
Error source	**Minimising strategy**
Equipment	Use of equipment often requires a laboratory setting.
Health and safety	Training is required when dealing with human fluids (handling of breathing masks).
Interpretation of results	Requires a subjective interpretation of data that requires a period of training.

Excess post-exercise oxygen consumption (EPOC) test

This term refers to the increase in oxygen consumption above rest and occurs after a bout of exercise in order to replenish ATP and PC stores. EPOC is also used to facilitate the breakdown of any lactate produced during a bout of high-intensity exercise for conversion to provide a further energy source of ATP. The degree of the anaerobic contribution to the bout of high-intensity exercise can be estimated by measuring the excess post-exercise oxygen consumption (formerly termed the oxygen debt). EPOC has been replaced generally by a maximal accumulated oxygen deficit or MAOD, as it is considered more accurate.

The test involves measuring the relationship between oxygen uptake (VO_2) and power (usually by means of a treadmill or cycle ergometer) during submaximal exercise. This type of testing is usually reserved for laboratory conditions by experienced testers although it can be done in a field environment if portable testing equipment is available.

Sources of error:

Table 16.3	SOURCES OF ERROR FOR EPOC TESTING
Error source	**Minimising strategy**
Equipment	Use of equipment often requires a laboratory setting.
Health and safety	Training is required when dealing with human fluids (handling of breathing masks).
Interpretation of results	Requires a subjective interpretation of data that requires a period of training.

Wingate anaerobic test

One of the most common laboratory *anaerobic capacity* tests is the Wingate anaerobic test (WAnT) in which the client is required to cycle at maximal effort for 30 seconds on a cycle ergometer. The test was designed at the Wingate Institute in Israel in the 1970s and has been used to develop field tests such as the running-based anaerobic sprint test.

Resources required:
Cycle ergometer, stopwatch

Test protocol:
1. The client performs a 5-minute standardised warm-up on the ergometer at 60W or 100W.
2. The client then begins pedalling as fast as possible without any resistance. Within 3 seconds, a fixed resistance is applied to the flywheel and the client continues to pedal 'all out' for 30 seconds.
3. This resistance is applied automatically using an electromechanically braked ergometer or manually when using a Monark cycle ergometer.
4. Clients should be encouraged to fight fatigue and cycle maximally throughout the 30 seconds.

Test results:
There are several parameters that can be measured using this test, such as absolute and relative peak power, and despite criticism, it is used as an indicator of anaerobic capacity. Energy supply during the test is typically 50–55% from anaerobic glycolysis, 23–29% from the phosphagen system and 16–25% from the aerobic system. Criticism suggests that the test is not long enough for full depletion of anaerobic energy sources but it is commonly used to estimate anaerobic capacity and is calculated as follows:

AC = force × total distance in 30 secs

Sources of error:

Table 16.4	SOURCES OF ERROR FOR THE WAnT TEST
Error source	**Minimising strategy**
Equipment	There are a wide range of ergometers that can be used, so the accuracy can vary. Use an ergometer with an associated validated protocol.
Training status	This is not a reliable test for deconditioned clients. Use for conditioned clients only.
Accuracy	Clients do not always reach maximum level, so encourage them to go to fatigue.

Running-based anaerobic sprint test (RAST)

Sprint speed can be used as an indication of the capacity of the anaerobic system and involves clients running linear distances of between 20 and 50m (22 and 55 yards). The RAST was developed at the University of Wolverhampton by Draper and Whyte. The test is typically used to measure fatigue index (FI), which is considered a reflection of the capacity of the anaerobic and aerobic systems.

Equipment required:
Stopwatch or timing gates (electronic timing devices), measuring tape, cones

Test protocol:
1. Complete a standardised warm-up appropriate to the environment.
2. The client should start at one end of the 35m (38-yard) track.
3. The client must sprint at maximal effort to the end of the track.
4. After the sprint there is a 10-second recovery.
5. During the recovery period, the client should get ready to perform the next 35m (38-yard) sprint.
6. Repeat this procedure for a total of six sprints (five 10-second recovery periods).

Test results:
Fatigue index is a measure of anaerobic capacity and indicates the rate at which the speed declines. A lower value indicates an ability to maintain performance. Calculate fatigue index using the following equation;

$$FI = [(\text{slowest sprint time} - \text{fastest sprint time})/\text{slowest sprint time}] \times 100\%$$

Sources of error:

Table 16.5	SOURCES OF ERROR FOR THE RAST TEST
Error source	**Minimising strategy**
Equipment	Use an electronic measuring device to reduce human error.
Training status	This is not a reliable test for deconditioned clients. Use for conditioned clients only.
Accuracy	Clients do not always reach cone level, so give warnings followed by elimination.

Take-home messages
- A variety of direct and indirect tests are available to measure anaerobic endurance.
- Practitioners should consider the population they are testing and the equipment available before considering which test is most appropriate to use.

Stabilisation //testing

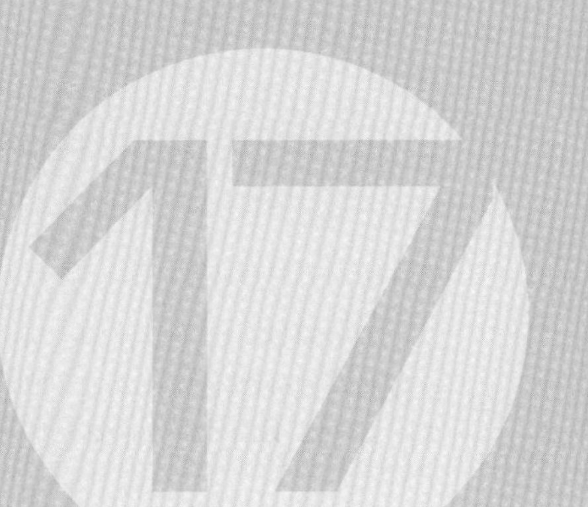

The areas covered in this chapter are:

- Typical field tests for stabilisation that are accessible for the S&C practitioner

- Typical sources of error associated with individual stabilisation tests

Introduction

Improvement in stabilisation has been linked to many benefits, such as improving balance and coordination. This is important not only in terms of athletic performance but for the general population, since good stability can reduce the risk of falls. Over the years, developing stability of the core has become one of the most important components of S&C programmes. The general understanding is that stability training can provide a strong foundation by increasing the strength of deeper muscles to allow the body to perform more powerful movements. Stability training is also linked to improvements in posture, which is beneficial for the entire population. This chapter looks at how to measure the progress of stabilisation using scientifically robust tests and investigates how they can be used for development of stabilisation.

Testing

Core stability is regarded as a complex interaction between local and global muscles and neuromuscular control in relation to the demands of specific tasks, which means that accurate assessment is challenging. Tests often measure an aspect of stability such as muscle recruitment, strength, postural control and movement patterns, although trunk endurance testing appears to be a commonly used method in sporting environments. Trunk extensor endurance testing first developed by Biering-Sorenson has since been adapted by McGill to include trunk flexion and lateral flexion endurance, which is performed as a test battery, as outline below:

Trunk flexion endurance

The test as described by McGill measures how long the client can keep the unsupported upper body in a 60 degrees supine position, with bent knees and the arms folded across the chest.

Equipment required:

Plinth, massage table or floor mat, stopwatch

Test protocol:

1. The starting position requires the client to be seated upright, with the hips and knees bent to 90 degrees, aligning the hips and knees. Arms are folded across the chest or out in front.
2. The practitioner can anchor the toes under a strap or manually stabilise the feet if necessary.
3. Instruct the client to lean back to a 60-degree position, as shown in figure 17.1 (clients can practise this position prior to attempting the test).
4. Record the time while the client maintains the 60-degree suspended position.
5. Terminate the test when there is a noticeable change in the trunk position: watch for a deviation from the neutral spine (i.e. the shoulders rounding forwards) or an increase in the low-back arch.

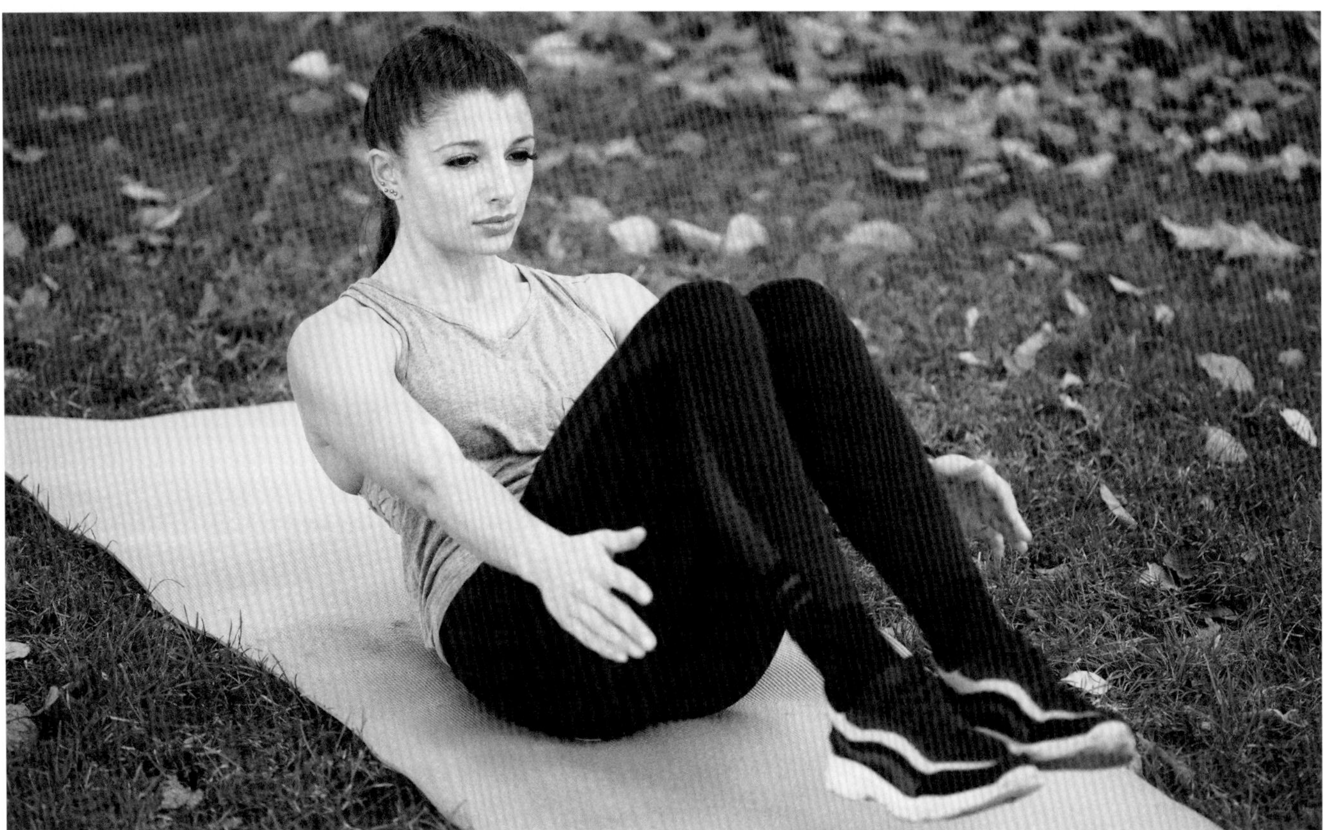

Figure 17.1 Trunk flexion endurance test

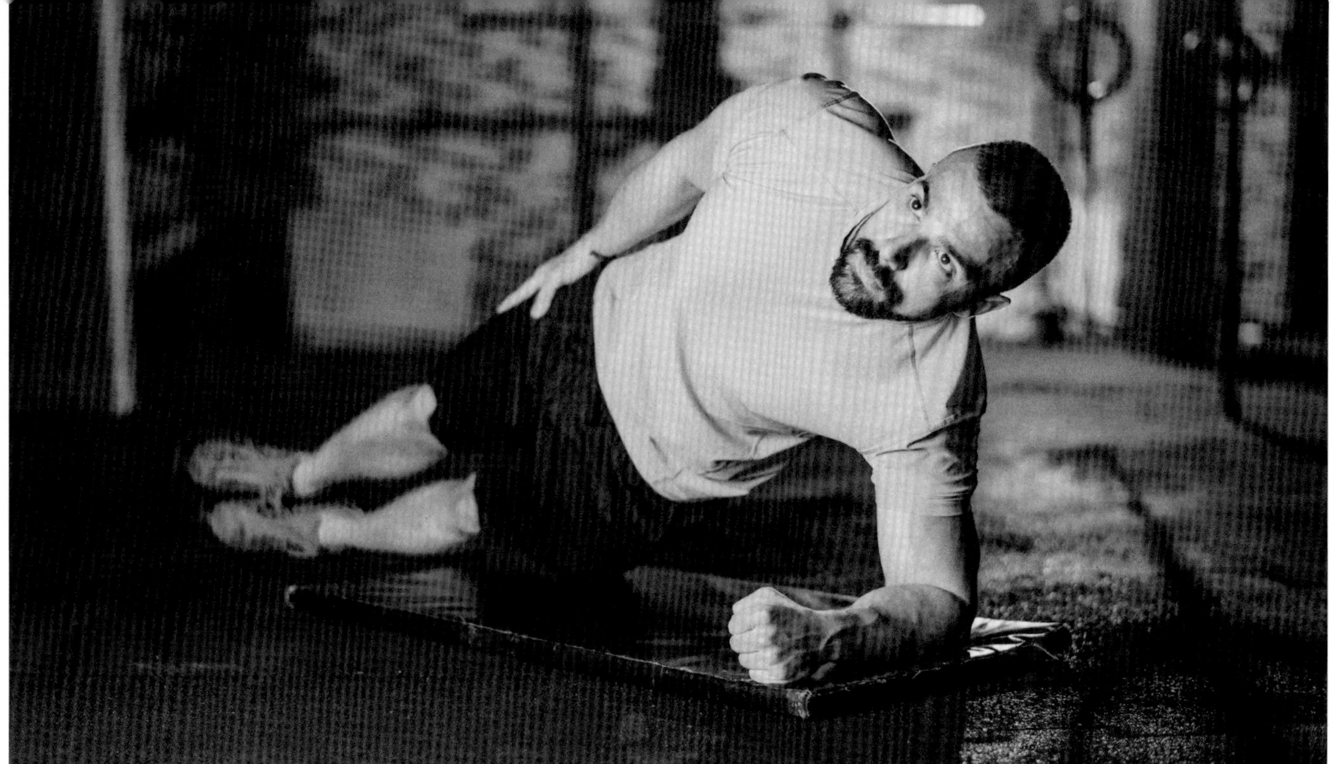

Figure 17.2 Trunk lateral flexion endurance test

Trunk lateral flexion endurance test

The test as described by McGill measures how long the client can keep the unsupported upper body in a side bridge position.

Equipment required:
Plinth, massage table or floor mat, stopwatch

Test protocol:
1. The starting position requires the client to be on their side with extended legs, aligning the feet on top of each other or in a tandem position (heel-to-toe).
2. Have the client place the lower arm under the body and the upper arm on the side of the body.
3. When the client is ready, instruct them to assume a full side bridge position, keeping both legs extended and the sides of the feet on the floor, as shown in figure 17.2. The elbow of the lower arm should be positioned directly under the shoulder with the forearm facing out (the forearm can be placed palm down for balance and support) and the upper arm should be resting along the side of the body or across the chest to the opposite shoulder.
4. The goal of the test is to hold this position for as long as possible. Once the client breaks the position, the test is terminated (clients can practise this position prior to attempting the test) and the time is recorded.
5. Terminate the test when there is a noticeable change in the trunk position, such as a deviation from the neutral spine (i.e. the hips dropping downwards) or the hips shifting forwards or backwards in an effort to maintain balance and stability.
6. Repeat the test on the opposite side and record this value.

Trunk extensor endurance test

The test as described by Sorenson measures how long the client can keep the unsupported upper body (from the upper border of the iliac crests) horizontal, while placed prone with the legs fixed to a plinth and the arms folded across the chest.

Equipment required:
Plinth or massage table, stopwatch

Test protocol:
1. The client lies prone on the apparatus with the upper edge of the iliac crests in alignment with the edge of the support as shown in figure 17.3.

2. With the arms folded across the chest, the client isometrically maintains the upper body in a horizontal position while time is recorded.

3. Once the client falls below horizontal, the test is terminated.

Test results:
Recorded times can be transferred to the trunk endurance test battery record sheet (*see* fig. 17.4) so that results can be assessed. A score of poor or good can be assigned depending on the relationship between extensor endurance time and flexion and lateral flexion times.

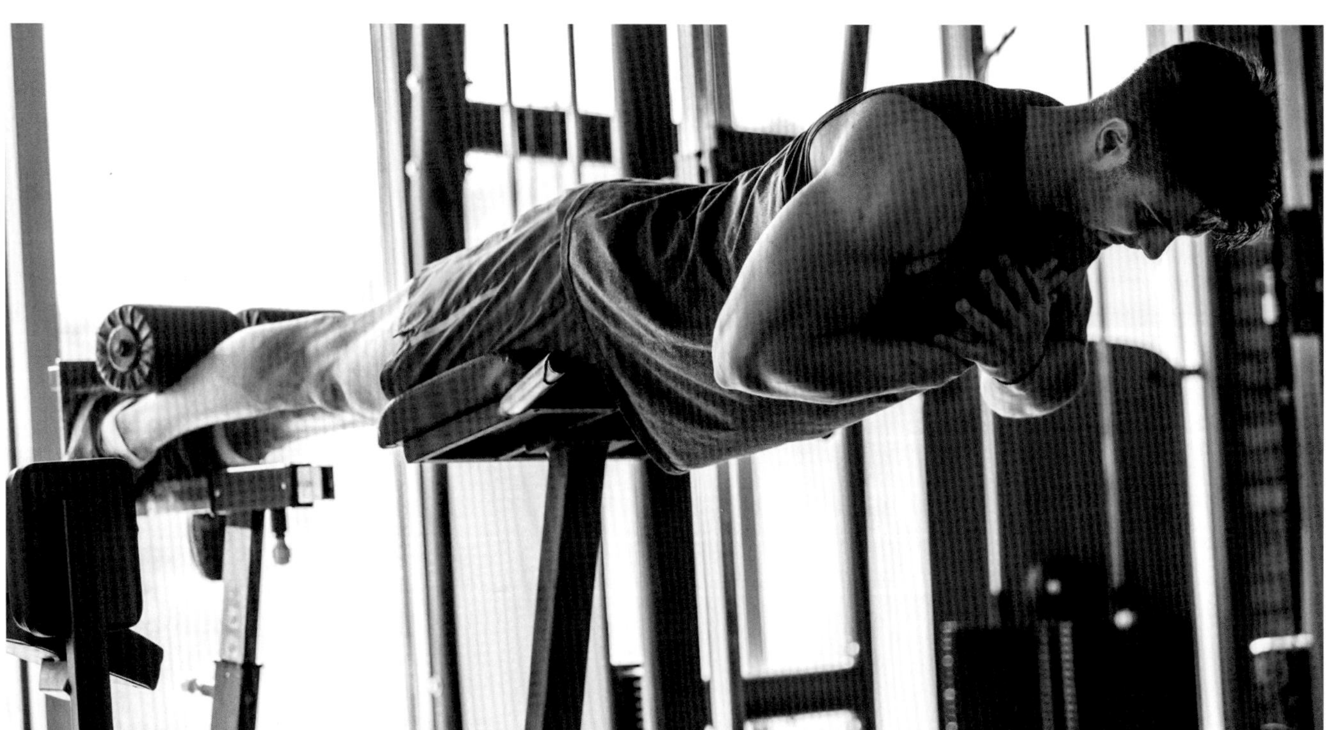

Figure 17.3 Trunk extensor endurance test

<table>
<tr><td colspan="2">Trunk flexor endurance test: Time to completion (s)_________</td></tr>
<tr><td colspan="2">Trunk lateral flexion endurance test:
Right side time to completion (s)_________   Left side time to completion (s)_________</td></tr>
<tr><td colspan="2">Trunk extensor endurance test: Time to completion (s)_________</td></tr>
<tr><td>Ratio of comparison</td><td>Criteria of good relationship</td></tr>
<tr><td>Flexion:extension</td><td>Flexion greater than 80% of extension</td></tr>
<tr><td>Right-side bridge:left-side bridge</td><td>Less than 5% asymmetry</td></tr>
<tr><td>Side bridge (each side):extension</td><td>Side bridge greater than 75% of extension</td></tr>
<tr><td colspan="2">Flexion:extension ratio   Rating: Good Poor</td></tr>
<tr><td colspan="2">Right-side bridge:left-side bridge ratio Rating: Good Poor</td></tr>
<tr><td colspan="2">Side bridge (each side):extension ratio Rating: Good Poor</td></tr>
</table>

Figure 17.4 Trunk endurance test battery record (adapted from McGill's torso muscular endurance test battery)

Sources of error:

Table 17.1	SOURCES OF ERROR FOR STABILISATION TESTING
Error source	**Minimising strategy**
Timing	Ensure a test administrator is available to record time, as the practitioner will be required to administer the test.
Technique	Ensure that the client shows good technique. The test must be terminated if technique is lost (*see* criteria for each test).

Take-home messages

- A variety of direct and indirect tests are available to measure stabilisation.

- Practitioners should consider the population they are testing and the equipment available before considering which test is most appropriate to use.

Muscular strength and endurance testing

The areas covered in this chapter are:

- Typical field tests for muscular strength and endurance that are accessible for the S&C practitioner

- Typical sources of error associated with individual tests

Introduction

Muscular strength and endurance are important for athletic performance and activities of daily life. The benefits of both muscular strength and endurance are very similar. In relation to athletic performance, benefits include improved balance, reduced risk of injury and improved body composition. Muscular strength and endurance can also enhance daily function by making everyday tasks easier and enhancing mood and sleep quality. This chapter looks at how to measure the progress of muscular strength and endurance using scientifically robust tests and investigates how they can be used for development of these components of fitness.

Testing

Both static and dynamic muscular strength and endurance can be measured. In static testing, dynamometers are used to measure how much force a client can exert isometrically at a particular joint angle. In dynamic testing, a client is required to move an external load (usually free weights or resistance machines). Some of the most common tests are the grip strength test, the full-body press-up test, the modified press-up test, the 1-minute half sit-up test, the multiple repetition maximum test and 1RM prediction using a barbell accelerometer. We will now look at each in detail:

Grip strength test

Testing of grip strength using a hand-held hydraulic dynamometer can be traced back to 1954. Grip strength is commonly used as a tool to predict total body strength, but it is also used to assess for sarcopenia as a proxy measurement for well-being, health and future mortality. As low grip strength is associated with reduced health-related quality of life in older age it can be a useful tool to identify those at risk of mobility limitations, such as difficulty walking or climbing stairs.

Equipment required:
Hand-grip dynamometer

Test protocol:
1. Ensure the dynamometer is set to zero.
2. Adjust the hand grip to suit the client. Adjust the base and handle until the handle rests on the middle phalange and the base on the first metacarpal of the *non-dominant* hand.
3. Raise the dynamometer above the head with palms facing inwards.
4. The client takes a deep breath and squeezes the handle as hard as possible while lowering the arm. Perform three trials with 10–20 seconds of rest between each trial to avoid the effects of muscle fatigue.
5. If the difference between results is within 3kg (6.6lb), the test is complete.
6. If the difference between any two measures is more than 3kg (6.6lb) then repeat the test once more after a rest period. Use the best three measurements.
7. If a fourth measurement is taken (when any of the three measurements are 3kg/6.6lb apart) the outlier (the *lowest* value) is discarded so that the three *highest* measurements are used.

Test results:
A hand-grip strength of 150N (approximately 15kg/33lb), equivalent to 20% of bodyweight for a 75kg (165lb) client, is considered a threshold for the performance of occupational tasks requiring a firm grip. For categorisation purposes, normative tables based on gender and age are available, such as those shown in table 18.1.

Note: Most published tables are for the non-dominant hand.

Sources of error:

Table 18.2	SOURCES OF ERROR FOR THE GRIP STRENGTH TEST
Error source	**Minimising strategy**
Hand grip	Allow clients several attempts using a different hand grip to find the one that is most appropriate for them.
Breathing	Encourage clients to breathe out on exertion.
Fatigue	Ensure clients are fully recovered between attempts to avoid fatigue.

Table 18.1	NORMATIVE VALUES FOR HAND-GRIP RATING (kg)				
Gender	**Excellent**	**Good**	**Average**	**Fair**	**Poor**
Male	>56	51–56	45–50	39–44	<39
Female	>36	31–36	25–30	19–24	<19

Full-body press-up test

This is an easy test to administer, as it uses body-weight rather than an external resistance. The test requires no equipment and is often used to assess muscular endurance in groups.

Test protocol:

1. Lie on an appropriate surface such as a mat, with hands shoulder-width apart and palms flat on the ground. Fully extend the arms to push the body away from the ground.
2. Lower the body until the upper arm is parallel to the floor (mid position).
3. Return to the starting position with arms fully extended.
4. Repeat. The push-up action is to be continuous with no rest.
5. Record the total number of full-body press-ups completed by the client before fatigue.

Test results:

The normative values in table 18.3 provide categories based on age for full-body press-ups.

Modified press-up test

Some clients are not able to complete full press-ups (or can only do very few), in which case the modified press-up test can be used.

Test protocol:

1. Start with hands shoulder-width apart, with bent knees and fully extended arms (*see* fig. 18.1a).
2. Lower the upper body until the elbows reach 90 degrees (mid position, as shown in fig. 18.1b).
3. Return to the starting position with the arms fully extended.
4. Repeat. The push-up action should be continuous with no rest periods.
5. Record the total number of modified press-ups completed by the client before fatigue.

Table 18.3	**NORMATIVE VALUES FOR FULL-BODY PRESS-UPS**									
Age	20–29		30–39		40–49		50–59		60–69	
Gender	M	F	M	F	M	F	M	F	M	F
Excellent	>54	>48	>44	>39	>39	>34	>34	>29	>29	>19
Good	45–54	34–38	35–44	25–39	30–39	20–34	25–34	15–29	20–29	5–19
Average	35–44	17–33	25–34	12–24	20–29	8–19	15–24	6–14	10–19	3–4
Fair	20–34	6–16	15–24	4–11	12–19	3–7	8–14	2–5	5–9	1–2

Table 18.4	NORMATIVE VALUES FOR MODIFIED PRESS-UPS					
Age	17–19	20–29	30–39	40–49	50–59	60–65
Excellent	>35	>36	>37	>31	>25	>23
Good	21–34	23–35	22–36	18–30	15–24	13–22
Average	11–20	12–22	10–21	8–17	7–14	5–12
Poor	2–10	2–11	1–9	1–7	1–6	1–4

Note: Norms are only available for female subjects

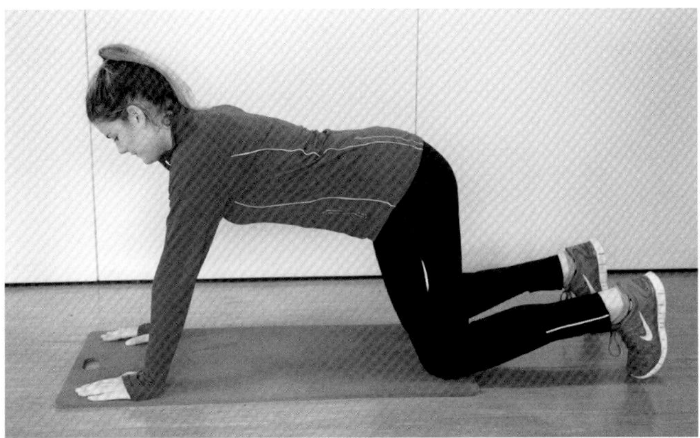

Figure 18.1a Modified press-up start

Sources of error:

Table 18.5	SOURCES OF ERROR FOR THE PRESS-UP TEST
Error source	**Minimising strategy**
Pacing	Clients often start too quickly. Allow clients several attempts to find the most effective pacing technique.
Technique	Ensure that clients achieve full range of movement as described in the protocol. Do not count attempts that have poor technique.

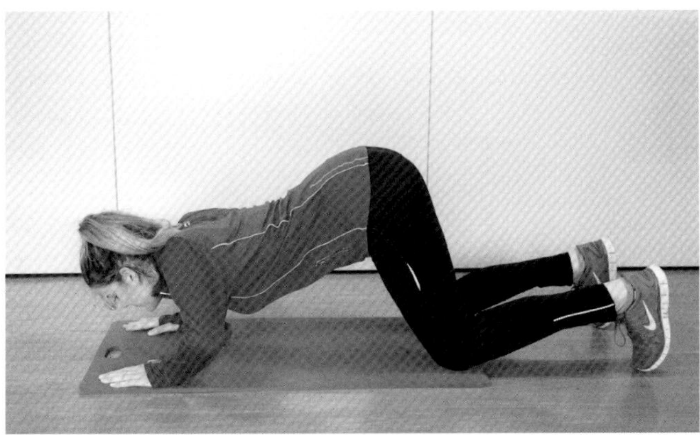

Figure 18.1b Modified press-up mid position

One-minute half sit-up test

Variations of the 1-minute sit-up test have been studied for their validity and reliability in assessing abdominal strength and functional capacity. The 1-minute half sit-up test has been proposed as a reliable measure of muscular endurance although the relationship to specific health outcomes such as low back pain is still a topic of debate.

Table 18.6 — NORMATIVE VALUES FOR 1-MINUTE HALF SIT-UPS (ADAPTED FROM GOLDING *ET AL.*, 1986)

1-minute half sit-up test (men)

Age	18–25	26–35	36–45	46–55	56–65	65+
Excellent	>49	>45	>41	>35	>31	>28
Good	44–49	40–45	35–41	29–35	25–31	22–28
Above average	39–43	35–39	30–34	25–28	21–24	19–21
Average	35–38	31–34	27–29	22–24	17–20	15–18
Below average	31–34	29–30	23–26	18–21	13–16	11–14
Poor	25–30	22–28	17–22	13–17	9–12	7–10
Very poor	<25	<22	<17	<13	<9	<7

1-minute half sit-up test (women)

Age	18–25	26–35	36–45	46–55	56–65	65+
Excellent	>43	>39	>33	>27	>24	>23
Good	37–43	33–39	27–33	22–27	18–24	17–23
Above average	33–36	29–32	23–26	18–21	13–17	14–16
Average	29–32	25–28	19–22	14–17	10–12	11–13
Below average	25–28	21–24	15–18	10–13	7–9	5–10
Poor	18–24	13–20	7–14	5–9	3–6	2–4
Very poor	<18	<13	<7	<5	<3	<2

Test protocol:

1. Perform a standardised warm-up and practise the half sit-up technique.
2. The client starts by sitting upright with their knees bent, feet flat on the floor, and the arms across the chest.
3. Start in the up position, with the back in a vertical position.
4. When the timing starts, lower the back so the shoulder blades touch the floor, then return to the up position, maintaining good form.
5. The total number of sit-ups completed with good form in 1 minute is recorded.

Test results:

The normative values in table 18.6 provide categories for 1-minute half sit-ups based on age and gender.

Sources of error:

Table 18.7	SOURCES OF ERROR FOR THE 1-MINUTE HALF SIT-UP TEST
Error source	**Minimising strategy**
Pacing	Clients often start too quickly. Allow clients several attempts to find the most effective pacing technique.
Technique	Ensure that clients achieve full range of movement as described in the protocol. Do not count attempts that have poor technique.

Multiple repetition maximum (RM) test

One repetition maximum (1RM) testing is not suitable for most clients, therefore repeated RM testing should be carried out as a safer alternative. The number of repetitions chosen should be based on the needs and goals of the client (for example, to determine a 10RM).

Equipment required:

Suitable resistance machine or free weights

Test protocol:

1. The client should perform a suitable warm-up, for example, 6–10 reps of 50% of their estimated 10RM, 8 reps at 70% and 5 reps at 90% with a 1-minute rest between sets.
2. Rest for 2–3 minutes before attempting an actual 10RM.
3. If successful, rest for 2–3 minutes then increase the weight by 2–5% and attempt another lift.
4. Keep increasing the weight until failure.

Test results:

It is possible to predict 1RM from multiple RM testing. There are a range of prediction equations, though, so the practitioner must select the most suitable for each client as the validation of the equations varies greatly in terms of client groups, number of repetitions and specific lifts used. In the examples below, the client's 5RM has been established. Prediction equations by Brzycki and Epley have been used to estimate 1RM.

Brzycki equation

$$1RM = \frac{W}{(1.0278-(0.0278 \times r))}$$

W = the amount of weight lifted; r = the number of repetitions performed

Example: if a client had a 5RM of 80kg then:

$$IRM = \frac{80}{(1.0278-(0.0278 \times 5))}$$

$$= \frac{80}{(1.0278-0.139)} = \frac{80}{0.88} = 91kg$$

Epley equation

$$IRM = (W \times r \times 0.033) + W$$

W = the amount of weight lifted; r = the number of repetitions performed

Example: if a client had a 5RM of 80kg then:

$$IRM = (80 \times 5 \times 0.033) + 80 = 93.2kg$$

Sources of error:

Table 18.8	SOURCES OF ERROR FOR REPETITION MAXIMUM TESTING
Error source	**Minimising strategy**
Fatigue	Allow clients sufficient recovery time.
Technique	Ensure that clients achieve full range of movement as described in the protocol. Do not count attempts that have poor technique.

1RM prediction using a barbell accelerometer

The prediction of the 1RM of a specific lift can be calculated using a barbell accelerometer. The accelerometer calculates the speed at which the bar is moving, so this data can be recorded at different weights and the 1RM can be predicted using either linear or quadratic formulas. Research has provided data for the speeds at which the 1RM occur for different lifts. These speeds are shown in table 18.9.

Equipment required:
Barbell, squat rack, gym bench

Test protocol:
1. The client should perform a suitable warm-up as prescribed by the practitioner.
2. The client is required to perform 4–5 repetitions of a specific exercise at three or four different weights (e.g. back squats ranging from 40 to 70kg in 10kg increments).
3. An accelerometer is mounted to the floor and on to the bar and the speed of each lift is recorded.

Table 18.9	BARBELL SPEEDS FOR NOVICE AND ELITE ATHLETES	
Lift	**Novice barbell speed (m/s)**	**Elite barbell speed (m/s)**
Back squat	0.35	0.20
Front squat	0.45	0.25
Deadlift	0.25	0.12
Bench press	0.30	0.15

4. An average (mean) is taken for each weight category and a scatter graph is created where bar speed is plotted on the x axis and weight is plotted on the y axis.
5. From here, a linear or quadratic line of best fit is plotted, and the equation of this line is used to estimate a 1RM that is predicted to be performed at the speeds quoted in the previous table.

Figure 18.2 shows an example of how a linear regression graph and equation can be used to predict a 1RM. This graph is plotted using mass (kg) on the x axis and barbell velocity (m/s) on the y axis. It shows the average velocity of 4 sets of barbell back squats performed with increasing increments of 10kg:

Set 1 = 40kg

Set 2 = 50kg

Set 3 = 60kg

Set 4 = 70kg

The linear regression equation $y = ax + b$ (y = mass, a = slope, x = velocity, b = y intercept) can be used to predict 1RM. This type of equation can be preformed in Excel and requires familiaristion. For the back squat, 1RM velocity is predicted to be 0.3m/s. So, inputting this figure into the equation of the graph ($y = -100.63x + 135$) gives a 1RM prediction of 104.8kg.

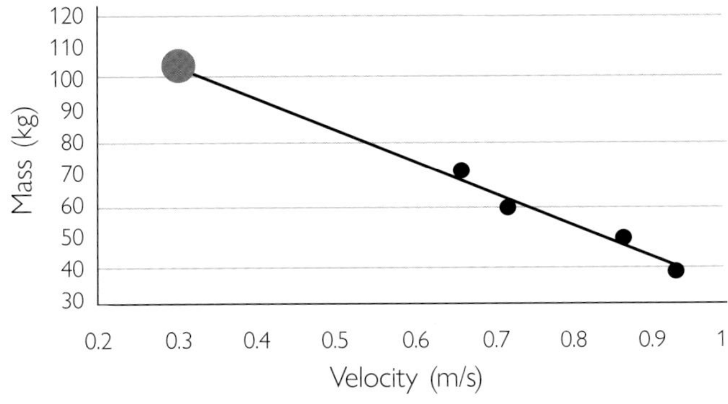

Figure 18.2 Linear regression for prediction of 1RM

Sources of error:

Table 18.10	SOURCES OF ERROR FOR 1RM PREDICTION TESTING
Error source	**Minimising strategy**
Fatigue	Allow clients sufficient recovery time between sets.
Technique	Ensure that clients show good technique. Do not count attempts that have poor technique.
Equipment	Ensure the accelerometer is correctly mounted and securely fastened to the barbell and on a flat surface on the floor.

As with the Brzycki and Epley prediction methods, using an accelerometer is a much safer method than the traditional method of a client performing their 1RM in a training session.

Take-home messages

- A variety of direct and indirect tests are available to measure muscular strength and endurance.

- Practitioners should consider the population they are testing and the equipment available before considering which test is most appropriate to use.

//Speed testing

Introduction

Speed can be tested in a range of sports such as cycling and swimming but are typically overseen by a specialist coach. This chapter will focus on running speed, with training mainly used for athletes since it can help to develop areas such as maximum speed and acceleration. Speed training can also help recreational runners, as it can improve running technique and efficiency, which will also benefit distance running. This chapter looks at how to measure the progress of running speed performance using scientifically robust tests and investigates how this can be used for development of this component of fitness.

Testing

Speed testing within a laboratory or field setting can target a variety of physical components depending on the needs of the client. These include change of direction at speed, speed endurance, maximum speed, acceleration and deceleration. One of the most used tests is sprint testing:

Sprint testing

Testing in sport is typically done between 10 and 60m (11 and 66 yards) depending on the nature of the sport. Stopwatches are commonly used, but, due to human errors incurred, electronic timing devices such as light gates can be used, although these can be expensive. Elite-level sprinters usually reach their maximal speed at approximately 50–60m (55–66 yards).

Resources required:

Stopwatch (or light gates), up to 60m (66 yards) of straight track or field depending on the distance being tested, tape measure

Test protocol:

1. Mark out a start and finish line of a distance that has been selected to be tested.
2. The client lines up (sprint or standing start) on the start line of the straight track.

Table 19.1	CLASSIFICATION OF 30M (33-YARD) SPRINT TIMES (IN SECONDS) FOR ADULTS				
Gender	Excellent	Above average	Average	Below average	Poor
Male	<2.6	2.6–2.9	2.9–3.1	3.1–3.3	>3.3
Female	<3.0	3.0–3.3	3.3–3.5	3.5–3.7	>3.7

Table 19.2	CLASSIFICATION OF 30M (33-YARD) SPRINT TIMES (IN SECONDS) FOR 16–19-YEAR-OLDS				
Gender	Excellent	Above average	Average	Below average	Poor
Male	<4	4.0–4.2	4.3–4.4	4.5–4.6	>4.6
Female	<4.5	4.5–4.6	4.7–4.8	4.9–5.0	>5.0

3. The tester gives the command to go and starts the stopwatch at the same time (not required for light gates).
4. The tester should record the time for the client to complete the distance.

Repeat the test several times and record the fastest time. Allow the client complete recovery between sprints. The client can have as many attempts as they choose.

Test results:

Results can be compared to previous tests or can be compared to published norms, such as those in tables 19.1 and 19.2

Sources of error:

Table 19.3	SOURCES OF ERROR FOR SPRINT TESTING
Error source	Minimising strategy
Fatigue	Allow clients sufficient recovery time between tests.
Equipment	Hand timing can be erroneous. Equipment such as electronic light gates are more accurate.

Take-home messages

- Practitioners should consider the population they are testing and the equipment available before considering which test is most appropriate to use.

- There are different protocols to test the effectiveness of speed, which are dictated by the event or sport of the client.

//Power testing

The areas covered in this chapter are:

- Typical field tests for power that are accessible for the S&C practitioner

- Sources of error associated with the individual tests

Introduction

Similar to speed, power is a component of fitness that is normally associated with athletic performance. However, research has shown that power training can help to make everyday activities easier to perform, such as going up and down stairs and even going for a walk. Power training has also been shown to improve balance, coordination and bone density, so is beneficial for all ages. This chapter looks at how to measure the progress of power performance using scientifically robust tests and investigates how this can be used for development of this component of fitness.

Testing

The ability to apply force rapidly is an important component of many sports and events and for this reason it is commonly tested. There are a range of lab-based tests, such as those that use isokinetic dynamometers, which are non-transportable and expensive. Field-based tests are also available. For example, there is a range of portable devices on the market that can be used to measure power. These devices can be fitted to cycles or even barbells. However, one of the most widely used power tests is the vertical jump test, as results can be compared to normative data.

Vertical jump test

The standing vertical jump is one of the most used methods to test the power of the lower limbs. It is sometimes referred to as the Sargent jump after the researcher who developed the first protocol in 1921. There are various protocols that can be used, such as countermovement, non-countermovement, arm swing and no arm swing. The choice of protocol should be related to the needs of the client.

Equipment required:

An electrical, pressure-sensitive jump mat that uses the length of time the client is in the air to calculate jump height (some devices such as force plates and infrared beam systems will calculate this, whereas others require the tester to calculate the jump height)

Test protocol:

1. The client stands in the middle of the jump mat or device.
2. The client jumps as high as possible and lands with slightly bent knees (performing the chosen protocol, such as countermovement, no countermovement, hands on or off the hips etc.).
3. The jump height should be recorded.
4. The test can be repeated several times. The highest height should be recorded.

Test results:

The normative values in table 20.1 are for male and female countermovement jumps with arms.

Sources of error:

Table 20.1	NORMATIVE VALUES FOR VERTICAL JUMP (COUNTER-MOVEMENT WITH ARMS)	
Jump height: male (cm)	Jump height: female (cm)	Rating
>70	>60	Excellent
61–70	51–60	Very good
51–60	41–50	Above average
41–50	31–40	Below average
31–40	21–30	Poor
<31	<21	Very poor

Table 20.2	SOURCES OF ERROR FOR THE VERTICAL JUMP TEST
Error source	Minimising strategy
Muscle temperature	Cold muscle tissue can negatively affect jump performance, so an appropriate warm-up is required.
Technique	Technique can affect performance. Allow practice attempts.
Test order	If done as part of a test battery, make sure the client is fully recovered before undertaking the jump test.

Take-home messages

- Jumping ability is considered important in terms of testing for power.
- There are various field tests that can be used to determine power.
- Practitioners should consider the population they are testing and the equipment available before considering which test is most appropriate to use.

//Agility testing

The areas covered in this chapter are:

- Typical field tests for agility that are accessible for the S&C practitioner

- Sources of error associated with the individual tests

Introduction

Agility is also a component of fitness that is mainly suited to athletes, as it can help to develop specific movement patterns for their chosen sport or event. Agility training is also performed at high intensity and often high impact so would not be suitable for beginners. This chapter looks at how to measure the progress of agility performance using scientifically robust tests and investigates how this can be used for development of this component of fitness.

Testing

Many agility tests have been designed to mimic the movement patterns of various sports. However, as the movements are all pre-planned and do not require a response to a stimulus they can be classed as closed skill tests and are commonly referred to as change of direction of speed (CODS) tests. These include the Illinois agility test, the 5-0-5 agility test, the T test and the use of electronic light device testing. As balance is considered a component of agility we also include static balance tests such as the Y-balance test and the Stork test. Below, we look at each in turn:

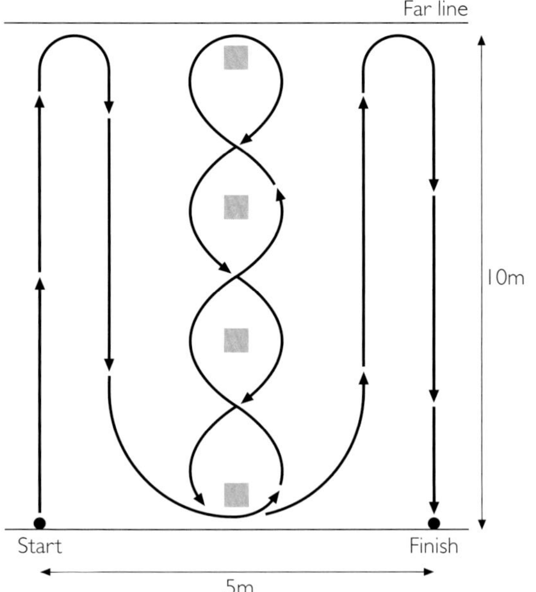

Figure 21.1 Illinois agility test

Illinois agility test

One of the more commonly used CODS tests is the Illinois agility test, as set out in figure 21.1. This test was developed in 1942 as a test of motor ability.

Equipment required:
Flat surface, tape measure, cones, stopwatch (or timing/light gates)

Set up:
The length of the course is 10m (33ft) and the width (distance between the start and finish points) is 5m (16.4ft). Four cones are used to mark the start, finish and the two turning points. Each cone in the centre is spaced 3.3m (10.8ft) apart as can be seen in figure 21.1.

Test protocol:
1. The client lies face down on the floor at the start point of the course behind the line and facing the direction of the course.
2. On the tester's command the client jumps to their feet and negotiates the course around the cones to the finish point as quickly as possible.
3. The tester should record the total time taken to complete the course.
4. The client must ensure that they go around the cones and don't step on any; this will result in that test run being cancelled.
5. The test can be repeated as many times as possible, but rest periods should be given between attempts.

Test results:
The normative values (measured in seconds) in table 21.1 are for male and female adults.

Sources of error:

Table 21.2	SOURCES OF ERROR FOR THE ILLINOIS AGILITY TEST
Error source	**Minimising strategy**
Equipment	Hand timing can be erroneous. Equipment such as electronic light gates are more accurate.
Course navigation	Ensure that clients navigate the course correctly. Use poles instead of cones if possible.
Familiarisation	Allow a practice attempt at submaximal intensity.

Table 21.1	NORMATIVE VALUES FOR THE ILLINOIS AGILITY TEST (ADAPTED FROM ROOZEN, 2004)				
Gender	**Excellent**	**Above average**	**Average**	**Below average**	**Poor**
Male	<15.2	15.2–16.1	16.2–18.1	18.2–18.3	>18.3
Female	<17.0	17.0–17.9	18.0–21.7	21.8–23.0	>23.0

The 5-0-5 agility test

This test was originally developed in 1985 for cricket players but has since been used for a variety of sports to test CODS ability.

Equipment required:
Flat surface, tape measure, cones, stopwatch (or timing/light gates)

Set up:
Markers and a timing gate are set up 10m (33ft) from the start and 5m (16.4ft) from a line marked on the ground, as can be seen in figure 21.2.

Test protocol:
1. The client starts 10m (33ft) from the timing gate.
2. On the tester's command the client will run, building up speed for 10m (33ft), pass through the timing gate and sprint to the line 5m (16.4ft) further on (at the 15m/49.2ft line).
3. The client will perform a 180-degree turn at the 15m (49.2ft) line and sprint 5m (16.4ft) back through the timing gate. Turns can be performed on the right and left legs.
4. The timing starts when the client runs through the timing gate at 10m (33ft) and ends when the client returns through the gate.
5. The test can be repeated as many times as possible, but rest periods should be given between attempts.

Table 21.3	NORMATIVE 5-0-5 TEST TIMES FROM A VARIETY OF SPORTS (ADAPTED FROM RYAN *ET AL.*, 2021)		
Sport	**Sex**	**Number**	**Average 5-0-5 times (mean ± sd [s])**
Basketball	Male	34	2.62 ± 0.21
Cricket	Male	37	2.32 ± 0.08
Lacrosse	Female	17	2.55 ± 0.20
Netball	Female	45	2.69 ± 0.14
Recreational	Male & female	64	2.38 ± 0.12
Rugby union	Male	22	2.51 ± 0.19
Rugby league	Male	57	2.43 ± 0.16
Football	Male	118	2.53 ± 0.26
Tennis	Male	6	2.49 ± 0.13

Note: The number column refers to how many participants took part in the testing.

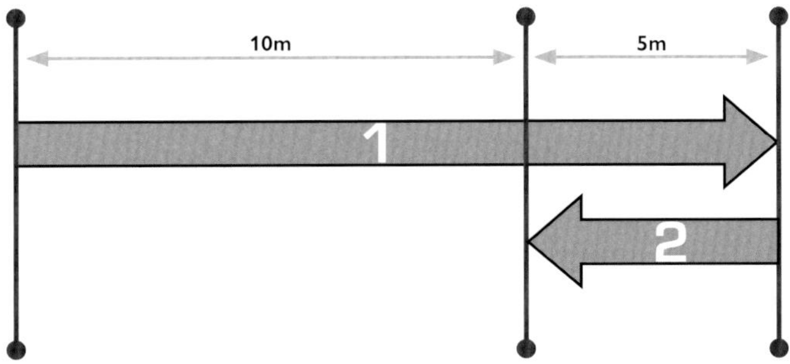

Figure 21.2 The 5-0-5 agility test

Test results:
See Table 21.3

Sources of error:

Table 21.4	SOURCES OF ERROR FOR THE 5-0-5 AGILITY TEST
Error source	**Minimising strategy**
Equipment	Hand timing can be erroneous. Equipment such as electronic light gates are more accurate.
Course navigation	Ensure that clients navigate the course correctly. Record turns on both legs. Swap start and finish sides.
Familiarisation	Allow a practice attempt at submaximal intensity.

Agility T-test

This test was developed to assess movement in a lateral direction (i.e. sidestep).

Equipment required:
Flat surface, tape measure, cones, stopwatch (or timing/light gates)

Set up:
The timing gate is set up at the start/finish line and a centre cone is placed 10m (33ft) in front and two cones 5m (16.4ft) either side of that, as can be seen in figure 21.3.

Test protocol:
1. The client starts at the start/finish line.
2. On the command of the tester, the client sprints to cone 1.
3. The client then sidesteps to cone 3.
4. The client then sidesteps to cone 2.
5. The client then sidesteps back to cone 1 and runs backwards to the start/finish line.

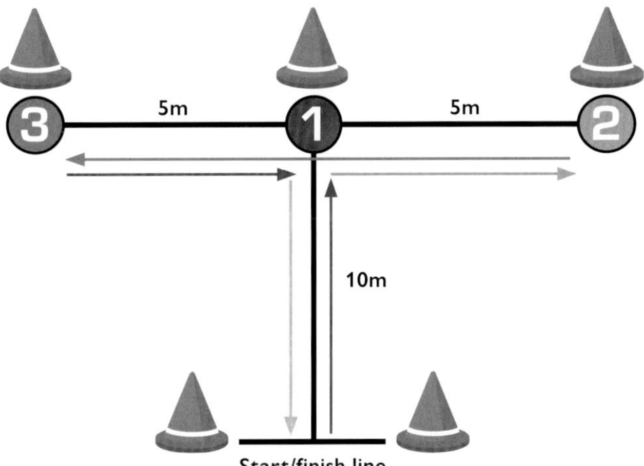

Figure 21.3 The T-test

Test results:

The normative values in table 21.5 are for male and female adults.

Table 21.5	NORMATIVE VALUES FOR THE AGILITY T-TEST	
Ranking	**Males (seconds)**	**Females (seconds)**
Excellent	<9.50	<10.50
Good	9.51–10.50	10.51–11.50
Average	10.51–11.50	11.51–12.50
Poor	>11.50	>12.50

Sources of error:

Table 21.6	SOURCES OF ERROR FOR THE AGILITY T-TEST
Error source	**Minimising strategy**
Equipment	Hand timing can be erroneous. Equipment such as electronic light gates are more accurate.
Course navigation	Ensure that clients navigate the course correctly.
Familiarisation	Allow a practice attempt at submaximal intensity.

ELECTRONIC LIGHT DEVICES

There are many devices available that can test the ability of a client to react to a random light source. Reaction training lights can be set up to represent sport-specific movement patterns whereby clients must turn off lights (with their hand or foot) as quickly as possible either in a random or predetermined sequence. Even though this type of testing device includes a reaction to a stimulus, it does not include sport-related perceptual and decision-making components.

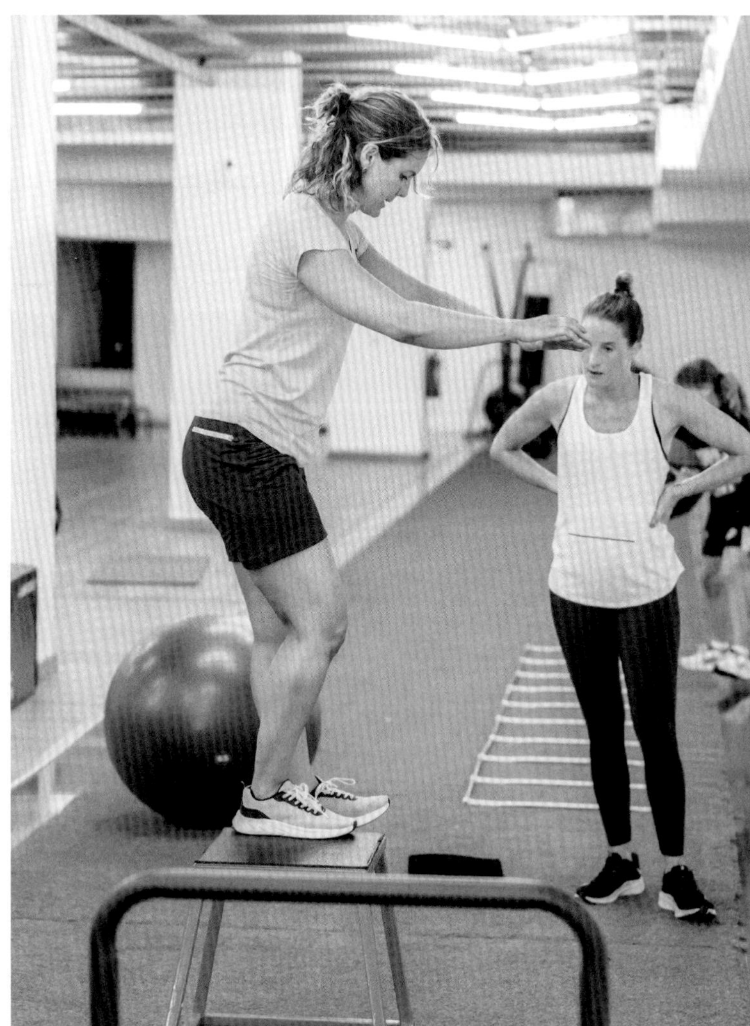

Y-balance test

The Y-balance is used typically as a test of dynamic balance. It is considered a measure of lower extremity neuromuscular control, which can be useful in the determination of physical readiness and injury risk identification (Lesch *et al.* 2024).

Equipment required:
Y-balance test kit, measuring tape

Test protocol:
1. The kit must be set up in accordance with the manufacturer's guidelines and placed on a suitable flat surface.
2. The client stands on the centre platform (behind the red line) with their footwear removed.
3. With hands outstretched the client is instructed to slide the left posterior box backwards as far as possible and then return to the start position.
4. The tester should record the furthest distance reached (to the nearest 0.5cm/$\frac{1}{5}$in).
5. The client should repeat this twice more.
6. The client then performs three attempts in the following order: right posteromedial, left posteromedial, right posterolateral, left posterolateral.
7. The tester should record the reach distance of all attempts to calculate the client's composite score.

Note: An attempt is failed for any of the following:

- Any part of the floor is touched before returning to the start position.
- The foot must stay in contact with the target indicator until the reach is complete. No flicking or kicking allowed!

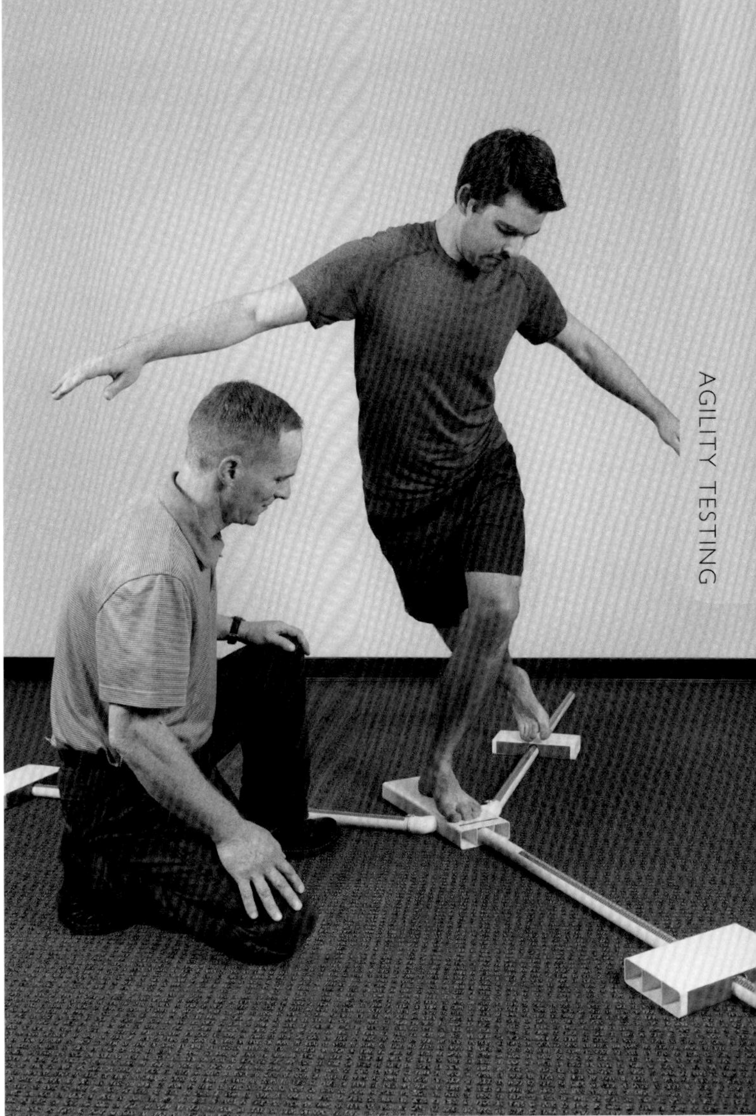

Figure 21.4 Y-balance end point

Test results:
Comparing scores between legs can be useful to help identify asymmetry. Although there is no consensus as to a cut-off value, Pliskey *et al.* (2006) found that an anterior reach asymmetry of greater than 4cm (1$\frac{2}{3}$in) indicated a higher injury risk.

Sources of error:

Table 21.7	SOURCES OF ERROR FOR THE Y-BALANCE TEST
Error source	**Minimising strategy**
Equipment	The equipment is not robust due to the material being plastic in type. Ensure the three arms are set correctly.
Execution	Ensure that clients are in control during performance of the test. Do not allow rapid movement.
Familiarisation	Allow a practice attempt at submaximal intensity.

Stork stand test

Static balance can be assessed using the Stork stand test, which requires no resources and is simple to administer.

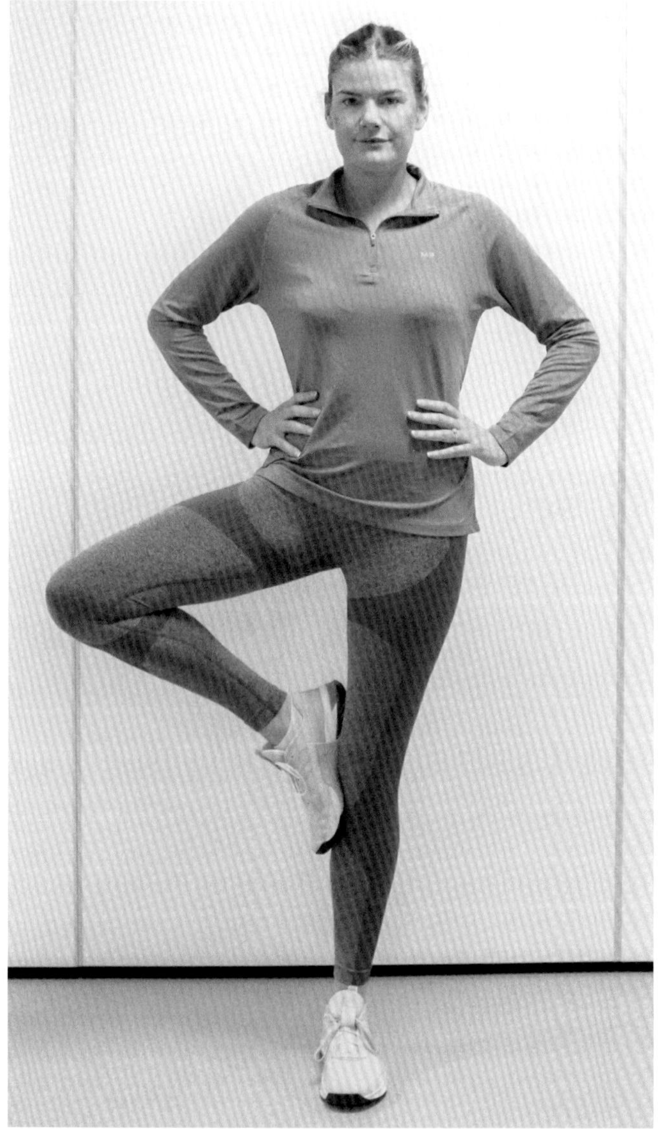

Figure 21.5 Stork stand test

Test protocol:

1. The client stands comfortably with both feet on the floor and with hands on hips.
2. The client then lifts one leg and places the sole of that foot against the inside of the knee of the other leg (*see* fig. 21.5).
3. On command, the client raises their heel.
4. Clients balance for as long as possible without letting either the heel touch the ground or the other foot move away from the knee. Repeat on the opposite leg. Have as many attempts as required.

Note: The test is stopped if any of the following occur:

- The hand(s) come off the hips.
- The supporting foot swivels or moves (hops) in any direction.
- The non-supporting foot loses contact with the knee.
- The heel of the supporting foot touches the floor.

Table 21.8	STORK TEST NORMATIVE VALUES FOR MALE AND FEMALE (ADAPTED FROM SCHELL & LEELARTHAEPIN, 1994)	
Classification	Score females (seconds)	Score males (seconds)
Excellent	27	>50
Above average	23–27	37–50
Average	8–22	15–36
Below average	3–7	5–14
Poor	<3	<5

Test results:

Table 21.8 provides classification based on gender. Practitioners may have to adapt the test for frail older adults in a way that minimises any risk of falling, such as holding a chair or the shoulder of the tester. If the test is adapted in any way the practitioner should be aware that any score should be treated as a baseline and not compared to any norms.

Sources of error:

Table 21.9	SOURCES OF ERROR FOR THE STORK STAND TEST	
Error source	Possible solution	
Tester perception	The height the heel is raised off the floor can be subjective, so use the same tester if possible.	
Technique	Ensure that clients place their foot on the inside of their knee and keep their hands on their hips.	

Take-home messages

- Agility testing should be dictated by the event or sport of the client.
- A variety of direct and indirect tests are available to measure agility.
- Practitioners should consider the population they are testing and the equipment available before considering which test is most appropriate to use.

//Flexibility testing

The areas covered in this chapter are:

- Typical field tests for flexibility that are accessible for the S&C practitioner

- Sources of error associated with the individual tests

Introduction

Flexibility is a component of fitness that is often developed for athletes and the general public alike, since flexibility can be important for athletic performance but also for carrying out a range of daily tasks. This chapter looks at how to measure the progress of flexibility using scientifically robust tests and investigates how this can be used for development of this component of fitness.

Testing

When the flexibility of each joint is assessed, it is known as *goniometry*. This involves the range of motion at each joint being measured and compared against normative data. It is considered the most valid and direct method of testing but requires a degree of training, so it is sensible to learn alternative methods, too, such as the indirect method of testing flexibility known as sit and reach. Let's take a look at both of these methods now:

GONIOMETRY

The term goniometry comes from the Greek words *gonia*, meaning angle, and *metron*, meaning measure. Electrical or manual devices known as goniometers measure static positions of limb segments with respect to the range of motion (ROM) available at a specific joint. Considerable experience is required for this type of measurement, as the tester must place the goniometer at precise landmarks so that angles can be compared to normative values. It is beyond the scope of this book to describe the testing method for each individual joint, though table 22.1 shows typical range of motion values for various joint movements.

Table 22.1	TYPICAL RANGE OF MOTION VALUES FOR VARIOUS JOINT MOVEMENTS	
Joint	**Movement pattern**	**Expected range of movement (degrees)**
Shoulder	Flexion	160–170
Shoulder	Extension	40–62
Shoulder	*Internal rotation*	60–70
Shoulder	External rotation	60–104
Hip	Flexion	90–155
Hip	Extension	9–29
Hip	Internal rotation	26–50
Hip	External rotation	26–70
Hip	Abduction	30–40
Hip	Adduction	10–30
Knee	Flexion	140–145
Knee	Extension	0–5
Ankle	Dorsiflexion	10–20
Ankle	Plantarflexion	30–50

Sit and reach test

The sit and reach test is simple to administer. To do it, a client sits with straight legs and reaches forwards to record the distance reached with the fingertips. This test is often performed as a measure of hamstring flexibility, but it should be noted that the test was originally described by Wells and Dillon in 1952 as a test of back and leg flexibility. In order to only measure hamstring flexibility, an adapted protocol can be used.

The sit and reach test can also be used by practitioners to identify asymmetry. For example, if the flexibility of one leg at a time is measured then it should be possible to identify if there is a discrepancy.

Equipment required:

A sit and reach table or a bench with a ruler

Test protocol (adapted):

1. The client should perform a standardised warm-up and hamstring stretch.
2. The client's legs should be fully extended with the feet (no shoes) flat against the vertical surface of the box.
3. The client should sit upright with a normal lumbar curve, palms down, arms shoulder-width apart and outstretched.
4. The client should lean forwards as far as possible, sliding their hands along the sit and reach box (if they reach it) while maintaining the normal lumbar curve.

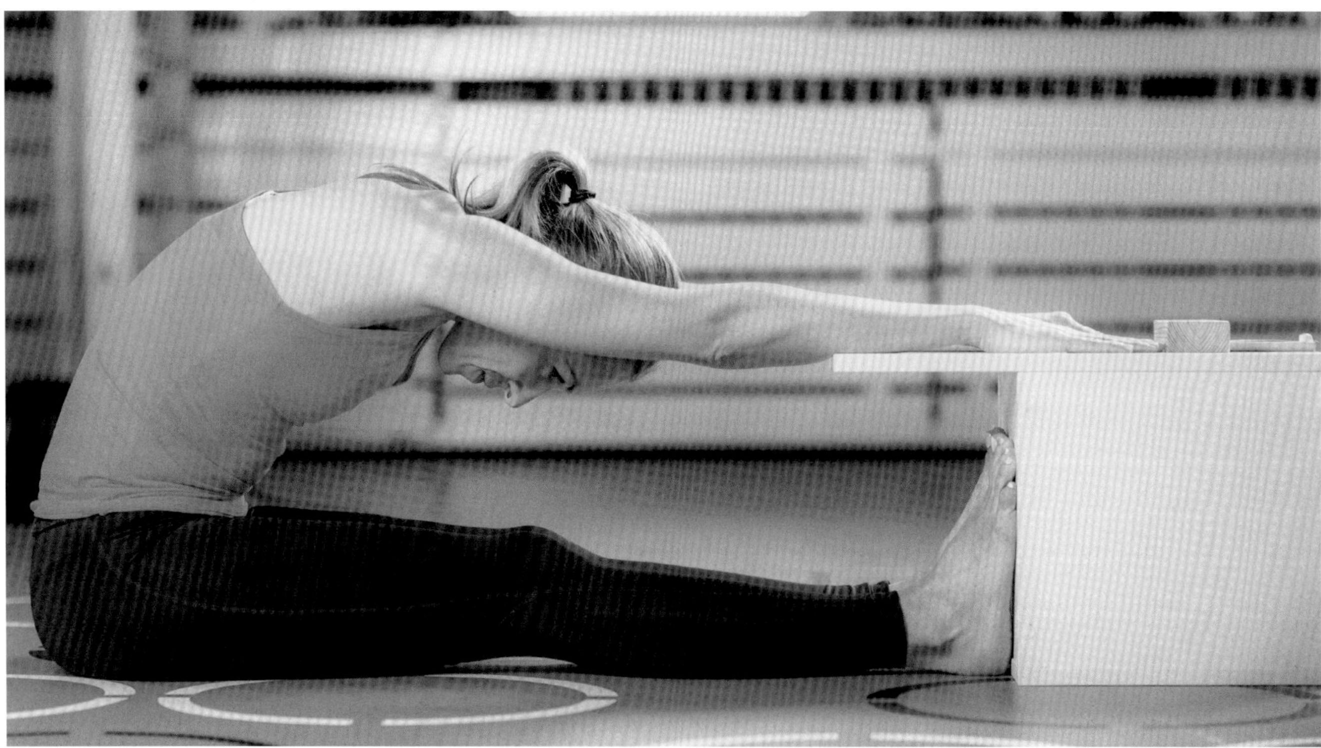

Figure 22.1 Hamstring flexibility

Table 22.2	NORMATIVE TABLE FOR 16-YEAR-OLDS AND ADULTS (VALUES IN CM)				
16-year-olds					
Gender	**Excellent**	**Above average**	**Average**	**Below average**	**Poor**
Male	>28	24–28	20–23	17–19	<17
Female	>35	32–35	30–31	25–29	<25
Adults					
Male	>29	26–28	22–25	19–21	<18
Female	>30	27–29	22–26	19–21	<18

5. The client should be stopped at the point where the upper back starts to arch or the normal lumbar curve is lost. This point should be recorded as the hamstring flexibility score.

6. The client is then allowed to continue to stretch as far as they can (*see* fig. 22.1). The maximal distance the fingers reach is recorded as the hamstring/back flexibility score.

7. The client must keep their hands parallel and should not lead with one hand.

8. Have several attempts and record the best score.

Test results:

There are no normative tables available for hamstring flexibility only. Table 22.2 can be used to classify the combined hamstring and back flexibility score for 16-year-olds and adults.

Sources of error:

Table 22.3	SOURCES OF ERROR FOR THE SIT AND REACH TEST
Error source	**Minimising strategy**
Muscle temperature	Cold muscle tissue is inflexible, so an appropriate warm-up and stretch are required.
Inertia	Clients tend to overreach by bouncing, so control the speed of the movement.
Asymmetry	If clients have an imbalance in hamstring flexibility, then measure one leg at a time.
Population	Differences in body size (for instance height and limb length) can affect scores.

Take-home messages

- There are direct and indirect methods of assessing flexibility that can be adapted for various populations.

- Practitioners should consider the population they are testing and the equipment available before considering which test is most appropriate to use.

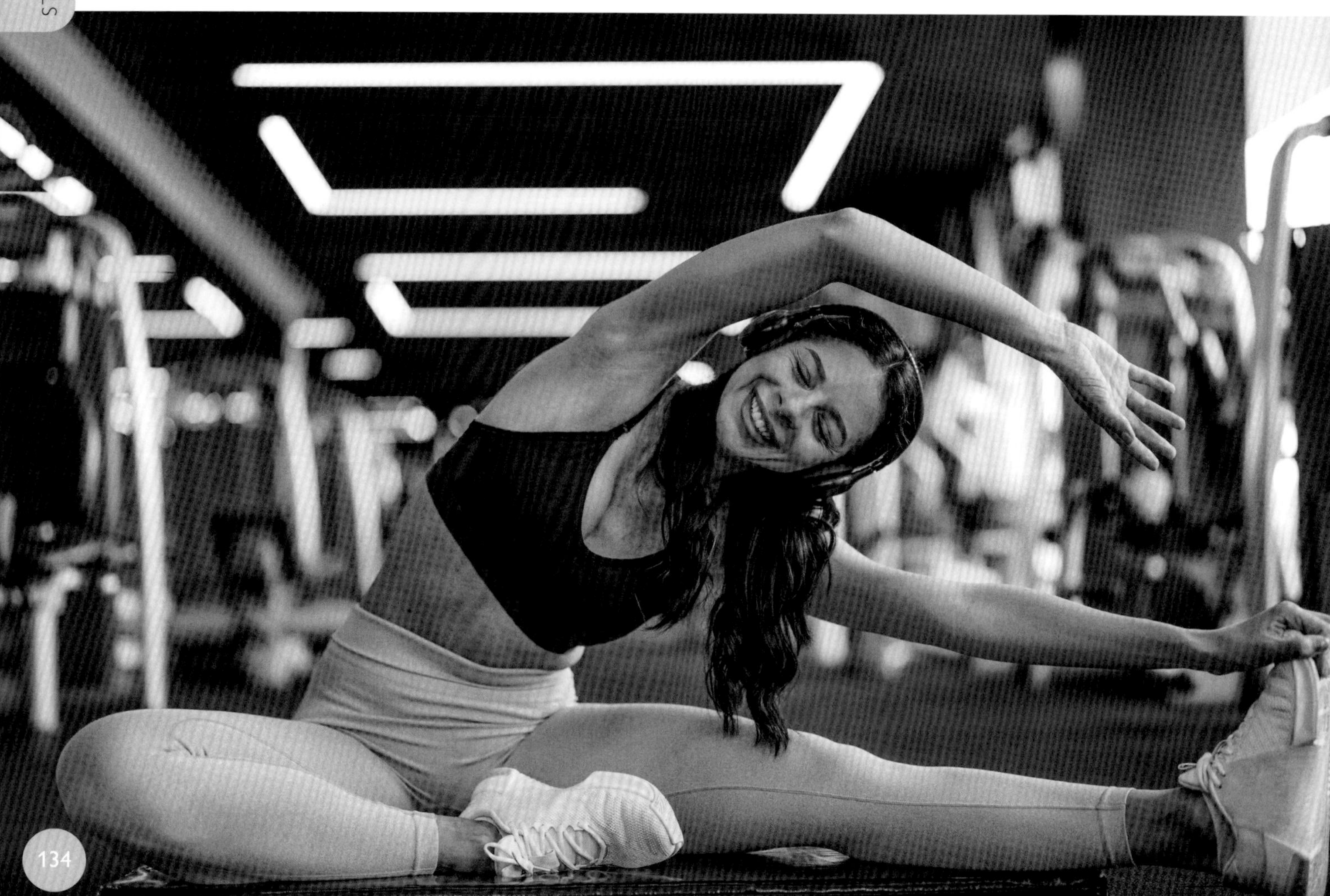

Body composition testing

The areas covered in this chapter are:

- Typical field tests for body composition that are accessible for the S&C practitioner

- Sources of error associated with the individual tests

Introduction

Body composition testing is important because it can give the practitioner an indication of the overall health of the client, as it can assess the proportion of fat mass as opposed to just weight alone. It also allows the tracking of changes in body fat, which can help to gauge the effectiveness of a training programme and therefore enable you to make informed decisions in relation to programme adaptations.

Testing

Body composition can be measured using several methods, including densitometry, plethysmography, body imaging, bio-electrical impedance and *anthropometry*, the latter including *body mass index* (BMI) and skinfolds. The validity and reliability varies between testing methods. A brief overview of each is given in table 23.1.

Many of these methods are not easily accessible for the S&C practitioner (densitometry, plethysmography and body imaging), as the equipment is prohibitively expensive. So, you might want to consider more accessible options such as BMI, waist circumference, electrical impedance and skinfolds. You may also want to consider your client's goals when selecting the most suitable method. For example, if your client has a goal to reduce overall body fat then electrical impedance would be the most suitable method whereas if the goal was more site specific then skinfolds and waist circumference could be more suitable methods. Now we'll look at some of the most common, and accessible, forms of testing:

Table 23.1	BODY COMPOSITION TESTING METHODS
Method	**Description**
Densitometry	For example, underwater weighing, where a measurement of density is converted to body fat percentage. It is based on Archimedes' principle that 'a body immersed in a fluid is balanced by a buoyancy force equivalent to the weight of fluid displaced'.
Plethysmography	The volume of air displaced by the body is converted to body fat percentage.
Body imaging techniques	Dual-energy X-ray absorptiometry (DXA) and nuclear magnetic resonance imaging (NMR). DXA passes X-rays through the body, which can identify the composition of the tissues. NMR uses powerful magnetic fields, which provide a clearer picture of soft tissues than X-rays do.
Bio-electrical impedance	This is based on the principle that an electric current flows more easily through water than fat.
Anthropometry	This uses metrics such as skinfolds, height, bodyweight, girths (such as waist circumference and waist-to-hip ratio), bone widths and BMI.

Body mass index (BMI)

Body mass index is an anthropometric index that is used to indicate the risk of certain diseases such as obesity, heart disease and diabetes. BMI was originally known as the Quetelet Index, named after a Belgian statistician in 1832. It is widely used but is a poor predictor for those with high muscle mass, as BMI is equally affected by gains in lean body mass as it is by fat mass. It is, however, a widely used, relatively quick and inexpensive method used to identify those with potential health risks, in particular by the NHS.

Equipment required:

Scales, stadiometer (height measure), calculator

Test results:

Body mass index can be calculated using the following formula:

Table 23.2	BMI CLASSIFICATIONS (ADAPTED FROM THE ACSM)
BMI classifications	**BMI score**
Underweight	<18.5
Normal	18.5–24.9
Overweight	25–29.9
Class I obese	30–34.9
Class II obese	35–39.9
Class III obese	40 or above

$$BMI = \frac{Weight\ (kg)}{Height^2\ (m^2)}$$

Once BMI has been determined, table 23.2 can be used to identify the classification. For example, a client with a body mass index of 26.7 would be categorised as overweight whereas a client with a body mass index score of 12.5 would be classed as underweight.

Sources of error:

Table 23.3	SOURCES OF ERROR FOR BMI MEASUREMENT	
Error source	**Minimising strategy**
Clothing	Ask the client to wear lightweight clothing and no shoes.
Weighing equipment	Scales are often not calibrated. Also, cheaper scales often give variable results.
Time of day	Standardise the time of the testing. First thing in the morning is a good time to measure weight.
Height measuring	Try to use a stadiometer (not expensive).

Waist circumference

The location of fat mass can increase disease risk. For example, central fat mass can increase the risk of cardiovascular disease. The ratio between waist and hip circumference (waist-to-hip ratio or WHR) can indicate body fat distribution and therefore give an indication of risk. Measurements of BMI and waist circumference in combination are considered a better predictor of risk than WHR alone. The National Institute for Health and Care Excellence (NICE) guidelines on prevention, identification, assessment and management of people who are in the overweight or obese categories suggest using a combination of BMI and waist circumference for those with a BMI of less than $35kg/m^2$ (those with a BMI over $35kg/m^2$ or above are assumed to be at risk regardless).

Equipment required:
Tape measure

Test protocol:
1. The client should stand erect, abdomen and buttocks relaxed, arms at the side and feet together.
2. Measure the waist at the end of normal respiration.
3. Waist circumference is measured twice, midway between the lower rib margin and the iliac crest in the horizontal plane (*see* fig. 23.1).
4. If the measurements are within 1cm ($\frac{2}{5}$in), the average should be calculated. If the difference between the two measurements exceeds 1cm ($\frac{2}{5}$in), the measurements should be repeated.

Test results:
According to the WHO, a waist circumference of greater than 102cm (40in) for males and 88cm (35in) for females is an indication of an increased risk of

Table 23.4	WHO RISK CATEGORIES FOR BMI AND WAIST CIRCUMFERENCE		
	Waist circumference		
	Low	**High**	**Very high**
Male: Female:	<94cm (37in) <80cm (31½in)	94–102cm (37–40in) 80–88cm (31½–34½in)	>102cm (40in) >88cm (34½in)
Normal weight	No increased risk	No increased risk	Increased risk
Overweight (BMI 25 to <30)	No increased risk	Increased risk	High risk
Obesity I (BMI 30 to <35)	Increased risk	High risk	Very high risk

developing type 2 diabetes, coronary heart disease and/or hypertension.

Note: The main source of error is related to clothing. If taking the measurement over clothes, make sure that the same clothes are used in repeat measurements.

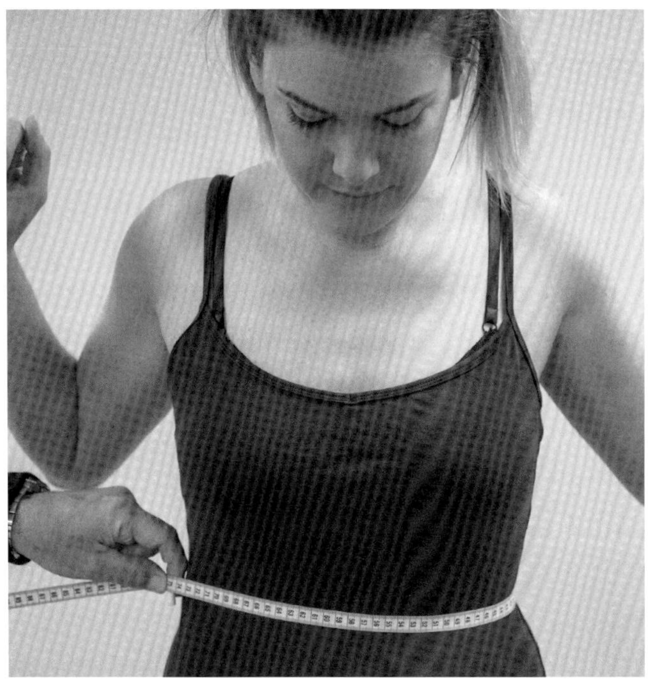

Figure 23.1 Measuring waist circumference

Electrical impedance (bio-impedance)

All bio-electrical impedance machines use the principle that the resistance to a current is inversely related to the fat-free mass (anything that is not fat) in the body. Fat-free mass contains most of the water and electrolytes in the body and so easily conducts electric current. Fat mass, however, is low in water and electrolytes and resists the flow of electric current.

Equipment required:
Electrical impedance machine, floor mat or bench

Test protocol:
1. Ensure that the analyser is calibrated before use.
2. The client should lie on a nonconductive surface such as a mat.
3. Position the electrodes with reference to the manufacturer's recommendations. This is usually relative to anatomical landmarks.
4. The electrode sites should be cleaned to reduce loss of signal and depending on the type of electrode used, a conducting gel should be placed between the electrodes and the skin.

5. The source electrode produces the current and the reference (detecting) electrode detects it. The drop in voltage between the two reference electrodes determines the impedance.

Test result:

There are classification tables available from various sources that describe body fat percentage classifications. Table 23.6 is adapted from the WHO's guidelines. Table 23.7 is adapted from the ACSM.

Sources of error:

Table 23.5	SOURCES OF ERROR FOR ELECTRICAL IMPEDANCE MEASUREMENT
Error source	**Minimising strategy**
Exercise	No exercise for 12 hours before the test.
Hydration	Food and fluid intake can affect hydration status. No eating or drinking in the 4 hours before the test. Urinate within 30 minutes before the test.
Timing	Standardise the time of the testing.
Diuretics	No diuretics such as coffee, tea or any other caffeinated drink should be consumed within 24 hours before the test.

Skinfolds

Between 50 and 70% of adipose tissue in adults is located under the skin (subcutaneously). A simple and inexpensive method of measuring subcutaneous fat stores is known as skinfolds. The location of the skinfold (point at which a skinfolds measurement is taken) differs depending on the protocol used.

Equipment required:

Skinfold calipers, tape measure, marker pen

Test protocol:

1. The tester's left hand should raise a skinfold between the thumb and forefinger at the marked site (depending on the protocol) in the required direction, following the natural cleavage lines of the skin (*see* fig. 23.2).

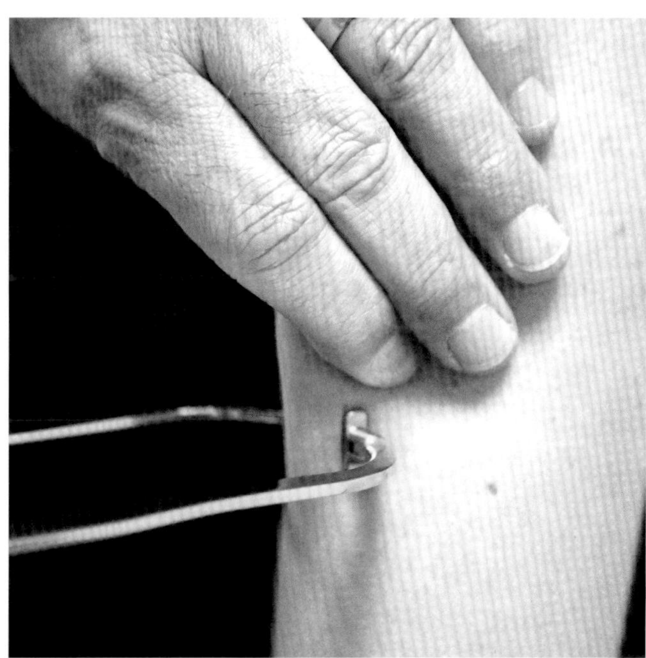

Figure 23.2 Skinfolds caliper placement

Table 23.6 — **BODY FAT PERCENTAGE CLASSIFICATIONS (ADAPTED FROM THE WHO)**

Female				
Age (yrs)	Underweight	Healthy range	Overweight	Obese
20–40	Under 21%	21–33%	33–39%	≥40%
41–60	Under 23%	23–35%	35–40%	≥41%
61–79	Under 24%	24–36%	36–42%	≥43%
Male				
Age (yrs)	Underweight	Healthy range	Overweight	Obese
20–40	Under 8%	8–19%	19–25%	≥26%
41–60	Under 11%	11–22%	22–27%	≥28%
61–79	Under 13%	13–25%	25–30%	≥31%

Table 23.7 — **BODY FAT PERCENTAGE CLASSIFICATIONS (ADAPTED FROM THE ACSM)**

Male	Age				
Category	20–29	30–39	40–49	50–59	60+
Excellent	7.1–9.3%	11.3–13.8%	13.6–16.2%	15.3–17.8%	15.3–18.3%
Good	9.4–14%	13.9–17.4%	16.3–19.5%	17.9–21.2%	18.4–21.9%
Average	14.1–17.5%	17.5–20.4%	19.6–22.4%	21.3–24%	22–25%
Below average	17.5%+	20.4%+	22.4%+	24%+	25%+
Female	Age				
Category	20–29	30–39	40–49	50–59	60+
Excellent	14.5–17%	15.5–17.9%	18.5–21.2%	21.6–24.9%	21.1–25%
Good	17.1–20.5%	18–21.5%	21.3–24.8%	25–28.4%	25.1–29.2%
Average	20.6–23.6%	21.6–24.8%	24.9–28%	28.5–31.5%	29.3–32.4%
Below average	23.7–27.6%	24.9–29.2%	28.1–32%	31.6–35.5%	32.5–36.5%

2. There should be a slight rolling and pulling action to separate the fold from the muscle beneath.

3. The caliper is held in the right hand and the blades are applied perpendicularly to the fold and 1cm (²⁄₅in) away from the thumb and forefinger.

4. Spring pressure is released, and value is recorded 2 seconds later to the nearest 0.2mm.

5. All skinfolds should be measured three times with a 2-second recovery to allow compression of the tissue to return to normal. Use the median (middle) value obtained.

Test results:

Normative tables for all protocols predict body fat percentage. Once this is established, results can be categorised using classification tables such as those in tables 23.6 and 23.7.

Sources of error:

Table 23.8	SOURCES OF ERROR FOR SKINFOLD TESTING
Error source	**Minimising strategy**
Equipment	Harpenden and Holtain calipers have better reliability than most other types.
Caliper placement	There are errors in placement between testers. Practise before using on clients and try to use the same tester.
Obesity level	Errors increase with obesity levels, so choose an alternative method for those who are morbidly obese.
Population	There are many norm tables available for use, so use norms appropriate to the client.

Take-home messages

- There are direct and indirect methods of assessing body composition.

- Practitioners should identify the most suitable technique for a client based on resources and goals.

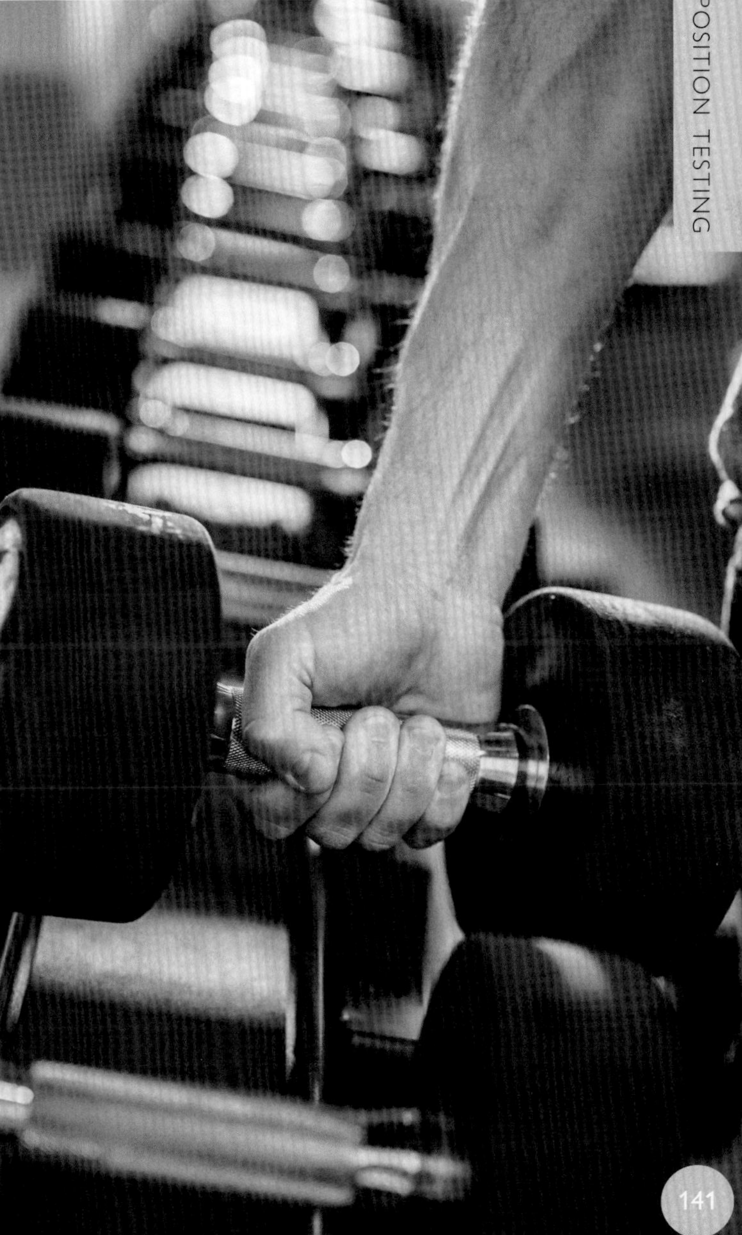

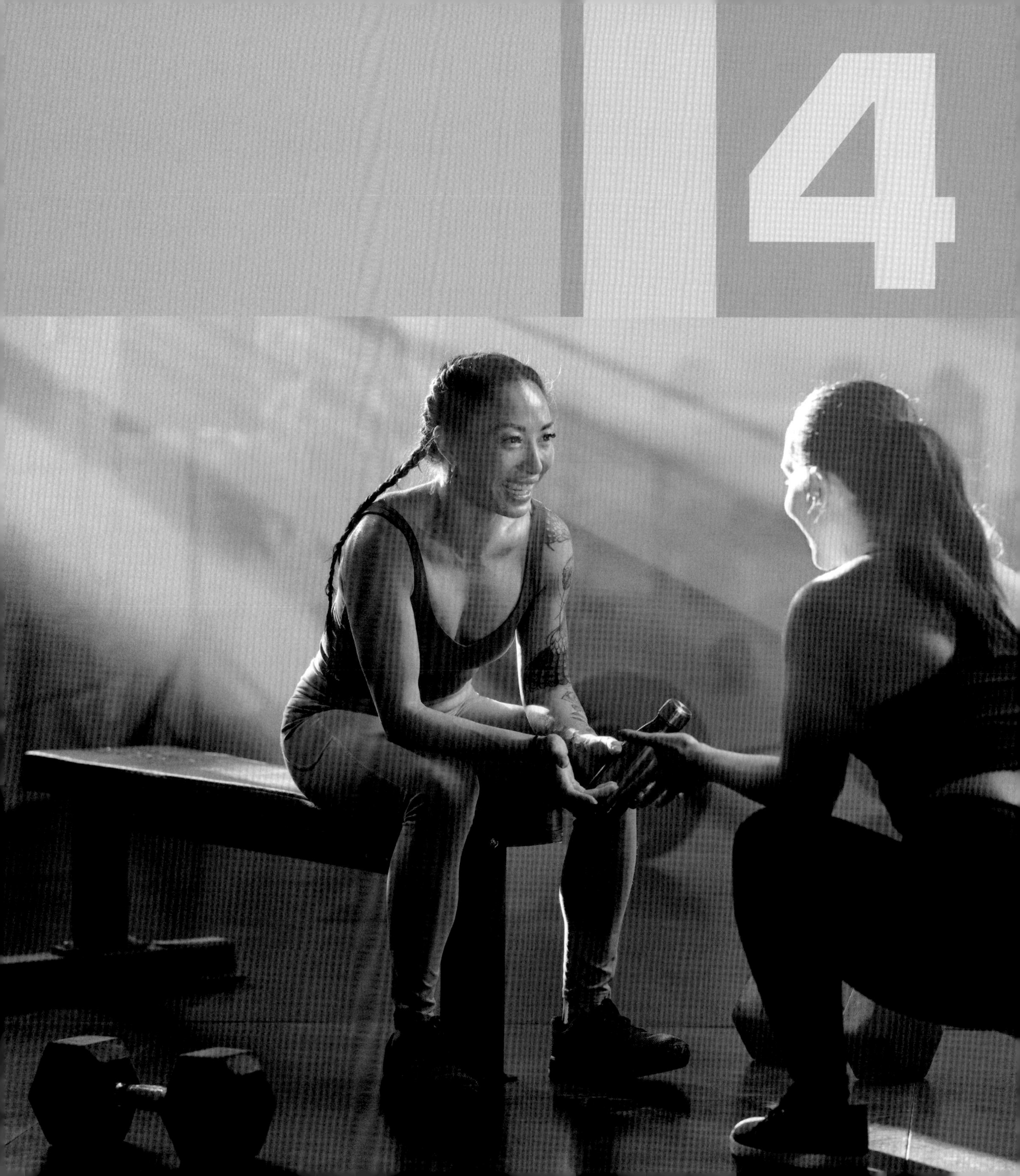
14

PART **FOUR**

GENERAL TRAINING STRATEGIES

Parts 1, 2 and 3 were designed to guide you through the process of designing S&C training programmes for a range of clients, which should help get you started on your journey as an S&C practitioner. There are, however, many other areas related to S&C that will help you further develop your knowledge and skills. We encourage you to use the chapters in part 4 to broaden your knowledge and maybe stimulate ideas for future professional development, because in the S&C environment we never stop learning!

The first chapter deals in more detail with how to manipulate a wide range of variables that can impact a training programme and then goes on to cover theory relating to a concept known as periodisation (which simply means how to programme in the long term). The next chapter looks at the mechanisms of fatigue and strategies to reduce the impact of this, which is important in the design of S&C programmes. The third chapter addresses skills required to be a good S&C practitioner, such as communication, observation, listening and feedback. We firmly believe that as an S&C practitioner you need a certain knowledge base, but you need to have a range of practical skills that enable you to be successful in an environment that can at times be challenging. For this reason, we have also included a chapter on motivation, which we hope will then encourage you to reflect on your own performance as a practitioner and continue your professional development. The final chapter in part 3 covers the legal and ethical information that you are required to understand and adhere to as an S&C practitioner.

Manipulation of training variables 24

The areas covered in this chapter are:

- The range of sports/events where variables are typically manipulated, i.e. team sports, endurance events, sprint events, and strength and power sports

- The importance of training load monitoring and exercise selection when designing programmes, taking into account factors such as client training age, training level, exercise complexity, type of exercise (compound or isolated) and the interference effect

- How to incorporate safe and effective warm-ups and cool-downs

- What periodisation is and how it can help in the design process of individual and team programmes, taking into account the performance calendar, the need for tapering and peaking and sport-specific requirements

- Client and logistical factors that can affect exercise programming, such as injury risks/history and the availability of time and resources.

Introduction

The previous chapters have explored different performance characteristics, how they can be trained and how they can be tested for. This next section will focus on how these performance characteristics can be developed through the manipulation of training variables. Different sports require the refinement of specific performance characteristics, so S&C practitioners must have the ability to tailor these characteristics to develop the desired performance outcomes that allow individuals or teams to excel in their sport.

Manipulation of training variables

Training programmes are designed to manipulate specific training variables to develop a client to elicit specific outcomes. The knowledge that the practitioner has gained from the consultation process and needs analysis should ensure that the content of any training programme should closely link to performance aims and goals. There is a plethora of ways in which training variables can be manipulated depending on the level of a client, their sport, injury history and training availability. Each performance component of a sport (technical, tactical, physical, psychological and social)

Table 24.1	TYPICAL SPORTS/EVENTS AND THE IMPORTANCE OF FITNESS COMPONENTS					
Sport or event	Aerobic endurance	Strength	Muscular endurance	Power	Speed / agility	Flexibility
Sprints	+	++	++++	++++	+++++	++
1500m	++++	+	++++	++	++	+
10,000m	+++++	+	++	+	+	+
Football	+++	+++	+++	+++	++++	+++
Boxing	+++	+++	++++	+++	+++	++
Long jump	+	++	+++	+++++	+++++	+++
Tennis	++	++	+++	++	+++	++++
Weightlifting	+	+++++	++	+++++	+	++
Recreational running	+++++	+	++	+	+	++
General body toning	+++	++	+++++	++	+	++

must be balanced to ensure clients possess the relevant level of competency in each area. More specifically, this is also true for the physical performance components of sport (strength, power, aerobic and anaerobic capacity, coordination etc.) where the development of each must be balanced to adequately prepare a client for their sport. Table 24.1 gives an example of fitness component importance relevant to various sports and events.

The importance of each performance component can differ depending on the type or nature of the sport or event such as team sport, endurance events, sprint events and strength and power sports.

TEAM SPORTS

The physiological demands and fitness requirements of team sports are variable, as match duration can range from 60 minutes in sports such as handball to several days in the case of test cricket. Intensity can also range from continuous to intermittent. For example, a midfield football player will normally cover 10–14km (6.2–8.7 miles) each match, at an average intensity of 80–90% of their maximum heart rate and perform 20–40 high-intensity sprints. By contrast, a batsman in cricket might only cover a distance of 1.7km (just over a mile) over the period of a 3-day test match.

ENDURANCE EVENTS

Performance in endurance-type events often relies on sustaining a relevantly high velocity for an extended period of time. Because of this, an ability to resist both peripheral and central fatigue is a vital component for this type of client. The range of events/sports considered to be endurance-based include running, swimming, cycling, triathlon, cross-country skiing, rowing, canoeing and kayaking. These can vary greatly in duration, for example from 10 to 20 minutes for some events up to an extremely demanding 23 days in the case of the Tour de France. Even though these events are considered to be primarily aerobic, anaerobic contribution can also be important in events of shorter distances or in events in which changes of pace occur frequently, for example in cycle races.

SPRINT EVENTS

Sprint events typically include 60–800m distances on a track, up to 1000m in cycling, and 50–100m in swimming. Acceleration and maximal speed are two of the most important components of fitness in sprint events. These events will mainly require anaerobic respiration through the ATP-PC system for approximately the first 10 seconds of activity, followed by the anaerobic glycolysis energy system for the remainder of the event.

STRENGTH AND POWER SPORTS

Sports such as Olympic weightlifting and powerlifting are mainly characterised by the ability to generate force rapidly. Muscular power and muscular endurance are components that are often addressed in sports such as these and are developed using resistance training.

Muscular power

Muscular power can be thought of as the application of force in a short time period. Typically, light to moderate loads lifted at speed are used extensively in training programmes to develop muscular power. A reduction in strength training is advised during muscular power training periods because it can have a detrimental effect on muscular power performance. It is recommended to have a good strength base before undertaking this type of training.

Muscular endurance (power endurance)

Muscular endurance (also called power endurance) can be diverse in relation to the number of repetitions and outcomes, so it is recommended that the training programme reflects the demands of the sport. As muscular endurance relates to resisting fatigue, training is associated with a high number of repetitions using a comparatively low weight or resistance. Slow twitch type 1 muscle fibres are predominantly used in this type of training, as the intensity required to stimulate the contraction of fast twitch type 2 muscle fibres has been estimated to be approximately 70% of maximum strength capability.

Resistance training intensity and volume selection

Resistance training intensity (otherwise known as the load) can be expressed as repetition maximum (RM) (maximum weight lifted for a specific number of repetitions, e.g. 3RM is the maximum weight that can be lifted for 3 repetitions). Intensity can also be expressed as a percentage of 1RM (e.g. 80% of 1RM). Training volume describes the total work performed per session and is typically calculated as:

$$\text{sets} \times \text{repetitions}$$

or

$$\text{sets} \times \text{repetitions} \times \text{load}$$

Training volume over the course of a week is simply the sum of the volume of each training session for that week. For example, for a client who performs 3 sets of 10 repetitions of 80kg, the volume can be calculated as 30 reps of 80kg, which is 2400kg. Training volume is one of the major factors affecting strength or muscle mass gains. During resistance training the intensity and volume of the load to be used depends upon many factors, including the aim or goal of the client.

Table 24.2	REPETITION MAXIMUM AND CORRESPONDING PERCENTAGE OF 1RM	
Repetition max		**%1RM**
14–15		65
12–13		70
10–11		75
8–9		80
6–7		85
4–5		90
2–3		95
1		100

Strength–endurance continuum

When designing resistance training programmes, it is useful to use the strength–endurance continuum (*see* fig. 24.1) to help establish repetition maximum related to the goal of the programme.

It can be seen in figure 24.1 that there is a degree of overlap with regards to repetitions and associated outcomes. However, as a general guide, increases in strength occur at about 40% of 1RM or more. The largest increases in maximal strength (1RM), however, occur near to maximal load. Increases in hypertrophy usually occur around 80% of 1RM, although intensity is only one factor that can determine hypertrophic response to exercise, with training volume, number of sets, choice of exercise and recovery also being important factors. Table 24.2 gives a general guide of repetition maximum and the corresponding percentage of maximal capability.

Training load monitoring

Training load must be finely balanced to ensure a training programme is adequate to prepare a client for the demands of their sport and ensuring they are robust without increasing injury risks through over- or undertraining. This process must be tailored for each

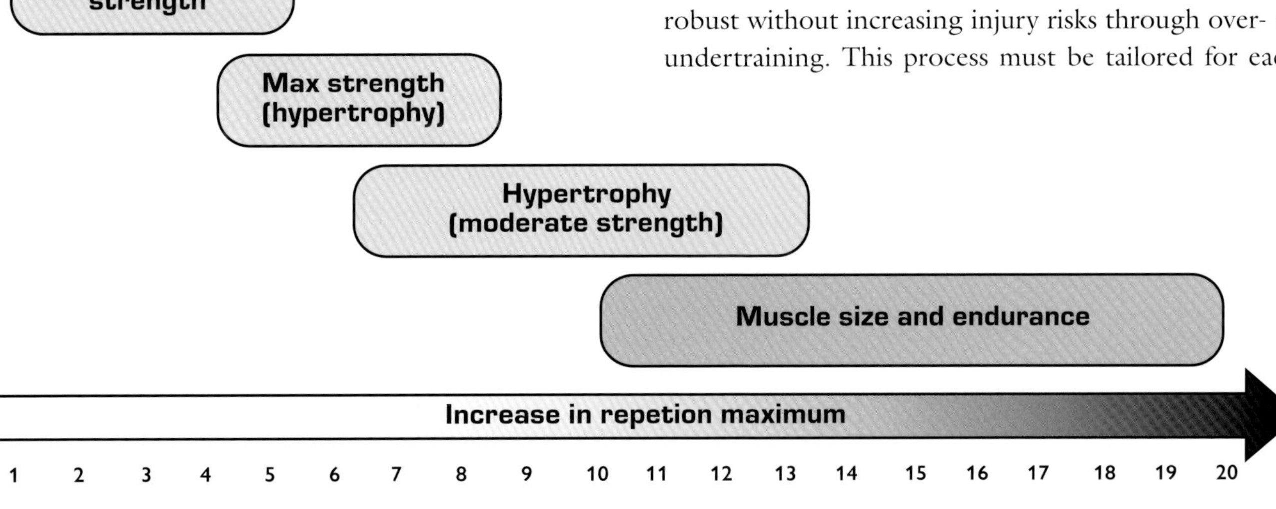

Figure 24.1 Strength–endurance continuum related to RM

client, as a one-size-fits-all approach may result in the overtraining of some clients and the undertraining for others completing the same programme.

Training load monitoring has become commonplace and provides a way to monitor the work done by the client (external load) and their response to the training load they are subjected to (internal load).

EXTERNAL LOAD MONITORING (REPS/ SETS RECORDING, GPS LOCOMOTOR VOLUME/INTENSITY)

External load is an objective quantification of the work done during training or competition. Markers of external load include recording exercise repetitions and sets, total running distance covered, sprint running distance and force or power output. These measurements are calculated using GPS devices, force platforms and power meters. The most basic form of external load monitoring is to track the mass, number of sets and repetitions of each exercise within a training programme. This method allows the recorded data to be tracked as a measure of progress and to ensure clients continue to develop.

GPS devices are commonplace in running-based individual and team sports. They are often mounted in a vest and worn on the upper back or as a wristwatch. They can track the volume and intensity of running-based training sessions through the calculation of total running distance and the speeds at which the distance is covered. Some GPS systems also contain integrated accelerometers that calculate acceleration and deceleration volume and intensity. Other methods to monitor external load include the use of force platforms and power meters. They are often used to track performance in specific tests and can be used to track longitudinal performance adaptations.

INTERNAL LOAD MONITORING

Internal load is how a client reacts and responds to the external load of a training session or competition. Internal load can be described as the response of biological stressors to physical exertion. Markers of internal load include heart rate responses, subjective scores such as ratings of *perceived exertion* (RPE), biomarkers measured through salivary or blood samples, and urine testing. Let's look at each of these in turn:

- **Heart rate response** – Tracking heart rate responses to certain training loads can help to ensure a client is training at the optimal intensity for the training aims. Heart rate zones (*see* fig. 24.2) are commonly used to programme training intensity and are calculated as a percentage of the predicted heart rate max. It is thought that training at intensities that elicit specific percentages of heart rate max will indicate that different energy systems will be targeted and developed.
- **Rate of perceived exertion** – RPE scores were originally developed by Borg in 1961 but there have been

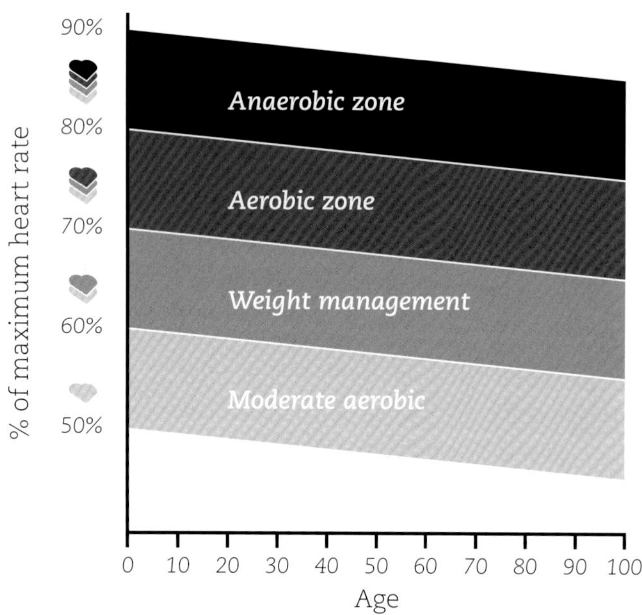

Figure 24.2 Cardio training zones

many variations to this scale, including the CR100 scale, RPE session load (RPE × training time) and differential RPE. All of these variations are designed to record a subjective measure of a client's perceived level of exertion to a training stimulus.

- **Biomarkers** – These are substances such as hormones, or by-products from biochemical reactions that are present in the blood or saliva. It is possible to measure the concentrations of biomarkers before, during or after exercise to provide an indication of the internal response to the exercise. For example, blood lactate levels can be monitored to identify when a client is respiring anaerobically. Also, salivary cortisol levels can provide an insight to the stress levels of the body following intense exercise.
- **Urine testing** – Urine concentration testing can be used to monitor the hydration levels of clients. This can be useful particularly within warmer climates or if clients are moving from a temperate to a warmer climate for training/competition. The requirement to modify fluid intake within warmer environments to maintain hydration levels can often be overlooked, in which case urine concentration tests provide the ability to quantify this and inform the client.

Internal load monitoring can also be used to gauge a client's readiness to train and pre-training condition. Readiness questionnaires may include information about how a client has slept (number of hours of sleep), their overall mood, muscle soreness, fatigue levels and desire to train. Some clients may be uncomfortable with questionnaires like these as they may feel invasive, or clients may feel that answers they give may impact their coach or manager's view of them. As a practitioner, it is important to build a working relationship with clients and ensure that the above monitoring techniques are used to protect them and not impact their opportunities to compete.

Exercise selection

Exercise selection is an important factor when designing training programmes. Practitioners must consider several factors when including specific exercises within a programme. These include:

- **Client training age** – Training age refers to the experience a client has within the training environment. A client who has a high level of experience and competency will likely be able to complete more complex exercises that recruit greater numbers of muscle groups while lifting greater loads.
- **Client training level** – Clients competing and training at a high level may be able to lift greater loads. However, they may require greater loads to elicit adaptations compared to lower-level, less-experienced clients.
- **Exercise complexity** – Is the time spent teaching correct technique and building the load worth it for the value that the exercise brings to the programme? Exercises such as Olympic lifting variations can have a high technical component to them that takes time for clients to become competent in. Furthermore, if performed incorrectly, they can increase the risk of injury. For this reason, a practitioner needs to identify if the pay-off from a complex exercise is worth the time required to teach a client the correct technique to perform it safely. Some machine-based exercises can be used as an alternative for general fitness goals as they require less time for teaching technique and also have a lower technical component.
- **Compound or isolated exercises** – Similar to exercise complexity, performing compound exercises that require the coordination of several muscle groups is more complicated than using isolated exercises that target specific muscle groups. However, compound exercises, due to their nature of recruiting multiple muscle groups within a system, may be more specific to movement patterns required in sport and so may provide more benefits than isolated exercises.

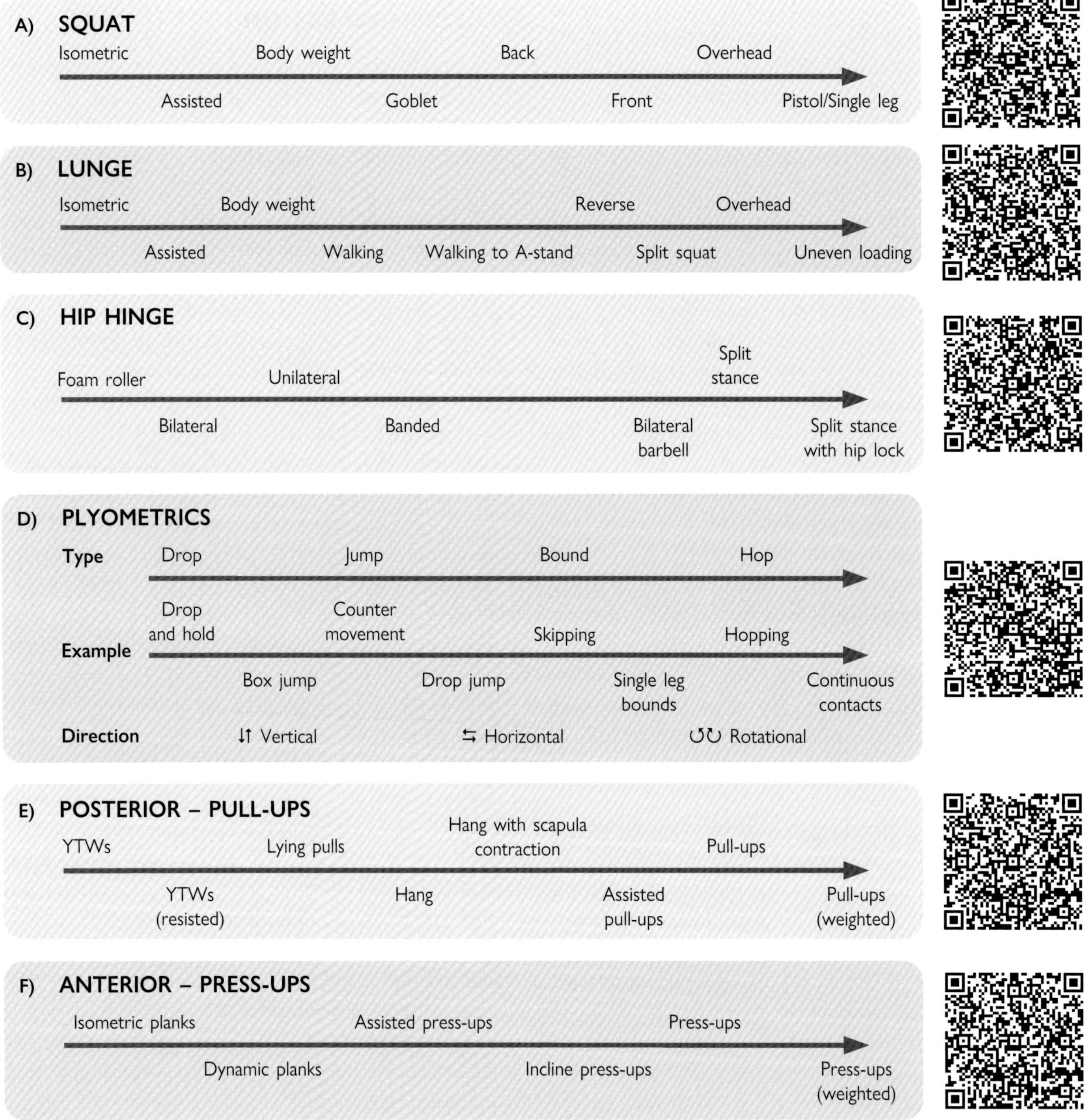

Figure 24.3 Compound exercise progressions: A) squat; B) lunge; C) hip hinge; D) plyometrics; E) posterior – pull-ups; F) anterior – press-ups

- **Interference effect** – This refers to the impact exercise choice may have on the ability of a client to perform subsequent exercises with the technique, volume and intensity required to elicit performance adaptations. The stimuli caused by one exercise may impact the performance of another exercise. For example, programming a leg extension followed by the Bulgarian split squat may inhibit the client's ability to effectively perform the Bulgarian split squat because the quadricep muscles may already be fatigued. The split squat is also a compound exercise, while the leg extension is isolated. So, depending on the rationale of programming these exercises, using the split squat in isolation may be viewed as being more beneficial to the client's development, since its use will result in the recruitment of multiple muscle groups in addition to the quadricep muscles.

Practitioners must use their expertise and experience to design training programmes that contain lifts and exercises that are suitable for the client being trained. Before lifts and exercises are included within a programme, a practitioner should evaluate their use and consider if the client is capable of completing them competently and if the exercise used will add value to their programme and aid their development.

Some examples of compound exercise progressions are shown in figure 24.3. These exercises increase in their technical requirement and perceived difficulty. Clients should be technically competent with the movement patterns and strength required to perform basic compound lifts before progressing through the exercise progression continuums.

Movement skills

S&C practitioners typically focus on the quality of movement (also known as movement mechanics or movement skills) of a client during the performance of any exercise. When choosing movement skills for your client programme, table 24.3 will help you to identify the difficulty level of those skills and any prerequisite ability (known as entry criteria) that the client should demonstrate before undertaking them. You will see in the table that many of the exercises classed as movement skills will be familiar to you, as they are commonly used to develop a range of fitness components. We have listed the skills in progressive order using the terms basic, fundamental, learning to train and train for performance. We chose these classifications because they are typically used in the S&C environment.

ASSESSING LIFTS AND EXERCISES SHOWN ON SOCIAL MEDIA

A common issue with programme design arises from the influence of social media. It is important to review lifts and exercises shown on social media before using them, as they may not necessarily be appropriate or safe to integrate into a training programme. There are very limited vetting processes used to police social media accounts, so people can post videos of exercises and lifts equipped with captions of their benefits regardless of their experience, expertise or education within this area. While there are no consequences for the people posting these videos, there may be for practitioners who use them to train clients, as they may increase the injury risk to the client or not provide them with a training stimulus that will promote performance development.

Warm-up

Research over the years has demonstrated that an appropriate warm-up can improve performance, positively affect mental preparedness, and reduce risk of injury, potentially due to decreased joint and muscle stiffness. However, the design of warm-up strategies can often involve a degree of trial and error. The manipulation of both intensity and duration should

Table 24.3	TYPICAL MOVEMENT SKILL PROGRESSIONS		
	Basic movement skills	**Fundamental movement skills**	
Goal	• Understand core movement mechanics • Develop coordination • Educate athletes	• Increase flexibility and mobility • Target basic movement mechanics • Develop functional strength • Develop closed chain eccentric strength	
Method	• Mostly bilateral (sub-max) to develop motor control and coordination	• Mostly bilateral (sub-max) to develop eccentric/motor control • Bilateral offset, asymmetrical and symmetrical	
Entry criteria	• Novices • For beginners to S&C	• Competent bodyweight bilateral squat technique • <20% asymmetry in loaded squat	
Skills	• Squat patterns • Lunge patterns • Hip hinge • Crawls/animal movements • Static balance • Hang • Press-up static hold • Push • Pull	• Skips in place • Bilateral squat jump (SJ) (in place, forwards) • Bilateral countermovement jump (CMJ) (in place, forwards) • Split jump (same leg land) • Step and land (forwards, lateral, standing and from running on spot) • Hop in place (forwards/lateral/angle) • Ladder and hurdle varied linear and lateral running drills • Sprint • Hang • Press-up	
Core	• Brace/resist • Weight transfer	• Abdominal hollowing • Supine and prone bridge • Supine foot slides • Superman (contralateral) • Donkey kicks	

Learning to train	Train for performance
• Develop bilateral power • Develop unilateral eccentric control • Address muscle asymmetry	• Develop closed kinetic chain power • Reinforce movement quality • Develop sport-specific movement skills
• Bilateral and unilateral to develop power and deceleration • Bilateral offset, asymmetrical and symmetrical. Unilateral (linear)	• Bilateral and unilateral to develop acceleration and explosive sport-specific performance • Bilateral offset, asymmetrical and symmetrical. Unilateral (multi-plane)
• Competent bilateral landing control • Competent bodyweight unilateral squat technique • Squat >1.25 × body mass (8RM) or 1.5 × body mass (1RM)	• Competent bilateral drop jump mechanics • Competent unilateral landing control • Squat strength >1.5 × body mass (8RM) or 2 × body mass (1RM) • Competent unilateral deceleration and COD
• Step-land-push back (forwards, lateral, standing and from running on spot) • SJ and CMJ to box • Step-up jump (same and alternating leg) • Bilateral drop jump (30cm/12in box) • Rotational jump and land • Tuck jump • Unilateral bounding • Press-ups • Pull-ups (assisted) • Push press (unilateral) • Single-arm rows (bear stance)	• Continuous UL SJ/CMJ to BL landing • UL SJ/CMJ to box • Continuous CMJ (hurdles) • SJ/CMJ weighted • Lateral hop (band/rope/med ball) • COD sport-specific drills with perturbation • Press-ups • Pull-ups • Push press • Rows
• Side bridge • Dead bugs, bear crawls, bicycle crunch • Superman (ipsilateral) • Superman donkey kicks	• Single-leg bridges • Jack-knife and V-sits

Table 24.4	RECOMMENDATIONS FOR WARM-UP STRATEGIES
Variable	**Recommendation**
Time between warm-up completion and game/event commencement	Between 9 and 20 minutes (slightly more if high intensity)
Warm-up duration	Approximately 15 minutes (intermittent protocols may offer additional benefits)

Table 24.5	RECOMMENDATIONS FOR COOL-DOWN STRATEGIES
Variable	**Recommendation**
Intensity	Gradually decrease dynamic activities from moderate to low intensity to prevent development of additional fatigue.
Impact	Employ low mechanical impact to prevent the development of muscular damage.
Duration	Less than 30 minutes to limit interference with glycogen resynthesis.
Exercise selection	Involve the same muscle groups as used in the session and also those that may be specific to the client's sport or event. For example, for a cyclist you might want to do the cool-down on a bike!

be considered when designing a warm-up strategy as well as the time between the warm-up and the event/match.

To further complicate matters, various methods of warm-up strategy are commonly employed, such as post-activation performance enhancing (PAPE) strategies and priming strategies (or a combination of both). The lack of consensus about the optimal warm-up strategy makes it difficult to recommend a one-size-fits-all strategy, although incorporating activities that closely mimic those performed in the event/sport seems sensible. Table 24.4 provides general recommendations relating to the manipulation of variables for warm-up strategies based on an overview of research in the area.

Cool-down

Most training sessions typically end with an active cool-down phase that incorporates a progressive decrease in intensity followed by a period of static stretching, as it is widely assumed that this will reduce delayed onset muscle soreness and increase range of motion. To date there is no consensus in the literature as to the benefits of a cool-down and indeed the inclusion post exercise has been questioned. However, although proposed benefits may not be supported by research it is recommended that cool-down strategies be incorporated into training sessions, as benefits may include the following:

- **Cardiorespiratory systems** – An active cool-down may result in a faster recovery of these systems.
- **Dizziness (syncope)** – A cool-down may help prevent the dizziness that some people experience post exercise.
- **Blood circulation** – The decrease in blood circulation may help prevent blood pooling.
- **Blood pH** – A low- to moderate-intensity cool-down can speed up recovery of pH to resting levels.
- **Psychological** – There may be psychological benefits to cooling down, especially if clients are familiar with the strategy employed.

As with warm-up strategies, it is difficult to recommend a one-size-fits-all approach but the authors suggest that cool-down strategies should follow the general guidelines shown in table 24.5.

Periodisation

Periodisation refers to the manipulation of training variables (frequency, volume and intensity) at regular intervals and is thought to have first been proposed by Russian physiologist Leo Matveyev in the 1960s. It is used to organise training programmes into more manageable periods, known as cycles, to achieve optimum adaptation and prevent overtraining. There are three types of cycle:

1. **Microcycle** – The shortest period of training, which is usually seven days.
2. **Mesocycle** – A repeating series of microcycles over a period of several weeks.
3. **Macrocycle** – A series of mesocycles, normally over a period of a few months to several years, which normally aligns with competition cycles.

Periodising a training programme can help clients to focus on short-, medium and long-term goals, which can impact positively on performance. There are many models that can be used when designing a periodised training programme, such as the linear, block and undulating models, as outlined below:

- **Linear periodisation** – Linear periodisation transitions from a volume focus to an intensity focus as the training programme progresses. For example, the volume (total number of reps) of an exercise may decrease while the intensity (total mass lifted) increases.
- **Block periodisation** – Block periodisation is organised into distinct sections of work, each with

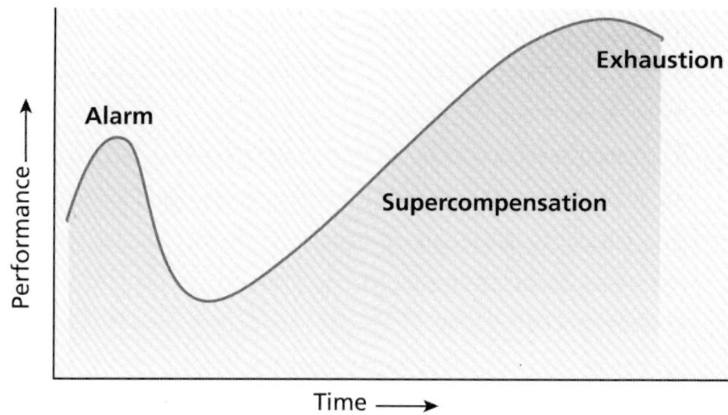

Figure 24.4 General adaptation syndrome (GAS)

a different focus. These blocks normally consist of general preparation, specific preparation, competitions and transition.

- **Undulating periodisation** – Undulating periodisation is alternatively known as non-linear periodisation. Unlike linear and block periodisation where the training periods are quite broad and may span multiple micro- and mesocycles, an undulating programme is much more varied and will include different training focuses within the same microcycle. For example, within one training week, there may be different training sessions, each one with a different training focus (e.g. hypertrophy, strength or power production).

Matveyev's general concept is that training should progress from high volume/low intensity to low volume/high intensity with respect to targeted fitness components. However, it should also be remembered that when a new training stress or stimulus (change in training intensity or volume) is introduced, there will be a typical response known as the general adaptation syndrome (GAS), which was first proposed by Hans Selye in 1936 and contains three phases:

1. **Alarm phase** – This is the initial response to a change in stimulus, which can last days to several

weeks. During this phase there might be a reduction in performance and increase in delayed onset muscle soreness.

2. **Supercompensation phase** – As training continues, increases in performance are typical. The length of this phase is dependent on the training status of the client and the increase in the training stimulus.

3. **Exhaustion phase** – If the stimulus continues to increase at a rate the body cannot adapt to, it could lead to a decrease in performance and possible overtraining.

General fitness component development

The development of fitness components is specific to the client and their goals but a model such as the fitness component pyramid as shown in figure 24.5 can be used for progression of typical components within various stages, as outlined below:

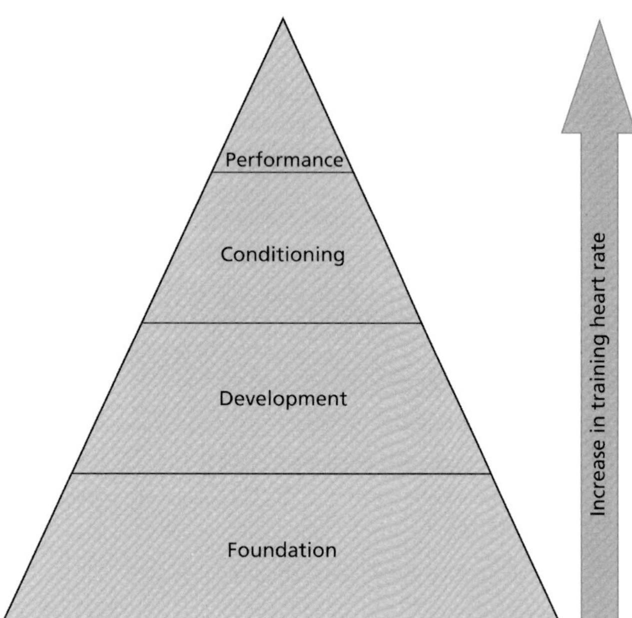

Figure 24.5 Fitness component pyramid

- **Foundation** – As with any progressive model there should be a foundation (base fitness level) prior to progression. Typical fitness components for this stage include flexibility, joint mobility (range of movement), joint stabilisation (posture awareness and static balance) and aerobic capacity.
- **Development** – Once a base level has been achieved, components such as movement coordination, dynamic balance, stability and aerobic conditioning can be developed.
- **Conditioning** – Depending on client needs, components such as muscular strength/endurance, hypertrophy, agility, anaerobic and aerobic capacity can be developed.
- **Performance** – For specific performance goals, components such as power, speed and skill can be developed.

Performance calendar – periodisation for specific sports/individuals

The periodisation of training can vary depending on the level of the client, the time required to prepare the client for competition, their sport and the competition schedule. Therefore, when creating a periodised programme, it should be planned in reverse from the competition period to the start date. Working back from the competition date will allow enough time to be planned for each stage of preparation, ensuring clients are prepared and resistant to injury. The type of periodisation used (linear, block, undulating – *see* p. 155) will depend on the aforementioned variables, which means all training programmes should be bespoke to the client.

ONE-OFF COMPETITION INDIVIDUAL (E.G. BOXING)

There are many sports in which clients compete in isolated competitions that do not follow a specific season or regular competition schedule (e.g. boxing and other combat sports). These clients are required to consistently train to maintain their physical condition within the foundation, development and conditioning phases of training. Upon the confirmation of a boxing match, the training will then elevate and shift into the performance phase to ensure the client is correctly preparing each of the physical components required for them to be at peak performance levels for the match. Often for boxers, the performance phase is seen when they start a training camp in the build-up to a boxing match. The length of time required for the training camp will depend on the physical condition of the client and how much adaptation is required to reach peak performance levels.

SHORT COMPETITION PERIOD CLIENTS (E.G. ATHLETICS' 2-YEAR AND 4-YEAR CYCLES)

Sports such as athletics, triathlon and gymnastics have relatively short competitive seasons and long periods of preparation. For elite clients, these sports are generally periodised using a 2- or 4-year programme in line with the Olympic Games or world championships schedule. The idea of these programmes is to allow a client to reach their peak for the biggest competitions while still being able to compete at smaller annual competitions. Training programmes for these clients may include a long general and specific preparation phase before entering competition phases in the lead-up to the big events. It is also important to note that often there are qualification competitions for these events that clients will be required to reach peak performance for, so this must be considered within the training programme.

LONG COMPETITION PERIOD INDIVIDUALS (E.G. TEAM SPORTS)

Team sports such as football, rugby and basketball have long competition periods and clients are expected to perform at their peak for 8–10 months of the year. For example, a football season may start in August and finish in May and in addition to this, some clients may represent their countries in international competition after the completion of the domestic season. Preseason would be regarded as the general and specific preparation stage while the off-season would be used for the transition and recovery phase of the training programme.

As the competition phase is long, an undulating periodisation programme would be considered the most appropriate method to use to maintain a client's performance levels throughout the season. An undulating programme would enable practitioners to focus on different components of performance (strength, power, aerobic and anaerobic capacity) on different training days within a training microcycle. Within some team sports, clients are expected to compete multiple times within one microcycle. For example, basketball teams may play three or four matches per week for a season lasting close to 200 days. With schedules as congested as that, a practitioner's main role is to maximise client recovery, reduce fatigue and minimise injury risks, as there is very little opportunity to train and elicit performance adaptations in season.

Tapering/peaking

Tapering refers to the period of active recovery and rest immediately prior to competition to ensure a client is not impacted by residual fatigue during competition from the performance training phase. A tapering period needs to be of adequate length to minimise any fatigue without being so long that a client may start to lose performance adaptations from training. Depending on the level of the client, sport and training schedule a taper may last anywhere between a few days to 2 weeks prior to competition. Tapering does not refer to a period of no training, rather a period of training that will not cause high levels of central

MACROCYCLE PLANNING SHEET

MACROCYCLE

Main goals: Increase aerobic and anaerobic endurance. Develop upper-body strength and core stabilisation. Maintain flexibility and body composition.

Tests: VO_2max (aerobic endurance). Onset blood lactate (anaerobic endurance). 5RM (strength). TA contraction (core stability). Sit and reach (flexibility). Skinfolds (body composition).

Jan				Feb				March				April			
Week				Week				Week				Week			
1	2	3	4	1	2	3	4	1	2	3	4	1	2	3	4

MESOCYCLES

Foundation	Development	Conditioning	Performance
• Baseline testing before week 1. • Introduce core stabilisation and flexibility exercises. • Introduce cardio training (aerobic). • Assess resistance training ability and start with light weights to develop ligament strength.	• Increase volume of core stability exercises. • Increase cardio volume. • Build up volume and intensity of weights for hypertrophy. • Develop flexibility as required.	• Retest at the end of week 4. • Increase challenge of core stability exercises. • Introduce anaerobic exercises to support aerobic programme. • Increase intensity of weights and decrease volume. • Maintain flexibility.	• Progress to using stability ball as the bench and introduce plyometric upper-body exercises. • Interval training at approximate swim distance times. • Maintain flexibility.

MICROCYCLES

Wk 1	Wk 2	Wk 3	Wk 4	Wk 1	Wk 2	Wk 3	Wk 4	Wk 1	Wk 2	Wk 3	Wk 4	Wk 1	Wk 2	Wk 3	Wk 4
CS1 UB1 LB1	CS1 UB1 LB1	CS1 UB1 LB1	CS1 UB1 LB1	CS1/2 UB1/2 LB1/2	CS1/2 UB1/2 LB1/2	CS1/2 UB1/2 LB1/2	CS1/2 UB1/2 LB1/2	CS2/3 UB1/2 LB1/2	CS2/3 UB1/2 LB1/2	CS2/3 UB1/2 LB1/2	CS2/3 UB1/2 LB1/2	CS1/4 WB	CS1/4 WB	CS1/4 WB	CS1/4 WB

CS = Cardio session   UB = Upper body   LB = Lower body   WB = Whole body
NB: Flexibility sessions dependent on testing

Specificity	Adaptation	Overload	Progression	Regression	Individuality	Recovery
= ✓	= ✓	= ✓	= ✓	= ✓	= ✓	= ✓

Figure 24.6 Example macrocycle plan for an elite swimmer (for a blank template, please visit: bloomsbury.com/uk/complete-guide-to-strength-and-conditioning-training-9781399421362)

and peripheral fatigue while still maintaining a client's performance capabilities.

Peaking is closely related to tapering and refers to the process of ensuring a client reaches optimum performance levels in time for competition. In the short term, tapering supports peaking by ensuring a client is not exposed to fatigue prior to competition, so that they can perform at their peak. In the longer term, peaking refers to the ability of the training programme and practitioner to efficiently move a client through the different stages of a training plan and induce performance adaptations so that the client can perform at their highest level in competition.

Periodised programming

There are many ways to develop a periodised programme. Practitioners should adopt a method that is suitable for them but it must also be in a format that can be understood by others in the team. Programmes can be developed for individuals or for sports teams.

CLIENT PERIODISED PROGRAMME

The following example is that of an elite sprint swimmer. Details have been gathered in relation to experience and goals with a view to designing a suitable training programme.

Client details

Gender: Male
Age: 23
Weight: 79kg
Height: 186cm

The client has reasonable experience of using the gym but he has never been on an individual programme and has always trained on his own. He is very enthusiastic about dry-land training to help his swimming performance. He has a full timetable as far as swim training is concerned and only has one full rest day per week.

Client goals

He feels he needs more strength, especially in his abdominal region and upper body. He wants a fuller chest and to improve strength in his arms and chest, as he feels they are his weak points. He has never trained his legs before and isn't sure if adding muscle to them would affect his swimming. He feels fit when sprint swimming but feels that dry-land cardio work would help his sprint endurance.

To develop a training plan, a macrocycle planning sheet such as that shown in figure 24.6 can be used. First, record the overall goals for the macrocycle period (in this case, approximately 4 months). Once this has been done, develop more specific objectives for each mesocycle (typically a period of a month). Microcycles can then be planned with information relating to client training sessions. In the example, each microcycle of 1 week contains cardio and resistance training codes (i.e. CS, UB, LB and WB), which relate to client training sessions that are planned separately.

Note: The bottom row of the macrocycle planning sheet includes principles of fitness that can be ticked if they are taken into consideration when planning the programme.

Each microcycle session can then be planned and recorded. Figure 24.7 shows a typical method of showing planned sessions for resistance training and core stabilisation across the 4-month period. Repetition maximum has been used to monitor resistance intensity. As the client wishes to increase upper-body size, repetitions in the hypertrophy range have been chosen. In relation to developing overall body strength, repetitions have been programmed that are in the power range, as the resistance offered by the water does not represent repetitions in the strength range. The weight programmed for each resistance exercise would be established during an initial training session, as would cardiovascular intensity.

Figure 24.8 shows planned sessions for cardiovascular training across the 4-month period. As can be seen,

MICROCYCLE RECORD SHEET

Client name:

Mesocycle: Microcycle week:

	Exercise	Intensity (RM)	Comment
Upper body 1	Bent over row	3 Sets (14, 14, 12)	Keep a neutral spine and tension in the TA.
	DB chest press – bench	3 Sets (14, 14, 12)	Limit descent so the upper arm is parallel with the floor.
	DB shoulder press	3 Sets (14, 14, 12)	DB no lower than shoulder level.
	Triceps over head (double)	3 Sets (12, 10, 10)	Keep the forearm in the swimming position.
	DB bicep curl (single)	3 Sets (14, 14, 12)	Avoid a twisting motion.
	Shoulder internal/external rotation	3 Sets (16, 16, 14)	Maintain a neutral spine.
Upper body 2	Cable cross fly standing	3 Sets (14, 14, 12)	Alternate between split and square stance.
	Single-arm cable pull through	3 Sets (14, 14, 12)	Mimic a swim motion.
	Seated row	3 Sets (14, 14, 12)	Use horizontal handles and keep elbows high.
	Shoulder shrug	3 Sets (14, 14, 12)	No rotation.
Upper body 3	Plyometric push-up	3 Sets (14, 14, 12)	Stop if form is lost.
	Plyometric standing med ball chest throw	3 Sets (14, 14, 12)	Keep a neutral spine throughout.
	Supine med ball overhead throw	3 Sets (14, 14, 12)	Keep a bend in the knees.
Legs 1	Alternating: Squat	5 Sets (12, 10, 10, 12, 12)	Full ROM. Contract the TA.
	Bounding	5 Sets (40m)	Quick land-to-take-off phase.
	Alternating: Split squat	5 Sets (12, 10, 10, 12, 12)	Set on one leg then set on the other.
	Box jump	5 Sets (6)	

Figure 24.7 Microcycle record sheet for resistance and core stabilisation (for a blank template, please visit: bloomsbury.com/uk/complete-guide-to-strength-and-conditioning-training-9781399421362)

Legs 2	Alternating: Single leg DB squat	5 Sets (12, 10, 10, 12, 12)	Use a low bench but maintain posture.
	Hopping	5 Sets (30m)	Quick land-to-take-off phase.
	Alternating: Dead lift	5 Sets (12, 10, 10, 12, 12)	Contract the TA and keep a neutral spine.
	Lunge drop	5 Sets (6 each leg)	Maintain posture at all times.
Whole body	Power clean	3 Sets (12, 12, 10)	Stop if form is lost.
	Split clean	3 Sets (12, 12, 10)	Stop if form is lost.
	Wood chopper	3 Sets (12, 12, 10)	Stop if form is lost.
	Med ball scoop	3 Sets (12, 10, 8)	Lie face down on the bench. Scoop the ball in a swim action.
Core 1	Supine foot slide Supine knee roll Superman	All stability exercises to be done to fatigue or loss of form.	There are many sources for core stabilisation exercises.
Core 2	Foot bridge roll Front bridge roll		
Core 3	Shoulder med ball drop Kneeling med ball throw		
Core 4	Single-arm row (ball as bench) Cable cross fly – Swiss ball Swiss ball hip crunch Swiss ball hamstring curl		

Figure 24.7 Microcycle record sheet for resistance and core stabilisation (cont.)

the cardio intensity starts at a lower level than the client is used to and progresses to levels that the client will experience in swimming training. The programme has been designed this way because the dry-land training will increase the amount of training volume, therefore progression should be incorporated.

Note: An alternative training programme template can be found in Appendix 2.

MICROCYCLE RECORD SHEET

Client name:

Mesocycle: Microcycle week:

	Exercise	Intensity (RPE 1–10)	Comment
Cardio 1	Warm-up: 3–5 min cycle/rower	3–6	The length of the main session depends on the ability of the client. Monitor this closely.
	Main: 20–30 min treadmill	6–8	
	Cool-down: 3–5 min cycle	8–3	
Cardio 2	Warm-up: 3–5 min cycle/rower	3–6	Increase the duration of the main session by about 15–20%.
	Main: 25–35 min treadmill	6–8	
	Cool-down: 3–5 min cycle	8–3	
Cardio 3	Warm-up: 3–5 min cycle/rower	3–6	Introduce periods of higher intensity. This is designed to take the client just into the anaerobic zone. Do not go to max at this stage.
	Main: 5–10 min 10–12 min 12–20 min 20–22 min 22–35 min	6–8 8–9 9–6–8 8–9 9–6–8	
	Cool-down: 5–10 min	8–3	
Cardio 4	Warm-up: 5–10 min	3–6	Number of high-intensity intervals depends on the ability of the client. After each interval, reduce intensity quickly then slowly build up in the next 4-minute period.
	Main: 5–10 min 10–11 min 11–15 min 15–16 min 16–20 min 21–22 min	6–8 8–10 10–7 7–10 10–7 7–10	
	Cool-down: 5–10 min	10–3	

Figure 24.8 Microcycle record sheet for cardio training (for a blank template, please visit: bloomsbury.com/uk/complete-guide-to-strength-and-conditioning-training-9781399421362)

TEAM PERIODISED PROGRAMME

The following is an example of what to consider for a team (in this case football) when developing a periodised programme across a full year in relation to the macrocyle, mesocycle and microcycle.

Macrocycle

Football is a sport with a relatively short preparation phase of several weeks (pre-season) followed by a long period of regular competition within a maintenance phase (season) and finally another relatively short off-season of a few weeks. All of these phases fall within one macrocycle, which takes place over 12 months.

Mesocycle

A typical mesocycle in football is made up of three distinct periods (not the same time period) across a full season.

Pre-season

Typically, in the European football schedule, pre-season will take place across 8–10 weeks during July and August. The main aim of pre-season is to prepare football players technically, tactically, physically and psychologically for the impending competitive season. This is done using testing batteries, a structured training programme to prepare players for the demands of competitive football and to make them robust with an aim to minimise injury risks.

In-season

The in-season programme will generally run from late August through to the end of May/early June, depending on competition progression and season schedules. This is a maintenance phase when the aim is to help players to compete as close to their peak level of performance as possible throughout the season. This incorporates different types of performance- and recovery-focused training sessions within a periodisation model that prepares players for each match. Further details about in-season training schedules are outlined in the microcycle section.

Off-season

The off-season signifies the end of the competitive season and is an opportunity for players to take time off and recover before pre-season starts. This normally takes place from the end of May until the beginning of July. Players should continue with some training that will ensure they do not return to pre-season training completely unconditioned. The off-season can also be an opportunity for players to focus on developing specific physical attributes that they may require within their sport and wouldn't be able to focus on within the season. For example, if a player is required to increase upper-body muscle mass to compete more in duels, then the off-season can be used to perform a hypertrophy programme that can develop these attributes.

Microcycle

In football, a typical microcycle will last one week, where a match would conclude the end of the microcycle. Typical training microcycles for a professional football team that includes one match and another that includes two matches are outlined below:

One-game microcycle

A one-game microcycle typically concludes with a match and the training week will be designed to optimise performance for the match. Following a game, match day +1 (MD+1) and MD+2 are focused on recovery for the players who started the match and top-up training for substitutes and players who didn't play, to maintain their fitness.

On MD-4 the focus is on intensive training, which refers to the use of small-sided games and training in small areas, which overloads the number of accelerations, decelerations and changes of direction compared to a match. These types of physical actions are associated with greater loads on the quadricep and adductor muscle groups. MD-4 training days also have a strength focus for S&C sessions, as they allow adequate time to recover from fatigue and DOMS before the next match.

Within English football, MD-3 is commonly a day off from training.

MD-2 has an extensive theme that incorporates training drills and games played in larger areas with a focus on exposure to higher running speeds. These training days are associated with greater loads on the hamstring and calf muscle groups. On MD-2, players should be exposed to two bouts of maximal speed exposure to minimise injury risks and condition them to maximal speed activities.

Finally, training on MD-1 is designed to minimise total running volumes and intensities but expose the players to low volumes of explosive and reactive activities to prepare them for the upcoming match without inducing neuromuscular fatigue that may impact match performance. An example of the physical and technical outputs within a one-game training microcycle is shown in figure 24.9.

Two-game microcycle

A two-game microcycle contains two matches that are typically separated by 3–4 days. For players who play both matches, it is important to utilise training days to maximise recovery while preparing the players tactically for the next match.

Following both games, as with the one-game microcycle, MD+1 and MD+2 are focused on recovery for the players who started the match and top-up training for substitutes and players who didn't play, to maintain their fitness. For the starting players, the matches are considered as their exposure to both the intensive and extensive training day qualities mentioned previously. However, for substitutes, they will need to be exposed

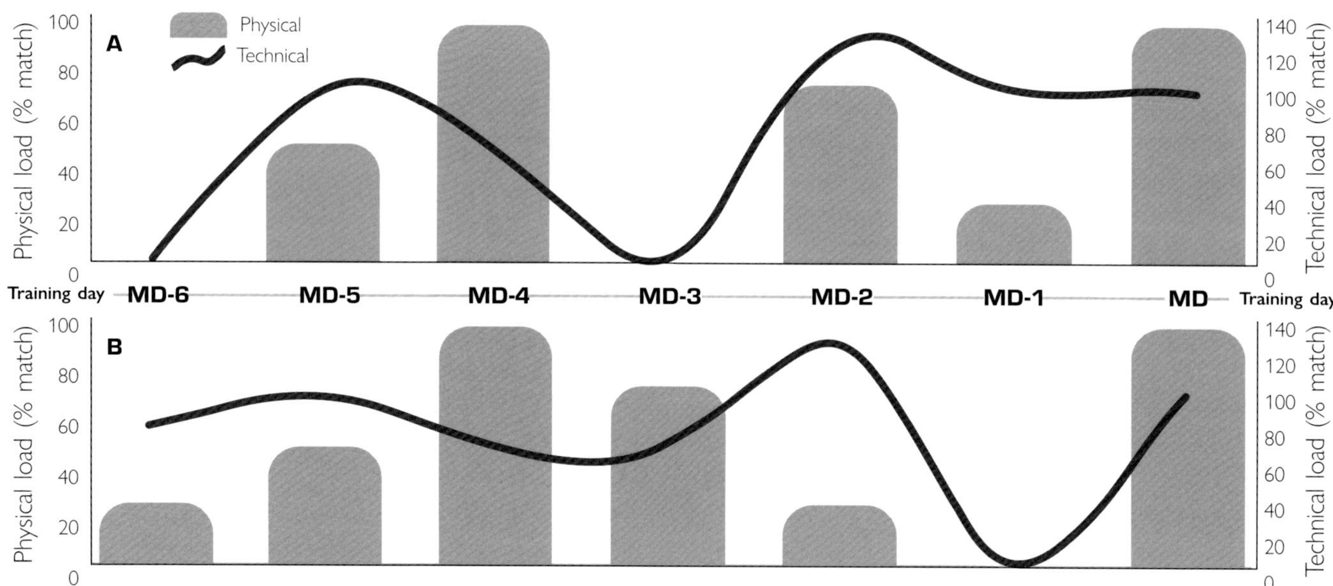

Figure 24.9 An example of different one-game training microcycles for a professional football team for both a physical and technical output compared to match demands. 'A' is a training week with rest and recovery days on MD-6 and MD-3. 'B' is a training week with a rest and recovery day on MD-1.

to these physical outputs within the training sessions or immediately after matches. MD-1 also has similar training themes as the one-game microcycle and will have a high tactical input to optimise preparation for the next match.

S&C microdosing

Often, because of the physical demands of competitive matches and congested fixture schedules, it can be difficult to deliver S&C training sessions for players without causing excessive DOMS that may affect performance. Therefore, microdosing is often used where players may perform small numbers of sets and reps of specific strength-based lower-body exercises immediately after training. For example, an extensive day will overload high-speed running outputs, which in turn will stress the hamstring and calf tissues more than the quadriceps and adductors. This is an opportunity to prescribe players with the Nordic hamstring exercise (e.g. 3 sets of 3 reps) or split-stance Romanian deadlifts (e.g. 3 sets of 5 reps per side) as an eccentric hamstring stimulus to increase the robustness of the hamstrings.

Likewise for intensive training days that overload accelerations, decelerations and changes of direction, which in turn stress the quadriceps and adductors, it may be beneficial to microdose the players with Copenhagen adduction exercises (2 × 20 seconds per side) and Bulgarian split squats (3 sets of 6 reps per side) to improve the robustness to injury of those muscle groups. This ensures players are still getting a stimulus and exposure to S&C training while minimising fatigue that may impact performance levels.

Factors affecting planning (individual)

There are many factors that the practitioner should consider when designing a training programme. Some of these are related to the client, as outlined below:

INJURY RISKS/HISTORY

A client's injury history will influence the planning and contents of a training programme. For example, if a client has a recurring soft tissue injury, then a programme needs to include a focus on developing and maintaining the mobility, strength, power and robustness to re-injury of the specific muscle group. It is important to take a full injury history from a client during the consultation stage (*see* part 1) before designing a training programme, to ensure steps can be taken to reduce any risks of re-injury.

Likewise, if a sport increases the risk of specific injury types, then the programme needs to pre-empt that and include training sessions/exercises to reduce the risks of those specific injuries. For example, hamstring strain injuries are more common in sprinters, as the demands of a maximal sprint require the hamstring muscle group to maximally contract to propel a client forwards. Therefore, a training programme needs to reflect this by including appropriate exercises that focus on developing eccentric hamstring strength at different lever lengths.

CLIENT TYPE – E.G. FULL TIME/PART TIME, AMATEUR/PROFESSIONAL

A professional client will often have multiple stakeholders involved in their programme design and training. It is important that all relevant parties (technical coaches, performance coaches, medical staff) are involved in creating the training programme so that everyone is in agreement on its contents before beginning. Furthermore, it is important that this process is transparent, and the client also has an input into the planning and periodisation of their programme so that they understand the requirements and aims of the programme before it begins.

An important factor to consider with part-time and amateur clients is the impact their daily lives will have on their ability to train and their fatigue levels. It is likely a part-time client will have an occupation, which, depending on the activity levels required, may impact their ability to train. For example, someone working in construction may have already spent a full day on their feet moving heavy building materials. These considerations need to be made when creating their programme – for example, is it possible to programme fatiguing training sessions on a client's day off work or do they have availability to train before work?

Factors affecting planning (logistical)

There are also logistical factors that should be considered when designing training programmes.

FACILITY/EQUIPMENT AVAILABILITY

It's important to consider and integrate into a training programme the availability of training facilities and equipment. This is rarely a problem for professional clients who have access to sport-specific training facilities, but for part-time and amateur clients, the contents of the programme must utilise the facilities and equipment available.

CLIENT AVAILABILITY

As mentioned above, programme design needs to take into consideration the availability of a client to train. This is particularly relevant for part-time and amateur clients, who will have other commitments that the training programme must work in tandem with. Planning a high-volume or high-intensity training session for a client who has just completed a full working day in an active job may not be beneficial for them, as it may compound fatigue levels and even increase injury risks.

Training programmes also need to be adaptable, since a client's training availability may change at short notice. For example, in a situation where someone was competing the previous day and only returned very late, it may be more beneficial for the client to sleep longer and for the planned recovery session to be moved to later in the day or cancelled for that specific microcycle.

Take-home messages

- The practitioner needs to manage delivery of training to minimise risk of injury by using an appropriate warm-up structure that will best capitalise on potential benefits.

- Be aware of best practice guidelines and evidence relating to session management variables such as activity/exercise selection and order, movement tempo, intensity, volume, work distribution/division and recovery periods.

- The practitioner needs to know the potential benefits of session-end cool-down activities and prescription to best capitalise on potential benefits.

- It is important to plan a structured and sequential strength and conditioning programme to support progression of performance.

- The practitioner should understand the implications of the performance calendar on the planning of training and the implications of the client's training and injury history on the planning of training.

- Strategies to monitor and evaluate training load retrospectively based on outcomes are important for success.

Fatigue and recovery strategies

The areas covered in this chapter are:

- Suggested theory related to the effects of overreaching and overtraining
- Typical tests for overtraining that are accessible for the S&C practitioner
- Suggested theory related to the effects of undertraining
- How and when training programmes may need to be modified, including to minimise injury risk
- The types of fatigue and the range of recovery strategies typically employed by practitioners
- What is meant by recovery and various strategies that can be used to improve it, including the three pillars of recovery
- The impact of alcohol on recovery

Introduction

To allow individuals or teams to adapt and develop from the training stimuli they are subjected to, they must have an opportunity to adequately recover and mitigate training-induced fatigue. Clients will not develop as effectively if they are consistently under-recovered. Therefore, S&C practitioners need to include ample opportunity for recovery within their periodisation models as well as instructing the individuals or teams they are training on the most appropriate recovery strategies that will aid this process.

Both overtraining and undertraining can be detrimental to performance, so it is essential that the prac-titioner understands the terms. Both are explored in detail below.

Overtraining and overreaching

In general, overtraining relates to physiological and/or psychological problems brought about by high levels of training usually over a long period. Overtraining syndrome (OTS) is thought to be a condition that can negatively affect the sympathetic and parasympathetic nervous systems.

The term overtraining is often used interchangeably with overreaching. Overreaching can be thought of as excessive amounts of training that if carried out regularly can lead to overtraining. Even though it is not the role of the practitioner to diagnose it, there are potential signs that are indicative of overtraining. Problems with overtraining tend to be grouped into three areas:

1. Movement or coordination problems
2. Physiological problems
3. Psychological problems

Table 25.1	TYPICAL SIGNS OF OVERTRAINING
Problem area	**Description**
Movement or coordination	• More frequent (than usual) coordination problems. • Loses concentration more often than usual. • More difficulty trying to correct technique or skills.
Physiological	• Decrease in cardio endurance. • Decrease in strength performance. • Decrease in speed performance. • Poor sleep quality. • Unusual muscle soreness post exercise.
Psychological	• Sudden dislike for competition. • Suddenly starts using different tactics to normal. • Has a negative attitude and starts giving up easily. • Behaviour becomes difficult and sometimes obstructive. • Becomes anxious and depressed. • Appears to lack any sort of motivation. • Starts becoming introverted.

Research agrees that the causes of overtraining are complex. Nevertheless, the practitioner should have an awareness of potential causes, which include those in table 25.2.

TESTING

There is no one test that can confirm OTS. Differential forms of diagnosis are often used, to rule out other conditions. Methods might include hormonal, blood, urine, pulmonary and immune system testing. A more common method, known as ergometry, measures decreases in workload, maximum heart rate and maximal blood lactate concentration to identify possible overtraining.

Questionnaires can also be used as a measure of overtraining. An example is the Profile of Mood States (POMS) questionnaire, which was originally developed in 1971 by McNair as an assessment method for people

Table 25.2	POSSIBLE FACTORS RELATED TO OVERTRAINING
Factor	**Reason**
Recovery	Insufficient time for recovery.
Frequency	Too many sessions per week, which affects recovery between sessions.
Intensity	Training intensity is increased too quickly or by increments that are too great.
Duration	Training sessions last too long, affecting energy stores for the next session.
Volume	Volume is increased by large increments.
Competition	Too many competitions may increase psychological and physiological stress.

undergoing counselling or psychotherapy but was then developed for use with people who participated in sport or exercise. As the POMS was a relatively long questionnaire (with 65 questions), a shorter questionnaire was subsequently developed. Clients are recommended to use the questionnaire on a daily basis by rating each statement on a scale of 1 to 5, as shown in figure 25.1, so that they keep a daily overall score.

If the score is 20 or above, then it is recommended that training can continue. If the score is below 20 then rest or an easy workout is recommended until the score rises above 20. When correctly used, the POMS questionnaire has been shown to be effective in providing an early indication of overtraining.

Undertraining

Undertraining can be described as a training load that will not adequately prepare a client for the physical, technical, tactical or psychological demands of competition within their sport. There are a number of ways in which undertraining may occur, includ-

SF-POMS questionnaire	
Please read the statements below and give a score of 1–5	
Statement	**Score**
I slept well last night	
I am looking forward to today's workout	
I am optimistic about future performance	
I feel vigorous and energetic	
I have little muscle soreness	
My appetite is great	
	Total =
Client name:	Date:
Mesocycle:	Microcycle week:
Yesterday's training intensity:	
Previous score:	Decision:

Figure 25.1 Short POMS questionnaire

ing an inadequate training volume or intensity, low training frequency or lack of compliance to a training programme. An avoidance of undertraining comes from an understanding of the demands of the sport and ensuring these demands are reflected in the training programme.

Modification of training programmes

It is quite common that a training programme will require modification. There may be a wide range of reasons why modification is required, including over- or undertraining as well as other factors such as client injury, illness or fatigue. Therefore, the ability to modify training programmes and tailor them to the needs of the client is a vital skill set to have as an S&C practitioner.

Modifications may take place on an acute (short-term) or chronic (long-term) basis depending on the reasons that modifications are required. There are different ways in which a training programme can be modified, some of which are outlined in table 25.3.

Note: Remember, training modifications can work to both increase and reduce the training load depending on how the client is responding to the original training programme. Clients will respond differently to the same training stimulus, so a one-size-fits-all approach to training programming will have different effects on different clients.

INJURY PREVENTION

Over- and undertraining can increase injury risk, which is why measures to prevent injury need to be considered when training programmes are created. As a reminder:

Table 25.3	ACUTE AND CHRONIC MODIFICATION OF TRAINING PROGRAMMES	
Factor	**Acute**	**Chronic**
Recovery	Increase recovery time between sets/exercises.	Increase the number of recovery days between training sessions.
Frequency	Reduce/increase the number of sets or exercises in a training session.	Reduce/increase the number of training sessions.
Intensity	The mass lifted or the number of repetitions of an exercise can be reduced/increased.	The intensity across a training week or month may be reduced/increased.
Duration	Training sessions' length may be modified.	The weekly or monthly workload can be modified.
Volume	The volume/training load can be modified within a training session.	The number of training sessions can be modified.
Competition	The expectations at competition can be managed (e.g. a fatigued client may be used as a substitute rather than starting a match).	The number of competitions a client is exposed to may be modified (e.g. a fatigued client may be removed from some competitions so that they can focus on the key ones within a season).

a training programme's key aim is to adequately prepare a client for the physical, technical, tactical and psychological demands of their sport/activity as well as developing robustness to and minimising injury risks. So, what are the risks posed by over- and undertraining? Let's take a look:

- **Overtraining injury risks** – Overtraining can have negative physiological, psychological and movement/coordination impacts on clients, which collectively can increase injury risks. Injuries such as repetitive strains, strains, tendonitis and cartilage tears can occur.
- **Undertraining injury risks** – Undertraining will not adequately prepare a client to cope with the demands of competition within their sport and will therefore increase their risk of injury.

ILLNESS

The general recommendation is that people *do not* train when they are ill. Depending on the nature of the illness it is prudent to consult a medical professional before undertaking any exercise.

FATIGUE

In a sports environment the term fatigue is associated with failure to maintain the force or intensity required to perform a particular task. Fatigue is a complex phenomenon that can occur as a result of training and in combination with appropriate recovery can result in physiological and cognitive function adaptation. It is thought that fatigue can occur in both a central and peripheral manner, but it must be stressed that there is currently no single conclusive marker of fatigue. Explanations of central fatigue and peripheral fatigue are provided below:

- **Central fatigue** – Also known as central nervous system (CNS) fatigue, central fatigue is induced by changes in the presence of different hormones that have an inhibitory effect on the firing of signals through the spinal cord nerves and therefore reduced neural activity at the muscular level. This type of fatigue can often be experienced by distance runners.
- **Peripheral fatigue** – This is also known as neuromuscular fatigue and refers to the decreased contractile strength of muscle fibres that has been induced by training or competition. Factors such as oxygen availability, presence of ions, energy (glycogen) availability and the presence of metabolites can impact peripheral fatigue. This type of fatigue is experienced in shorter-duration events of high intensity, such as sprint events.

What is recovery and why is it necessary?

Recovery in sport is an umbrella term for the reduction of exercise-induced fatigue and return to optimum performance outputs, while an adaptation process takes place following the demands of training/competition a client is exposed to. Two of the main factors that recovery is needed for are replenishing energy stores and muscle repair, which are explored below:

REPLENISHING ENERGY STORES

Exercise depletes glycogen stores within the muscle. Glycogen is broken down into glucose to provide the muscle with energy in a process called glycogenolysis and so it is important to replenish glycogen stores within muscles post exercise; carbohydrates are required to replace the depleted intracellular energy stores within the muscles. Exercise also induces protein breakdown within the muscles, so it is important to also replenish protein stores post exercise. It is advised to eat protein-rich food sources almost immediately after exercise completion and then at regular intervals of 3–4 hours to provide the body with adequate levels of *amino acids* for protein synthesis and muscle repair.

MUSCLE REPAIR

Intense exercise induces muscle damage, which is why muscle soreness is often experienced 24–72 hours post exercise. This is known as delayed onset muscle soreness. Intense exercise will cause microtears in muscles, which in turn elicits an inflammatory response as the body aims to heal any muscle destruction. The inflammatory response delivers proteins and satellite cells to the affected muscles so that the muscle repair process may begin.

There are a wide range of recovery strategies that are designed to optimise post-exercise recovery and return clients to pre-exercise performance levels without muscle soreness or fatigue. However, many of these strategies currently have conflicting evidence regarding their benefits or offer few benefits to a client when they are administered.

Recovery strategies

The three pillars of recovery refer to sleep, nutrition and hydration. These three processes are widely regarded as having the greatest impact on recovery rates and practitioners and clients should aim to optimise these in order to maximise recovery before considering other less impactful recovery strategies. Other recovery strategies (water therapies, compression, flexibility/mobility, foam rolling etc.) may also aid recovery but their benefits will not be able to counteract poor attention to the three pillars. They are more the stud walls to a house's foundations: they offer some support, but the house will collapse without the foundations in place. Figure 25.2 shows a representation of the importance of different recovery strategies and the impact they can have.

SLEEP

Sleep is a key contributor to sport performance and development. Tissue repair, growth and the embedding of skill acquisition into long-term memory occur at greater rates during sleep. It is recommended that clients get at least 8 hours of sleep to account for the additional tissue repair and recovery they will require. An internal clock called the circadian rhythm controls biochemical processes to induce sleep and waking. The key hormone that induces sleep is melatonin. The disruption of the circadian rhythm and the release of melatonin can impact sleep quality, as can these factors:

- Blue light (most commonly emitted by electronic devices) inhibits melatonin release, as it can be perceived as daylight.
- Room temperature should be between 16°C and 18°C (61°F and 65°F) to allow for the reduction of internal biomechanical systems, which helps induce sleep.
- Caffeine is a stimulant that increases the activity of the nervous system. Caffeine consumption should stop 6–8 hours before sleep.
- *Adrenaline* can inhibit sleep, which is why it can be difficult to sleep after sporting events that occur in the evening. Calming activities around bedtime can help to reduce these effects.

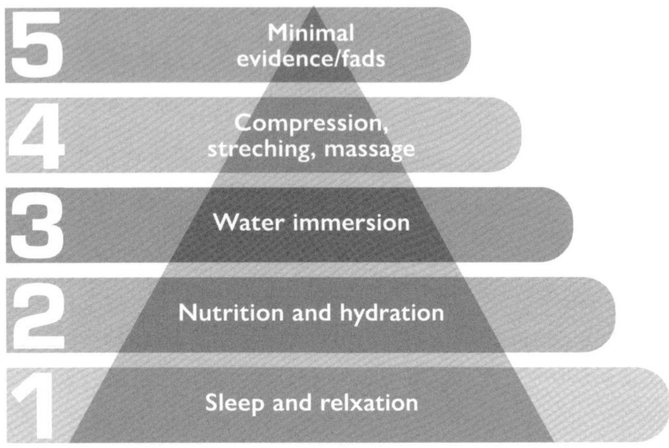

Figure 25.2 The recovery pyramid (adapted from Halson, S., 2021)

NUTRITION

As previously mentioned, exercise depletes intramuscular glycogen energy stores, induces protein breakdown and depletes fat stores. Therefore, it is vital that post-exercise nutrition is optimised to replenish macronutrients to provide the required materials for recovery. Further in-depth information on the importance of nutrition for performance and recovery can be found in chapter 29.

HYDRATION

Clients should aim to begin exercising in a state of *euhydration* (being in a state of water balance, e.g. not dehydrated or hyperhydrated). A 2% bodyweight loss in water can result in reduced aerobic capacity and muscular power production by 10–30%. A simple way to measure water loss is to weigh yourself before and immediately after exercise. The weight lost will roughly equate to the volume of fluids needed to help rehydration. Water is more readily absorbed by the body in the presence of salts and sugars, so electrolyte drinks can help to improve the rate of water uptake and rehydration.

ACTIVE RECOVERY

Active recovery refers to the action of performing a low-intensity workout after a competition or intense workout. Examples of this may include a slow-paced short run, swimming, cycling or walking. Low-intensity exercise will promote greater blood flow to the muscle groups that are likely fatigued and may have some soreness (caused by previously performed intense exercise) without causing further muscle damage. Improved blood flow to these muscle groups will bring oxygen, protein and satellite cells to the area while removing lactic acid from the muscles and transporting it to the liver so gluconeogenesis can occur to create glucose and replenish energy stores.

COLD-WATER IMMERSION (ICE BATHS, CONTRAST-WATER THERAPY, CRYOTHERAPY ETC.)

There are still some conflicting views and evidence surrounding the potential benefits of cold-water immersion (CWI), contrast-water therapy (switching between hot and cold baths) and cryotherapy. Applying ice/cold compresses globally (e.g. a whole-body ice bath) or locally (e.g. an ice pack applied to an affected area) causes vasoconstriction, which reduces blood flow to the extremities (arms and legs) and returns blood flow to the organs. This may offer some temporary relief from muscle soreness, as it will effectively inhibit the normal inflammatory response to the fatigued/damaged muscles. However, by doing this it may in fact inhibit overall recovery because the inflammatory response is required for muscle repair and recovery. This is because the inflammatory response delivers key proteins and satellite cells that aid recovery and promote muscle repair so by inhibiting this process, the recovery process may be slowed.

However, some clients may still find benefits in CWI or cold compress therapy. The acute (short-term) reduction in muscle soreness may be useful in competition. For example, a rugby player may find it beneficial to use an ice pack on a sore muscle at half time so that they can continue to play in the second half with reduced levels of pain. There may also be a placebo effect of using ice for recovery/pain reduction, which may be beneficial for clients in the short term too.

Contrast-water therapy (CWT) is a recovery technique that uses CWI in conjunction with warm-water immersion. A client may subject themselves to CWI for a predetermined time frame (normally >10 minutes) followed by immediate transfer to warm-water immersion for a similar time frame. Warm-water therapy acts as an antagonist to CWI. It causes vasodilation and an influx of blood flow to the extremities. In turn this increases the delivery of proteins and satellite cells to the muscle to promote repair.

It has been found that CWT improves the rate of recovery compared to passive recovery/rest after exercise but there is conflicting evidence on its effectiveness compared to other recovery strategies (compression, foam rolling, flexibility/mobility etc.).

Whole-body cryotherapy is a high-cost, specialised recovery solution that exposes athletes to temperatures of -110°C to -190°C (-166°F to -310°F) for short periods (2–3 minutes). This recovery strategy may reduce muscle soreness and inflammation post exercise. However, current evidence does not provide conclusive results regarding its effects.

COMPRESSION CLOTHING

Compression clothing comes in different forms, including calf sleeves, arm sleeves and leggings. As a recovery tool, their mode of operation is to compress a localised area of the body with an aim to increase *venous return* of the blood in order to reduce swelling and improve removal of waste products and delivery of oxygen and nutrients to the compressed area. While no negative effects of using compression garments have been reported, it is important to understand that to date, the majority of research investigating the potential benefits of using compression garments is of low quality, with underlying bias. Therefore, it is not yet possible to comprehensively confirm the reported benefits for use in recovery protocols.

FLEXIBILITY/MOBILITY

Flexibility and mobility are closely linked but are two different entities. Flexibility is a passive activity that involves stretching soft tissues (muscles, tendons, ligaments) whereas mobility is the ability of a joint, using its attached muscle systems, to actively move through its complete range of motion. Flexibility can involve using hands/equipment (e.g. a resistance band) to aid with the passive stretching of soft tissue whereas mobility is an active process that is done without assistance.

For example, a gymnast who can do the front splits would be described as flexible whereas a martial artist who can strike a target with a kick that is above their head height would be described as mobile, as the limb is actively moving to strike the target.

Stretching can be described as the process of applying force to musculotendinous structures to change their length with an aim of improving flexibility (joint range of motion). There are different types of stretching outlined in chapter 12 but the most commonly prescribed type to perform post exercise is static stretching.

Static stretching post exercise acts to reduce muscle soreness, increase muscle range of motion and modify blood flow to the stretched muscle. Studies have shown that static stretching improves range of motion compared to passive recovery. In addition, it has been reported that the use of pre- and post-exercise static stretching can reduce muscle soreness between 0.5% and 4%, which is minimal but within elite sport, a 1% advantage that will boost performance is often enough for success. Therefore, while the reduction may be small, it can be significant in terms of recovery. While there is limited research on this topic, it is thought that daily static stretching may increase parasympathetic nervous system activity (responsible for relaxation) and improve heart rate variability, so it may have wider health benefits other than those associated with sport performance.

FOAM ROLLING

Foam rolling is a recovery strategy that involves massaging muscle groups repeatedly with a foam roller device. As with other recovery strategies, foam rolling is thought to reduce muscle soreness, increase range of motion and improve neuromuscular performance. This recovery strategy has been shown to improve muscle group range of motion. Greater ranges have also been observed when foam rolling was combined with static stretching. Reviews have been

performed to assess the claimed benefits of foam rolling. For example, it was found that pre-training foam rolling was more beneficial for performance compared to post-training foam rolling. However, performance improvements for both strategies were negligible. Post-training foam rolling also reduced muscle soreness perception by ~6%.

Regarding the dosage required for foam rolling to be effective, foam rolling a muscle group for 90–120 seconds seems to be optimal to improve range of motion. Other methods for self-massage are also becoming more commonly used, such as massage guns and textured massage balls.

Things to avoid

As outlined above, the three pillars of recovery are widely considered the most important factors for reducing recovery times, so should be the focus for any client or practitioner to optimise before exploring other recovery strategies. It may be of benefit to work on a case-by-case basis to identify which recovery strategies are preferred. For example, a client may find CWI uncomfortable and prefer to use other recovery strategies while another client may prefer CWI as their mode of recovery strategy. Regardless of the strategies employed, there are several factors to consider that could negatively affect recovery rates, such as alcohol consumption and overtraining (*see* p. 167).

ALCOHOL

Drinking alcohol can negatively affect the rate and quality of recovery from exercise. For this reason, a complete avoidance of alcohol is recommended to ensure it does not cause inhibitions of performance or recovery. Mechanisms of impact include the following:

- The presence of alcohol inhibits calcium ion (Ca^{2+}) availability, which is required for muscle contrac-

tion. Therefore, alcohol can reduce the contractile strength of skeletal muscle.

- Alcohol is both a diuretic (promotes removal of fluids as urine) and a vasodilator (increases the surface area of the blood vessels to allow more fluid to be lost through the skin surface as perspiration), which collectively will result in greater loss of fluids and dehydration.

- Alcohol impairs metabolic pathways including protein synthesis, muscle uptake and storage of glycogen, and reduces gluconeogenesis.

- Sleep quality is disrupted in the presence of alcohol because it reduces the time spent in REM sleep phases and increases the time spent in lighter sleep stages. Skill acquisition, embedding memories and protein synthesis are all prevalent during deeper stages of sleep, so these will all be impaired by alcohol.

- As a depressant, alcohol inhibits the excitability of the central nervous system. This can impact balance, reaction time and fine motor skills.

Take-home messages

- The interaction between training activity, intensity, volume and the need for recovery are essential considerations in planning.

- The mechanisms of fatigue and implications for delivery of training stress and demand for recovery should be considered as important factors.

- Evidence and accepted best practice regarding strategies and interventions to optimise recovery and adaptation following training should be adopted.

//Practitioner skills 26

Introduction

A vital aspect of being an S&C practitioner is understanding the scientific theory and application that underpin the industry. However, it is equally as important to possess so-called soft skills that allow S&C practitioners to communicate effectively, present feedback and empathise with individuals and teams within the training and testing process. This chapter will outline these key areas and provide in-depth detail of how they can be developed in order to enhance the reader's effectiveness as an S&C practitioner.

Practitioner skills

There are many skills that a practitioner can develop that will help improve all aspects associated with the role, and research suggests that these can be crucial to coaching success. Skills such as communication, obser-

vation, listening and giving feedback are examples of areas in which the practitioner should aim to improve. Below, we look at each in turn.

COMMUNICATION

There are several different methods of communicating with clients, including verbal, paraverbal and non-verbal. These should not be viewed as discreet components but as methods that should be used in combination where appropriate.

Verbal communication

Practitioners should try and keep verbal information to a minimum, to avoid information overload. The ability to process verbal information can be limited, as demonstrated in the following task:

Table 26.1	**VERBAL COMMUNICATION TEST**
TASK	
You will need pens and paper enough for a small group of people.	
What to do	Read out a seven-digit number, get the group to wait for 5 seconds, then ask them to write down the number. Do this again but use an eight-digit number and ask them to write it down after 5 seconds. Most will recall the seven-digit number but not the eight-digit number.
Why does it happen?	This is a phenomenon called 'chunking'. Very simply, if the brain thinks it will be overloaded it will tend only to remember the first and last bits of a piece of information.

Paraverbal communication

This is related to the use of words and the structure of sentences. Placing stress on different words in a sentence can change the meaning of the sentence. Varying such things as the tone, pitch, delivery speed and volume can help to reinforce or convey emotions. For example, when leading a group training session, the practitioner will need a steady, firm tone, which displays confidence and authority, but may need to switch to an energetic pacing strategy to create a dynamic atmosphere followed by a more relaxed pace to encourage calmer approaches.

Non-verbal communication

This refers to the transfer of information without speaking and is also known as body language. Early research by Albert Mehrabian published in 1971 suggested that communication is 7% verbal, 38% para-verbal and 55% non-verbal. Even though this model has been challenged and adapted over the years, it is thought that over 70% of communication is achieved through non-verbal means. There are subcategories of non-verbal communication, as shown in table 26.2.

OBSERVATION

In relation to observation skills there are three main areas that the practitioner could focus on:

Table 26.2	**CATEGORIES OF NON-VERBAL COMMUNICATION**
Subcategory	**Strategies**
Role model	The way you look and dress can influence clients. Performing demonstrations with good technique can also inspire clients to improve their performance.
Body position	The way you position yourself with clients is important. Don't get too close (in their personal space), as it could be intimidating. Also, do not turn your back, as this is often construed as having been given the cold shoulder.
Body movements	Simple gestures with the eyes, hands, head, etc. can be very effective. For example, a tilt of the head to the side with furrowed eyebrows can easily say, *Why did you do that?*
Voice	You may have heard the saying, 'It's not what you say but how you say it.' People easily pick up on how we say things, so avoid sarcasm. You also need to speak with enough volume to be heard, and slowly but not too slowly. Try to articulate so there is no confusion with translation.

1. **Safety** – The most important aim of any training session is to maintain the safety of the client. There are many potential hazards and dangers in an exercise environment, and it is crucial that the practitioner always remains attentive. It helps to be positioned so that all performers are in view in group scenarios and if possible, to see the faces to monitor for signs of any undue distress in order that the exercise can be stopped as soon as possible if necessary.

2. **Performance** – During any training session the practitioner needs to observe client performance at all times to ensure good technique. It may be necessary to move around to view the client from different angles to see how different body segments are positioned either statically or in motion.

3. **Reinforcement** – When observing client performance, it may be necessary to reinforce good technique. This can be done either by performing demonstrations or using the mirroring technique, where the practitioner performs the exercise so that the client can mirror the action.

LISTENING

There is a difference between hearing and listening. For example, if you meet someone for the first time and within a few minutes forget their name, you'll likely have heard them say it but not really listened. This can occur because people often place more importance on what they have to say rather than on what others have to say. There are two types of listening, passive and active:

1. **Passive listening** – This can be described as listening without any response, which is appropriate in some situations, such as watching a film or listening to music.

2. **Active listening** – This requires a response to show understanding. For example, in the following scenario there is a typical question with a response that demonstrates understanding:

Scenario: 'Do you think I will have a good session today?'

This may seem like a straightforward question, but it could suggest a need for reinforcement and encouragement due to low confidence. A response that demonstrates understanding could be, 'As long as you try your best then I will be really happy.' This shows an understanding of the question but reinforces that it is effort and participation that are important.

GIVING FEEDBACK

Generally speaking, feedback can be provided in two ways:

1. **Extrinsic feedback** – This type of feedback is related to receiving information from external sources, such as a coach, practitioner, S&C coach, sports scientist etc. This can come in the form of verbal, video or written feedback.

2. **Intrinsic feedback** – Intrinsic feedback is related to the physical feelings and senses of the client during performance of movements as they occur, such as the kinaesthetic feedback from muscles, joints etc.

Details of how to give feedback to clients and teams is covered in depth in chapter 14, but below are some general strategies that are useful to bear in mind:

Correction

In a group situation, if corrective feedback is required, try to avoid singling out any client. In this situation the GET approach can be used:

- **G** – Make a **G**eneral comment to the whole group without looking only at the client that the comment is directed at.

- **E** – Make **E**ye contact with the client the feedback is targeted at.
- **T** – If there's no response then **T**alk directly to the client concerned and instruct them on a one-to-one basis.

The criticism sandwich

Feedback can often be perceived as criticism, so it is useful to complement correction points with positive praise. This is known as the criticism sandwich, as shown in figure 26.1. For example, start with the positive statement: 'You tried really hard today,' followed by, 'But I really need you to focus on running on your mid-foot,' and end with another positive statement: 'However, you are ahead of your short-term goal, so I am very pleased.'

OBTAINING FEEDBACK

It is important that you give feedback to your client but also that you obtain feedback from them, so that you can use this to adapt training programmes if necessary. This can be done by written, verbal or visual means.

For example:

- **Questionnaires** – Sometimes clients are reluctant to give verbal information, therefore you could construct your own questionnaire in which you ask the client open questions such as: 'What did you like about the session?' 'Are there any exercises that you don't like? Why?' 'Was the level of intensity suitable?' Questionnaires can provide a tangible record, but you might need to seek clarification on certain points.
- **Review** – You can organise a meeting with the client in which you would review the previous session/s. You can do this by informal discussion or take notes using your written questionnaire. Review sessions can help to build rapport and establish trust, so active listening skills and empathy are crucial to this process.
- **Observation** – With experience you can sometimes tell if a client is enjoying the session or not. You can also judge their intensity levels by their physical appearance (such as facial expression and technique performed) which gives an indication of the effort level of the client.

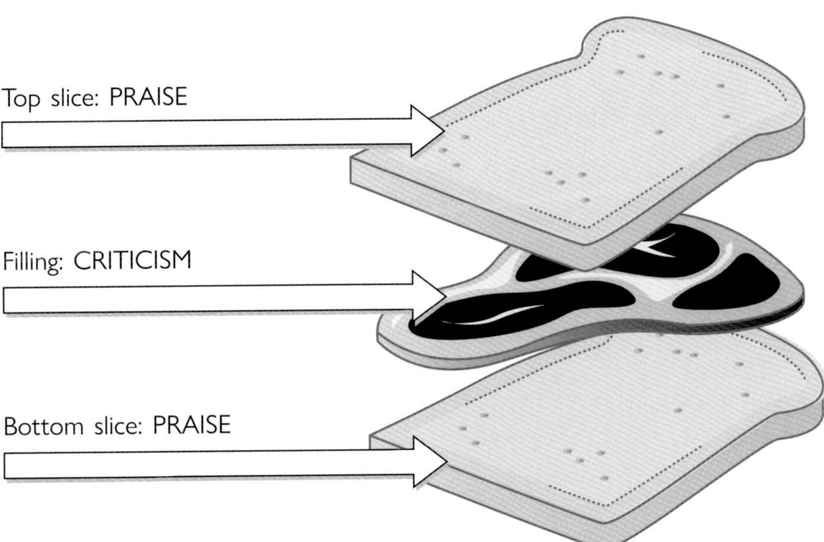

Figure 26.1 The criticism sandwich

Once you have obtained feedback in relation to a session you need to decide if any changes need to be made to the training programme. This can be by way of a change of type of exercise or a manipulation of variables such as the frequency, intensity, duration and rest periods. There is no specific way to do this, as changes depend on the feedback obtained, so practitioners should rely on their knowledge and experience for this process.

Take-home messages

- There are a range of communication skills that can improve practitioner performance.

- It is important to interpret client responses, including body language and other forms of behaviour, especially when undertaking physical activity.

- There are different ways of giving feedback, including the criticism sandwich.

- Feedback from clients should be interpreted to inform programme design.

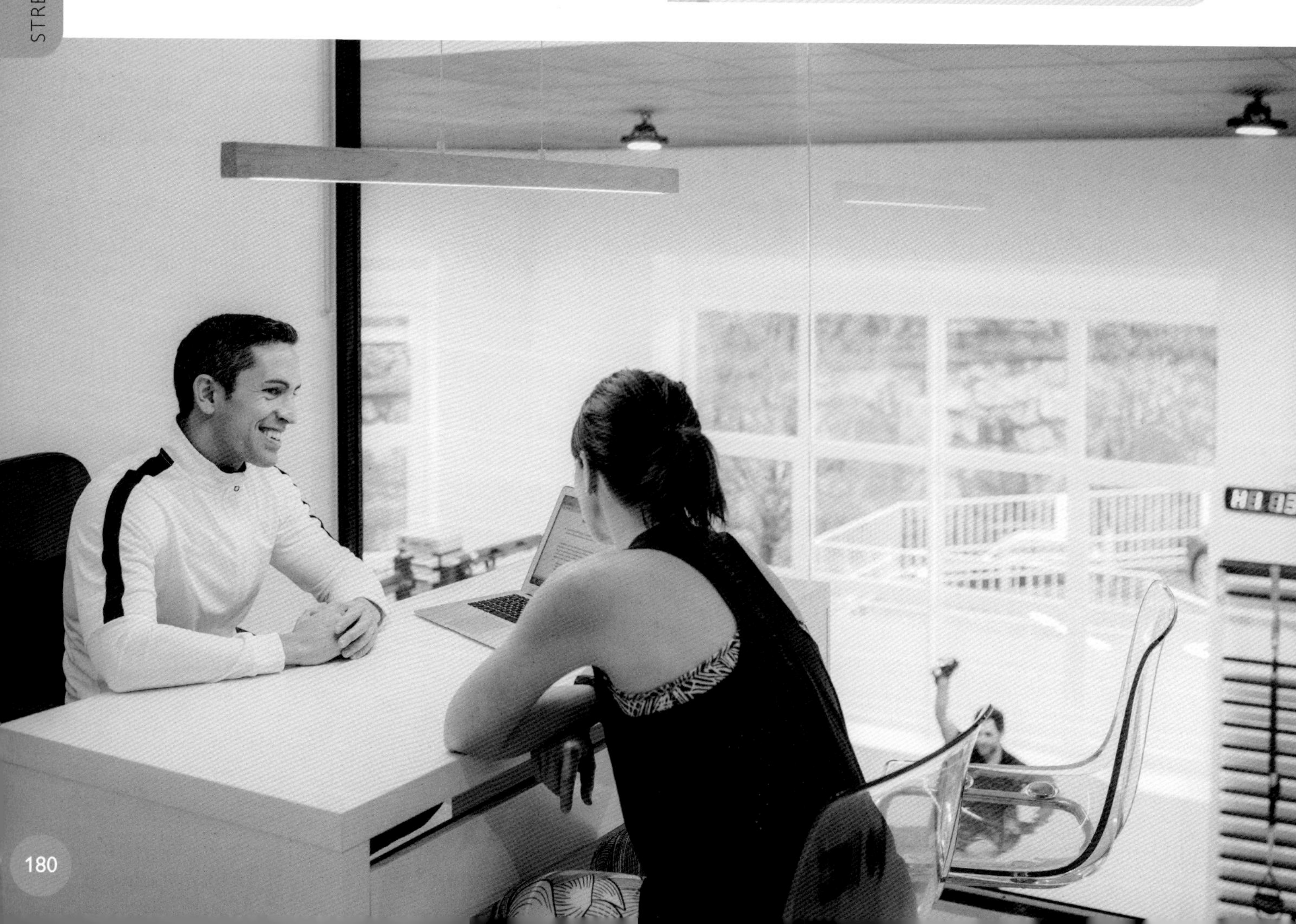

//Motivation

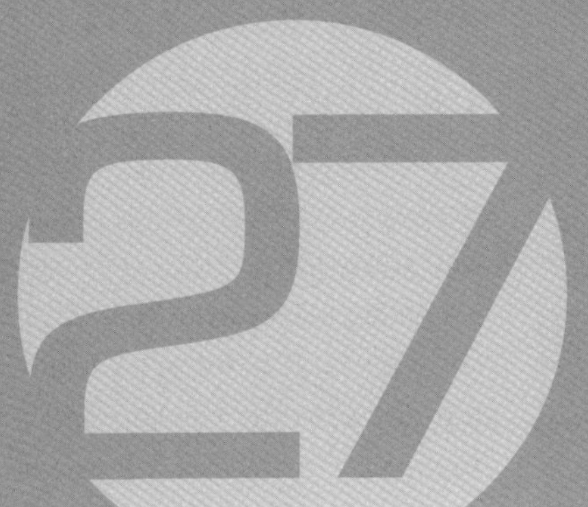

The areas covered in this chapter are:

- Understand the role of intrinsic and **extrinsic motivation** in exercise adherence
- Typical models and approaches that can motivate adherence to exercise
- How **self-efficacy** can influence performance and the methods typically used to measure it

Introduction

Similar to the previous chapter, this chapter focuses on more soft skills, specifically exploring motivation and how it can drive training programme adherence. S&C practitioners should learn to harness an individual's or teams' motivation to create buy-in to their programme and maximise the development of the performance outcomes that are being strived for. The way in which programmes are delivered can directly affect client adherence, which can be crucial to the success of the programme. Research suggests that there are a number of factors that can affect adherence to programmes, including motivation and self-efficacy, which will be explored in detail in this chapter.

What is motivation?

There is no agreed definition, but in general, the term motivation can be described as the internal mechanisms and external stimuli that arouse and direct our behaviour, often towards a particular goal. One of the earliest and most influential theories relating to motivation was the hierarchy of needs theory proposed in 1943 by Abraham Maslow. There have been many proposed models over the years since, but in the context of sports performance, it is broadly agreed that motivation can come from extrinsic and intrinsic sources:

- **Extrinsic motivation** – This is when clients are motivated by external rewards such as certificates, T-shirts, medals and trophies. It is also important to make sure that clients are not over-reliant on external rewards but focus on internal motivational factors as well.
- *Intrinsic motivation* – This is when clients are motivated by factors such as enjoyment, fun or self-satisfaction. This type of motivation can be linked to outcome goals: for example, when a performance goal is achieved it could promote a feeling of self-achievement and this is thought to be a more sustainable and long-term form of motivation.

THE ARCS MODEL

One way of promoting motivation is the ARCS Model of Motivational Design Theory. The ARCS stands for attention, relevance, confidence and satisfaction. Developed by John Keller in 1987, the model suggests that materials, such as training programmes, should be designed to meet the motivational needs of learners. The ARCS model consists of four components, as shown in figure 27.1. Although this model wasn't designed specifically for sports performance it can be used as a guide when designing training programmes. Let's look at each of the components in turn:

1. **Attention** – The materials must capture the attention of the learners by being interesting, novel and relevant to their needs and interests. Try to link current sessions to previous ones or to recent competition/games. It is also useful to introduce new techniques/drills on a regular basis.
2. **Relevance** – The materials must be relevant to the learners' needs, interests and goals, and must be presented in a way that connects to the learners' previous knowledge and experiences. Explain to clients how the session is linked to goals. Try to promote intrinsic motivation.
   Note: Strategies in this chapter can be implemented with the knowledge from chapter 14.
3. **Confidence** – The materials must provide the learners with a sense of confidence and self-efficacy by providing clear instructions, the appropriate level of difficulty, and feedback. Positive reinforcement and the opportunity for reflection can help to build autonomy.
4. **Satisfaction** – The materials must provide the learners with a sense of satisfaction and achievement by providing opportunities for success, problem-solving and creativity. Design meaningful assessments to help foster a sense of accomplishment.

Figure 27.1 Adaptation of the ARCS model

MOTIVATIONAL INTERVIEWING

Establishing a relationship of trust between practitioner and client can impact positively on adherence, which is why the development of interpersonal skills of the practitioner can be considered important. A technique known as motivational interviewing (MI) is a skill that can help to build rapport. This can be done by asking open-ended questions (allow the expansion of a point rather than a yes or no answer) or closed questions (yes or no response) when appropriate. The OARS model (table 27.1) can be used to help with the motivational interviewing process.

EMPOWERMENT

Another factor that can impact motivation is empowerment. Empowering clients to take responsibility and make choices for their own training programme is related to self-determination theory (SDT). According to SDT there are three key psychological needs that can contribute positively to motivation:

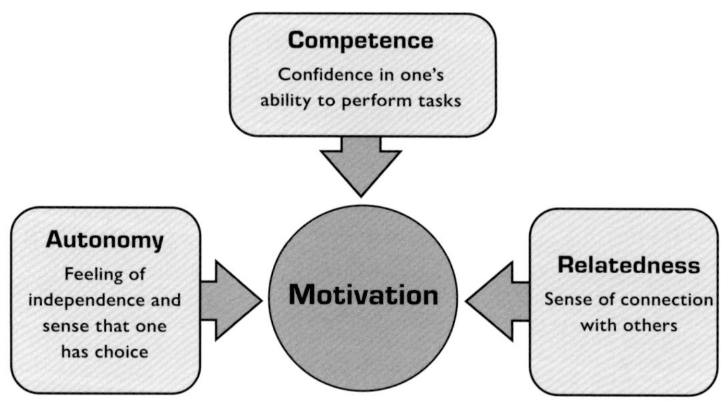

Figure 27.2 Self-determination theory (adapted from Deci and Ryan, 2017)

Table 27.1	OARS MOTIVATIONAL INTERVIEWING
Ask open-ended questions The practitioner says little Can help you learn about client values and goals	**Example** You mentioned you have concerns about the impact of training on your weight. Can you tell me about them? **Versus** Are you concerned about your weight?
Make affirmations Compliments, empathy, understanding Helps develop rapport	**Example** It must be difficult to discuss your weight concerns. Well done. I appreciate your honesty.
Use reflections Helps to understand motivation Used to reinforce reasons for change	**Example** You think that increasing your calorie intake will make you put on weight, which will impact your performance.
Use summarising Can identify a plan for future goals Can demonstrate client understanding	**Example** Can we just check the understanding so far. You are worried about your eating habits because you are aware of the health and performance issues. Am I on the right lines?

1. **Autonomy** – By building independence (autonomy), clients are more likely to adhere to new behaviours. When clients are internally motivated, they are more likely to achieve their goals.

2. **Competence** – Clients who feel more task-competent generally have higher self-esteem and autonomy. Providing regular appropriately challenging exercises and giving consistent and timely positive feedback can promote competence.

3. **Relatedness** – Supportive others (friends, family, training partner etc.) can be instrumental in helping to increase self-determination. Encouraging a sense of camaraderie and friendship by introducing training buddies or creating training groups can help foster a positive environment, which positively impacts motivation.

Self-efficacy

A client's belief in their capacity to execute behaviours necessary to produce specific performance attainments is known as self-efficacy. As part of the social cognitive theory proposed by Bandura in the 1980s, it was shown that high levels of self-efficacy expectations tend to foster a more positive outlook, which can lead to positive outcomes. It has been demonstrated that clients with high self-efficacy are more likely to adhere to exercise programmes. Any failure is often attributed to lack of effort, and they therefore try harder. On the other hand, clients with low self-efficacy may attribute failure to low ability, rather than lack of effort, and are more likely to give up. Goal setting on a regular basis is considered important especially if self-efficacy is low.

MEASURING SELF-EFFICACY

One of the most common measurement tools is the self-efficacy for exercise (SEE) scale (*see* fig. 27.3), which is used to assess perceived self-efficacy. The SEE scale consists of situations that might affect current participation in exercise. For each situation, the client rates themselves on a scale from 0 (not confident) to 10 (very confident) to describe their current confidence to

SELF-EFFICACY FOR EXERCISE SCALE

How confident are you right now you could exercise 3 times per week for 20 minutes if:	Not Confident										Very Confident
1 You were worried the exercise would cause further pain	0	1	2	3	4	5	6	7	8	9	10
2 You were bored by the programme or activity	0	1	2	3	4	5	6	7	8	9	10
3 You were not sure exactly what exercises to do	0	1	2	3	4	5	6	7	8	9	10
4 You had to exercise alone	0	1	2	3	4	5	6	7	8	9	10
5 You did not enjoy it	0	1	2	3	4	5	6	7	8	9	10
6 You were too busy with other activities	0	1	2	3	4	5	6	7	8	9	10
7 You felt tired during or after exercise	0	1	2	3	4	5	6	7	8	9	10
8 You felt stressed	0	1	2	3	4	5	6	7	8	9	10
9 You felt depressed	0	1	2	3	4	5	6	7	8	9	10
10 You were afraid the exercise would make you fall	0	1	2	3	4	5	6	7	8	9	10
11 You felt pain when exercising	0	1	2	3	4	5	6	7	8	9	10
Client name:											
Date:					Stage of change:						

Figure 27.3 Self-efficacy for exercise scale (for a blank template, please visit: bloomsbury.com/uk/complete-guide-to-strength-and-conditioning-training-9781399421362)

exercise three times a week for 20 minutes each time. A baseline measurement should be taken prior to the start of the programme to establish the confidence levels at that point in time. Subsequent tests would then show if self-efficacy had improved, and if so, goals could be set or adjusted in relation to this.

Take-home messages

- The manner of delivering instruction is important to foster development of a motivated client who is engaged in the strength and conditioning programme.

- Practitioners should be able to manage and maintain engagement of individuals and groups.

Legal and ethical // considerations

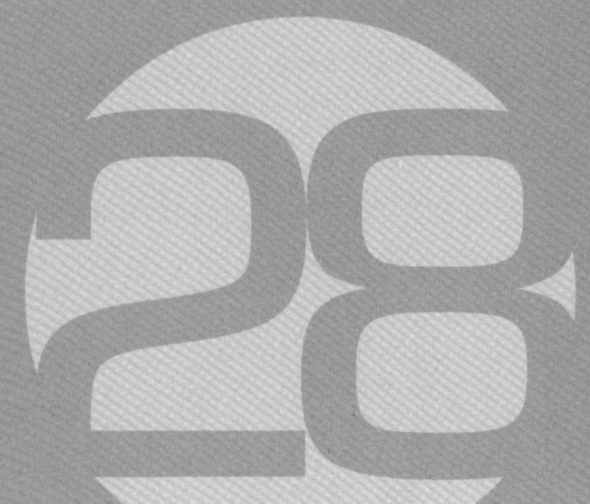

Introduction

S&C practitioners should be aware of legal and ethical implications in relation to training environments because it is their responsibility to always ensure the safety and well-being of clients. The areas that practitioners should focus on include health and safety at work, equipment management, risk assessment, emergency procedures, accident and incident reporting and child and vulnerable adult protection. This chapter will examine each of these in turn.

Health and safety at work

As in any work environment, the area of health and safety is an important issue for practitioners in relation to the delivery of training programmes. The statutory framework relating to health and safety (and to risk management) is, in the main part, covered by the Management of Health and Safety at Work Regulations (MHSWR) 1999 and the Health and Safety at Work Act (HSWA) 1974 (updated to include the Deregulation Act 2015). The HSWA 1974 outlines the role of a practitioner (as well as those appointed persons for all areas of health and safety) in relation to prevention of accidents. The act outlines the following areas:

- Taking responsible care for their own safety and that of others.
- Cooperating with employers in matters of safety.
- Interference with or misuse of anything provided for safety.

Organisations, should, by law, make a health and safety policy statement available to all staff and provide employees with relevant training. Organisations provide normal operating procedures (NOPs), which often include such things as security procedures and day-to-day operations and emergency operating procedures (EOPs) such as fire and medical emergency to help minimise the occurrence of accident or injury. Whether self-employed or employed, the practitioner should remain up to date with all areas related to health and safety.

Equipment management

Practitioners have at their disposal a wide range of equipment that can be used during training sessions, so it is important to address safety issues. Equipment should be checked regularly for wear and tear or malfunction. If operating equipment within a facility, manufacturers' guides should provide information on the type and frequency of maintenance required. Guidelines are usually found in NOPs, which include information such as gym maintenance and faulty equipment reporting.

Risk assessment

If practitioners do not make appropriate efforts to minimise the risk and injury occurs, it could be classed as negligence. If practitioners do what is reasonable to make people safe then there will be little chance of successful negligence claims. (*Note*: The Compensation Act 2006 gives a full explanation relating to negligence legislation.) If self-employed, then practitioners are directly responsible for any negligent act, but if they are employed while a negligent act is committed then the employer is said to be vicariously liable and as such responsible for the act. The statutory framework relating to risk management and health and safety at work in the UK is mainly covered by the Management of Health and Safety at Work Regulations (1999), which states that all self-employed persons should carry out risk assessments to identify health and safety risks to themselves and clients.

A risk assessment can help to identify hazards such as incorrect surfaces or cleaning substances not stored

Table 28.1	EXAMPLE RISK ASSESSMENT FORM		
Potential risk	**Method of minimising risk**	**Action to be taken**	**Done**
Recovery from shoulder injury.	Limit range of motion and weight.	Set the pec dec range to start at limited range of motion.	✔
Trips due to free weights on the floor in the training area.	Ensure users return free weights to storage when finished.	Put up signs around the training area to instruct members to return free weights to storage.	✔
Slippage on the floor space around a water fountain.	Wipe the floor regularly with paper towel.	Add this to the daily cleaning rota.	✔
Heat-related issues for an outdoor session.	Have a hydration strategy and timing consideration.	Ensure water bottles are available throughout. Avoid training sessions during the middle of the day.	✔
Falls on a grass surface.	Use correct footwear.	Brief clients about correct footwear for the session.	✔

correctly (Control of Substances Hazardous to Health Regulations [COSHH] provides guidelines for this). Although risks cannot be eradicated completely, they can be identified and minimised. It is advisable therefore to complete a risk assessment prior to any training session using a template such as that in table 28.1.

Emergency procedures

Emergency procedures are provided by organisations and should be located by practitioners at the earliest convenience. There are many types of emergency situation, but as a first-aider arriving at the scene of an incident, a primary survey should be carried out. The acronym DR ABC can be used to help make this survey easier to remember:

D	**Danger** – Assess the situation for danger. Approach quickly but remain calm. Identify any risks to yourself, the casualties and bystanders. Only when you have assessed there is no danger, approach and assess casualties.
R	**Response** – Can the casualty respond and give information about the situation?
A	**Airways** – If the casualty is unresponsive, you must check the airways and carry out appropriate manoeuvres to open them.
B	**Breathing** – Check for signs of normal breathing for 10 seconds. If the patient is not breathing normally or is breathing abnormally then go to the next step.
C	**Call 999/circulation** – If the casualty is not breathing, call 999 then start CPR immediately.

Note: Practitioners must have a valid first-aid qualification. First-aid courses will cover the above procedures in detail.

If the casualty is breathing normally and you are waiting for emergency responders, then it is important to give the casualty comfort and reassurance in a calm, controlled manner, since this is the best way to support them. Reassure the casualty that you are qualified and experienced in these situations. In addition:

- Keep the casualty warm and comfortable.
- You may need to ensure the safety of children, old people and disabled people.

In situations where you are the one to contact emergency services, it is important that clear and accurate information is given as calmly as possible. Information should include the following:

- Keep calm and speak clearly.
- Give your full name and state which service you require.
- Give the full name, address and telephone number of the club or facility where the session is being held.
- Give the exact location details and time of the accident/incident.
- Give the number and condition of any casualties and details of any treatment that is or has been given.
- Give the access point for the ambulance.
- Instruct someone to meet the ambulance, which will help them to reach the casualty as quickly as possible.

According to the Health and Safety (First-Aid) Regulations 1981 (hse.gov.uk), employers must provide adequate equipment and facilities to enable first aid to be carried out on sick or injured employees. This does not by law extend to customers using the facility, although first-aiders should make every attempt to administer first aid, should the situation arise.

ACCIDENT AND INCIDENT REPORTING

Any accident or incident during a training session supervised by the practitioner must be recorded (as a legal requirement) using an appropriate format such as an accident/incident report form. It is important to record an accident/incident at the earliest available opportunity so that an accurate recall can be made.

Note: It is a statutory requirement to keep records for at least 3 years.

Accident/incident report forms should contain a minimum amount of information, such as the example template in Appendix 4. Forms should always allow for additional information and be treated as confidential. When completing the form, practitioners must not draw conclusions or infer blame.

Child and vulnerable adult protection

Any adult who works with children or vulnerable adults has a responsibility to keep them safe and protect them from sexual, physical and emotional harm and failure to do so could lead to prosecution.

> A vulnerable adult is defined by the UK government as: 'a person aged 18 years or over who is in receipt or need of community care services by reason of mental or other disability, age, or illness and who is unable to take care of themselves or protect themselves against significant harm or exploitation.'

The UK Protection of Children Act 1978 was established to identify persons unsuitable to supervise children. Anyone wishing to deliver or supervise children's activities is required to carry out a disclosure check via the Criminal Records Bureau. On successful completion of a disclosure check, practitioners then have a responsibility to safeguard children and vulnerable adults by:

- reviewing their own practice in situations to ensure that they are complying with recognised codes of conduct;
- recognising the signs and symptoms and indicators of abuse and the impact this has on children and vulnerable adults;
- responding in an appropriate way and taking appropriate action if concerns are raised.

Areas relating to safeguarding include physical contact, confidentiality, sexual conduct, social contact, communication and comforting, as outlined in table 28.2.

Situations can arise where a child divulges sensitive information about potential abuse by another adult. Such incidents must be reported immediately but confidentially using the following guidelines:

- Stay calm throughout.
- Reassure the person you will take them seriously.
- Explain that you may have to follow a reporting procedure and do not promise anything.
- Encourage the person to tell the whole story but do not probe or ask closed questions (yes, no etc.).
- Listen carefully and do not comment on the allegation.
- As soon as possible, record the event and either speak to a colleague for advice or follow reporting procedures.

Table 28.2	SAFEGUARDING AREAS	
Area	**Main points**	**Advice**
Confidentiality	Treat all information as confidential.	Refer to the Data Protection Act 1998.
Sexual conduct	ALL sexual activity is a criminal offence. Special attention can be construed as grooming. Report any concerns about infatuation.	Never make sexual remarks, jokes or discuss your own relationship. Always make contact by email or phone through the parent or guardian. Avoid favouritism and giving special attention. Refer to the Sexual Offences Act 2003 and Working Together to Safeguard Children: 2006 HM Government.
Social contact	Social contact between trainers and vulnerable clients is not encouraged.	Make supervisors aware of any social contact with vulnerable clients and their families.
Communication	This includes phones, emails, websites and cameras.	Always communicate through the parent or guardian. Always get written permission before taking photos or videos.
Physical contact	Physical contact is often required in instructing, and this is fine so long as it is appropriate.	Get permission from vulnerable clients and parents/guardians before making any contact. Report any issues immediately.
Comforting	Vulnerable clients can become distressed and seek comfort.	Never comfort in a one-to-one situation unless another trainer or parent/guardian is present. Record any issues you may be unsure about.

Take-home messages

- S&C practitioners should be aware of legal and ethical implications in relation to training environments.

- Practitioners should make themselves aware of important documents relating to health and safety.

- Risk assessment is an important part of session delivery.

- Practitioners should have an understanding of emergency procedures.

- Any adult who works with children or vulnerable adults has a responsibility to keep them safe and protect them from sexual, physical and emotional harm.

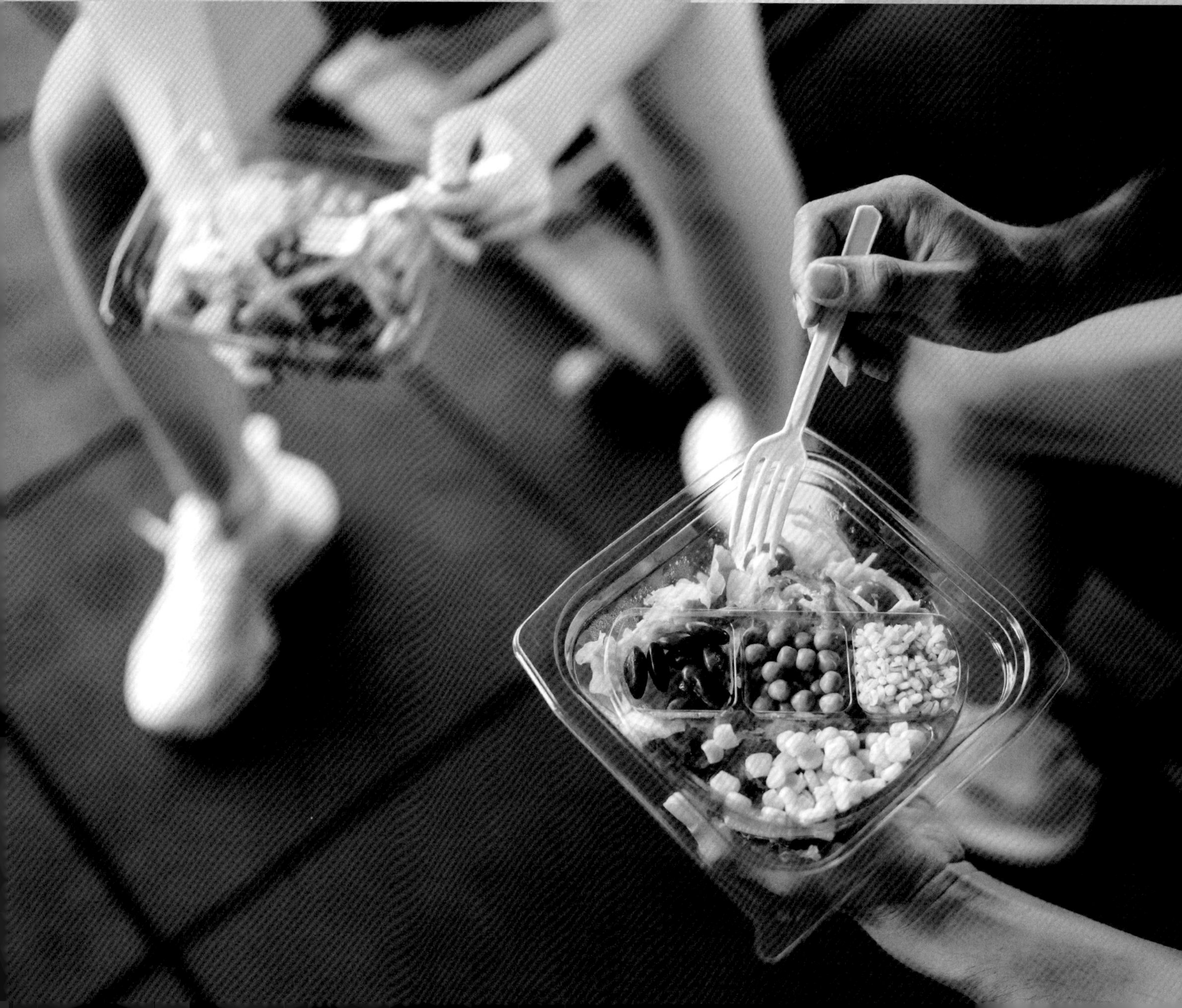

5

PART **FIVE**

NUTRITION FOR STRENGTH AND CONDITIONING

So far in parts 1, 2, and 3 we took you through a systematic process of gathering client information to design an S&C programme based on relevant components of fitness. We also looked at a range of available test protocols designed to assess these components of fitness. In part 4 we considered other factors that would be important to S&C practitioners, including the manipulation of key variables and practical skills considered important in the environment. In part 5 we are going to discuss the area of nutrition for strength and conditioning.

Nutrition is considered an essential component of strength and conditioning because it can provide fuel for optimal performance and the nutrients for muscle growth and repair, and recovery from exercise. As well as being important for athletic performance, the link between good nutrition and good health is also well established. The information in this part deals with areas of nutrition that are within the scope of practice of an S&C practitioner and the boundaries relating to the advice you are able to give to clients.

//**Nutrients**

29

> **The areas covered in this chapter are:**
>
> - The main recommendations and dietary issues associated with macronutrients
>
> - The role of micronutrients and conditions associated with deficiency
>
> - The importance of hydration and relevant guidelines
>
> - The professional role and scope of practice in relation to other relevant specialists when offering health and well-being advice and guidance
>
> - The nationally recognised healthy eating recommendations
>
> - How to understand food labelling
>
> - Cultural and religious dietary practices
>
> - How to seek evidence-based/reputable health and well-being advice

Introduction

Nutrition and its association with sport and S&C is a complex subject where a wide foundation of knowledge is required before practitioners can be considered competent in this area. Furthermore, while S&C practitioners can offer advice, it is important to understand that nutrition plans and dietary interventions should not be undertaken unless the practitioner has a nutrition or dietician qualification that certifies them to do so.

This chapter will provide a nutritional foundation that will focus on the variety of nutrients required to maintain health and a state of homeostasis. Furthermore, it will look at healthy eating protocols and insights into how to maintain a balanced diet.

Nutrients

Chemical substances in food, known as nutrients, are essential for the body to function. Nutrients needed in larger quantities are called macronutrients or macros (the main ones are proteins, fats and carbohydrates) and these act as a source of energy. Nutrients needed in small amounts are called micronutrients (*vitamins* and *minerals*) and play essential roles in metabolism (they have no energy content).

MACRONUTRIENTS

There are various guidelines in relation to the recommended average daily amounts of macronutrients. For example, the UK government's recommendations for protein, fats, carbohydrate and fibre can be seen in table 29.1. These recommendations are based on population averages and as such should be adjusted for training purposes.

Protein

Proteins can help to regulate processes in the body, such as enabling the function of vital organs and immune cells, and can also provide a source of energy if required. A protein is made up of chains of individual amino acids, which are the building blocks for growth and repair (the body is about 20% protein by weight).

There are about 20 types of amino acids, of which there are two main groups: non-essential and essential. Non-essential amino acids can be produced by the body (even if not ingested), whereas essential amino acids can only be ingested; they cannot be synthesised. Protein comes from animal sources, such as meat, fish, milk and eggs, and vegetable sources, such as pulses, nuts, seeds and beans. (*Note*: Vegetable sources may not contain all essential amino acids.)

Protein requirements for individuals

The Department of Health at the International Conference of Food, Nutrition and Sports Performance suggest the following guidelines:

- 1.2–1.8g/kg/day for those who engage in regular endurance activities
- 2.0–2.4g/kg/day for those who engage in regular strength and power activities

Table 29.1	GOVERNMENT ADULT RECOMMENDATIONS FOR PROTEIN, FATS, CARBOHYDRATES AND FIBRE					
	19–64 yrs		**65–74 yrs**		**75+ yrs**	
Gender	**Male**	**Female**	**Male**	**Female**	**Male**	**Female**
Energy (Kcal/day)	2500	2000	2342	1912	2294	1840
Protein (g/day)	55.5	45.0	53.3	46.5	53.3	46.5
Fat						
Total: (<g/day)	97	78	91	74	89	72
Saturated: (<g/day)	31	24	29	23	28	23
Polyunsaturated: (g/day)	18	14	17	14	17	13
Monounsaturated: (g/day)	36	29	34	28	33	27
Carbohydrate: (at least g/day)	333	267	312	255	306	245
Free sugars: (<g/day)	33	27	31	26	31	25
Dietary fibre: (g/day)	30	30	30	30	30	30

Dietary issues

A typical UK diet contains between 11% and 14% of foods from protein sources. Insufficient protein has been linked to low energy levels, reduced resistance to infection and decreased rate of healing. A healthy balanced diet is generally considered to contain enough protein without the need for supplementation. Excessive protein intake has been linked to adverse effects of insulin action and increased risk of developing type 2 diabetes.

Fat

The correct term for fat is **lipid**, which comes from the Greek *lipos*. Fat is the main source of stored energy in the body. Dietary fats are transported in the bloodstream as triglycerides and are either stored or burned as fuel. Triglycerides contain many forms of fatty acid chains, in which the structure of the chain determines if the fat is saturated or unsaturated. Saturated fats are normally solid at room temperature, while unsaturated fats are liquid. Unsaturated fats can be configured in a cis-orientation (a natural formation) or in a trans-orientation (a processed formation). Fat has a number of important roles in the body:

- As an energy source (predominantly in aerobic exercise)
- In cell membrane structure
- Protection for the nervous system
- Production of hormones
- Transportation of fat-soluble vitamins A, D, E and K
- As a source of essential fatty acids (these are fats that cannot be synthesised by the body so must be obtained in the diet in sources such as seeds, grains and oily fish)

Fat requirements

Guidelines typically recommend an average daily fat intake between 30% and 40%. Recommendations also state that less than 10% should come from saturated fat.

Calculating average daily fat intake

Example: if a client's energy requirements are 2400Kcal per day, and the target intake is about 30% (roughly one-third) then the calculation would be as follows:

Step 1: 2400 ÷ 3 (approximately ⅓) = 800Kcal

As 1g fat = 9Kcal of energy then:

Step 2: 800 ÷ 9 = 88.88g of fat per day

Dietary issues

Fat contains more than twice the number of calories per gram compared to carbohydrate or protein. A diet high in saturated fat can increase the risk of obesity and other conditions such as diabetes, coronary heart disease, high blood pressure and various cancers. There is also a link between high levels of saturated fat and high levels of **cholesterol**, which is a type of lipid.

Cholesterol

Produced in the liver, cholesterol is an essential compound needed for various roles, such as cell structure and hormone production. Like triglycerides, cholesterol is transported in the bloodstream. To do this, it must combine with protein to form various lipoproteins, which are then transported through the blood. The main types of lipoproteins are:

- **Very low-density lipoprotein** (VLDL), which is the main carrier of triglyceride.
- **Low-density lipoprotein** (LDL), which is the 'bad' carrier of cholesterol.
- **High-density lipoprotein** (HDL), which is known as the 'good' carrier of cholesterol.

Table 29.2 shows the classification of cholesterol

Table 29.2	UK CHOLESTEROL CLASSIFICATIONS ADAPTED FROM THE NHS (UNITS ARE mmol/l OF BLOOD)		
Lipoprotein	**Desirable**	**Borderline**	**Abnormal**
Total cholesterol	<5.2	5.2–6.5	>6.5
LDL cholesterol	<3.0	3.0–5.0	>5.0
HDL cholesterol	>1.0	0.9–1.0	<0.9

in the blood. High levels of LDL cholesterol are associated with atherosclerosis or hardening of the arteries. This is where plaque can form on the inside walls of the arteries. As a result, arteries can narrow and stiffen, which in turn can reduce the blood flow and lead to consequences such as angina, stroke and heart attack. Regular exercise can increase HDL levels, thereby reducing the risk of developing atherosclerosis.

Carbohydrates

Carbohydrates are the primary source of energy for humans and are made up of *saccharides* (or sugars). Carbohydrates are ingested in the form of monosaccharides, which are single sugars such as glucose, fructose and galactose, and disaccharides, which are two sugars such as lactose, sucrose and maltose.

Note: Complex carbohydrates can also be ingested in the form of oligosaccharides and polysaccharides.

Fibre

Another category of carbohydrate is fibre or non-starch-polysaccharide (NSP), which is indigestible and considered to play an important role in gut health and immune function. Fibre moves through the digestive system where it absorbs water and toxins to be excreted from the body and helps get rid of cholesterol and fats (by absorbing and excreting them), thus reducing the

risk of heart disease.

Glucose

Glucose is the most common source of energy and is vital for the following functions:

- The brain and nervous system (require 500–600 Kcals daily)
- The liver and digestive system (require 300–400 Kcals daily)
- Muscular contractions (requirement depends upon activity level)

When glucose is stored in the liver and muscles it is called glycogen. The body is capable of storing about 1600Kcals of energy as glycogen (about 1200Kcals in the muscles and 400Kcals in the liver), which is sufficient for the short term only (about 24 hours), which is why carbohydrates are important in the daily diet.

Carbohydrate requirement

Approximately two-thirds of total energy intake should come from carbohydrate but those who are active will require a higher intake to cater for the higher energy expenditure. The following is a quick method to calculate an average daily carbohydrate intake.

> ### Calculating the average daily carbohydrate intake
>
> Example: if a client's energy requirements are 2,400Kcal per day, then the calculation would be as follows:
>
> **Step 1:** 55–60% of 2400 = 1320–1440Kcal
>
> As 1 gram of carbohydrate = 4Kcal of energy then:
>
> **Step 2:** 1320–1440 divided by 4 = 330–360g of carbohydrate per day

Dietary issues

Carbohydrates that are digested quickly are referred to as simple carbohydrates (such as refined foods like cakes, soft drinks and sweets) and those that are digested slowly are referred to as complex carbohydrates. A diet high in simple carbohydrates has been linked to conditions such as diabetes. Regular exercise can help to reduce the onset of diabetes by regulating blood sugar and obesity levels and increasing insulin sensitivity.

MICRONUTRIENTS

There are two sources of micronutrients: 1) vitamins, which are organic compounds; 2) minerals, which are inorganic.

Vitamins

A vitamin is an organic compound (meaning it contains carbon) that is essential for metabolic function. They can be categorised as fat-soluble (such as vitamins A, D, E and K) and water-soluble (such as vitamins B and C). Water-soluble vitamins cannot be stored in the body whereas fat-soluble vitamins can be stored for future use. Healthy balanced diets are usually sufficient for vitamin intake but those who are deficient may require supplementation. Deficiencies of specific vitamins are linked to potential health issues, as shown in table 29.3.

> ### Glycaemic index
>
> The ***glycaemic index*** (GI) is a rating system for foods containing carbohydrate (ranging from 0 to 100). The index shows how quickly blood sugar levels are affected. Foods that have a high GI are absorbed into the bloodstream quickly (and produce a significant insulin response) whereas foods that are low GI are absorbed at a slower rate and produce a lesser insulin response. A GI of 85 or over is classed as high; a GI between 60 and 84 is moderate and low GI is less than 60. Low-GI diets are often recommended for diabetics because this can inhibit the sense of hunger after eating and increase endurance during exercise. Prolonged eating of foods that are high GI is linked to type 2 diabetes and obesity.
>
> *Note:* There are many available web sources for GI food lists.

Minerals

A mineral is a naturally formed substance (inorganic) formed in the earth but can be derived from the digestion of certain foods. Minerals that are required in amounts greater than 100mg per day are classed as macro-minerals and include calcium, phosphorous, magnesium, sodium, potassium and chloride, whereas those that are required in amounts less than 100mg per day are classed as micronutrients and include iron, copper, zinc, selenium and iodine.

Minerals lacking in the diet can lead to various health issues, such as ***osteoporosis*** (lack of calcium) and anaemia (lack of iron). Other minerals such as sodium tend to be over-consumed, which is a concern because high sodium intake has been linked to hypertension.

Table 29.3	HEALTH ISSUES RELATED TO VITAMIN DEFICIENCY AND SOURCES		
Vitamin	**Main use**	**Deficiency**	**Sources**
Vitamin A	**Retinol**: Essential for vision in dim light. It is required for skin, mucous membranes and growth.	Night blindness (xerophthalmia)	Legumes, vegetables and fruit
Vitamin B	B1: **Thiamine**: Required for the release of energy from carbohydrates. It is especially important for the brain and nerve function.	Beriberi (nervous system disorder)	Whole grains, legumes, pork
	B2: **Riboflavin**: Required for the release of energy, especially from protein and fat.	Problems with lips, tongue, skin	Whole grains, dairy, leafy vegetables, beef
	B3: **Niacin**: Required for energy release from nutrients.	Pellagra	Whole grains, milk, meat, eggs
	B5: **Pantothenic acid**: Utilised in metabolic pathways.	Fatigue	Widespread across food groups
	B6: **Pyridoxine**: Mainly required for amino acid metabolism.	Skin problems	Widespread across food groups
	B7: **Biotin**: Required for cell growth and fat metabolism.	Hair loss, dermatitis	Egg yolk, soybeans, whole grains
	B9: **Folic acid**: Needed to protect the foetus.	Diarrhoea, anaemia	Fortified grains, leafy vegetables, legumes
	B12: **Cyanocobalamin**: Required for folate metabolism.	Pernicious anaemia	Animal products
Vitamin C	**Ascorbic acid**: Required for the immune system. It also aids wound healing and iron absorption.	Scurvy (sickness and skin disorders)	Fruit and vegetables
Vitamin D	**Calciferol**: It promotes calcium absorption from food.	Rickets (bone softening)	Fish oils, exposure to sunlight
Vitamin E	**Tocopherol**: It has a protective effect for cell membranes.	Malabsorption of fats, anaemia	Grains, nuts, leafy vegetables
Vitamin K	**Menaquinone**: This is especially required to produce blood clotting proteins.	Poor blood clotting, internal bleeding	Leafy vegetables, soybeans

Table 29.4	MAIN FUNCTIONS AND SOURCES OF MINERALS	
Mineral	**Main function**	**Sources**
Calcium	Component of teeth and bones. Muscle and nerve activity. Blood clotting.	Dairy, cereals, legumes, vegetables
Chloride	Metabolism (the process of turning food into energy).	Meat, milk, eggs, vegetables, processed foods
Copper	Oxygen transportation.	Organ meats, nuts, seeds, chocolate, shellfish
Fluorine	Strengthening teeth.	Fluoridated water, canned shellfish, oatmeal, raisins
Iron	Transporting oxygen in red blood cells. Protein metabolism.	Animal sources
Iodine	Thyroid function, metabolism, growth and energy production.	Meat, plant foods (based on soil content)
Magnesium	Used in enzyme activity and muscle function. Protein building.	Fruits, vegetables, whole grains, legumes, nuts, dairy, meat
Manganese	It has a role in the body's antioxidant defences.	Whole grains, shellfish, nuts, leafy vegetables, legumes
Molybdenum	Involved in the metabolism of DNA.	Whole grains, legumes, dairy, beef
Phosphorus	Present in bones and teeth. A component of all cells.	Milk, dairy, meat, poultry
Potassium	Important for brain and nerve function.	Fruits and vegetables
Selenium	Antioxidant, growth and metabolism, pancreas function.	Grains and vegetables (based on soil content)
Sodium	Regulating body water content and nerve function.	Meat, milk, eggs, vegetables, processed foods
Zinc	Growth and repair, taste perception, antioxidant, foetal development.	Shellfish, red meat

Water

Water constitutes between 40% and 70% of the total body mass depending on age, gender and body composition. Metabolic processes in the body require water, especially digestion and absorption of nutrients, and this can be affected if the body becomes too dehydrated. An excess loss of water or insufficient intake can lead to a state of dehydration. Effects of dehydration can include:

- Decreased ability to sweat
- Reduced kidney function
- Decrease in muscle glycogen
- Increased risk of heat stroke
- Impaired cardiac function
- Reduced strength and power performance
- Altered cognitive performance

Note: Water is continuously lost through processes such as urination, exhalation and evaporation through the skin, so replenishment is vital to avoid dehydration.

DEHYDRATION

Typical symptoms of mild dehydration include headaches, decreased blood pressure (***hypotension***), dark-coloured urine or decreased urine volume, tiredness and dizziness. If dehydration increases, urine output can cease, and fainting can occur. If dehydration becomes severe, the heart rate can increase, leading to delirium and in some instances, death, especially in elderly clients who are at higher risk of dehydration due to a decrease in thirst sensation and reduced kidney capacity. It is also important to note that children are more susceptible to dehydration for reasons such as renal immaturity and large skin surface area.

HYDRATION GUIDELINES

The recommended daily water intake amount can vary due to factors such as temperature, humidity, altitude, activity level and diet. General guidelines for hydration before, during and after training sessions are as follows:

- Do not rely on thirst as an indicator to drink, as this could be dangerous.
- Wear breathable exercise clothing and NO sweat suits.
- Cut down on the intake of drinks such as tea, coffee and alcohol since they are all diuretics, which cause the body to lose water.
- Check the colour of urine on a regular basis. It should be pale in colour rather than a dark yellow/orange, which indicates possible dehydration.
- Before exercise (pre-hydration), drink approximately 5–6ml/kg.
- Drink 100–200ml every 15 minutes during the session.
- Take regular sips in the hour after the session.
- For exercise sessions of less than 60 minutes, water is recommended.
- For exercise sessions of more than 60 minutes, sports drinks that contain 5–10% glucose polymers are recommended.
- After exercise, approximately 1.5 litres should be consumed for each 1kg (23fl oz per 1lb) of bodyweight lost. It is generally recommended to rehydrate within 6 hours following exercise.

Note: Daily fluid intake relates to the amount of water consumed from foods as well as drinking water and other beverages.

Guideline daily amounts

In the 1990s in the UK, Guideline Daily Amounts (GDAs) were produced as a guide to help people understand what they could consume each day for a healthy, balanced diet. However, Dietary Reference Values (DRVs) for food, energy and nutrients have since replaced GDAs. DRVs are estimates of the energy and nutrients needed by a *healthy* UK population and were set by the Committee on Medical Aspects of Food and Nutrition Policy (COMA), which used the values:

- **Estimated Average Requirement (EAR)** – This indicates an average level of energy or nutrients that would be sufficient for about 50% of the population.
- **Reference Nutrient Intake (RNI)** – This is the amount that would be sufficient for 97.5% of the population.
- **Lower Reference Nutrient Intake (LRNI)** – This level of intake would only be sufficient for 2.5% of the population.

Notes: Guidelines for DRVs can be found in *Department of Health, Report 41: Dietary reference values for food energy and nutrients for the United Kingdom. London HMSO.*

COMA has been replaced by the Scientific Advisory Committee on Nutrition (SCAN).

Food labels

In 2021, Natasha's Law came into effect. It is legislation that requires all food that is pre-packed for direct sale to list all ingredients (pre-packed food is any food that is put into packaging before sale and cannot be altered without opening or changing the packaging). The mandatory

Table 29.5	**TRAFFIC LIGHT SYSTEM VALUES**			
	Food levels per 100g			
Food	**Green (low)** **grams/100**	**Amber (medium)** **grams/100**	**Red (high)** **grams/100**	**Red (high)** **Per portion**
Fat	≤3.0	>3.0 to ≤20.0	>20.0	>21.0
Of which saturates	≤1.5	>1.5 to ≤5.0	>5.0	>6.0
Sugars	≤5.0	>5.0 to ≤12.5	>12.5	>15.0
Salts	≤0.3	>0.3 to ≤1.5	>1.5	>2.4
Drinks	**Green (low)** **grams/100ml**	**Amber (medium)** **grams/100ml**	**Red (high)** **grams/100ml**	
Fat	≤1.5	>1.5 to ≤10.0	>10.0	
Of which saturates	≤0.75	>0.75 to ≤2.5	>2.5	
Sugars	≤2.5	>2.5 to ≤6.3	>6.3	
Salts	≤0.3	>0.3 to ≤1.5	>1.5	

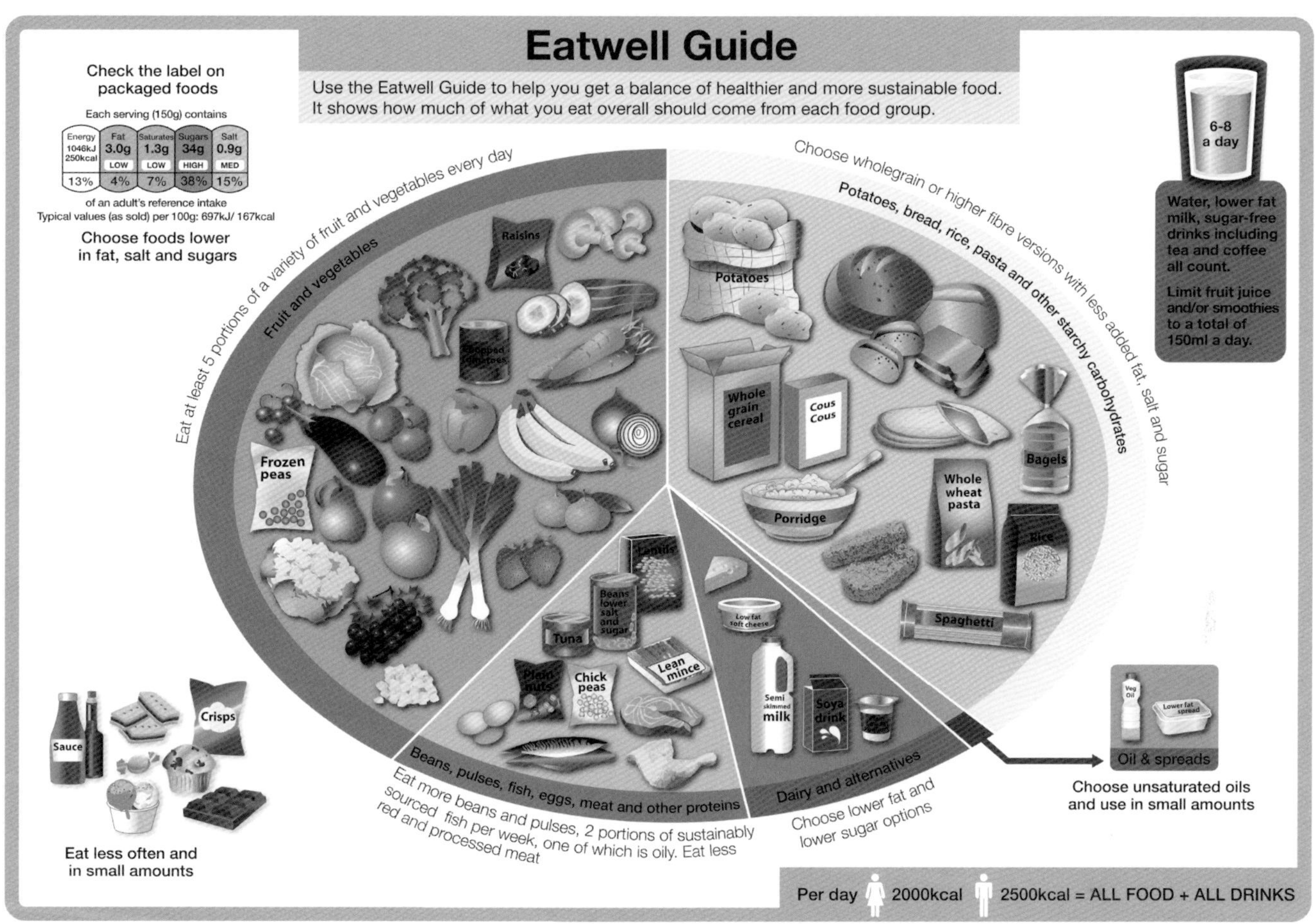

Figure 29.1 The Eatwell Guide (nhs.uk/live-well/eat-well/food-guidelines-and-food-labels/the-eatwell-guide)

information should include the name of the food, quantitative ingredients declaration, weight or volume, a list of ingredients (including allergens), the best before or use-by date, date and storage conditions, preparation instructions, and the name and address of the food business operator responsible for the food information.

Additional information can be added optionally, such as the amounts of specific nutrients, often as a percentage of the Dietary Reference Value. As an alternative to GDAs, the Food Standards Agency (FSA) developed a system for front-of-pack labelling that provides simple visual information on labels about the nutritional content of food and drinks called the traffic light system, which uses a logo of traffic light colours to indicate low, medium and high amounts of fat (of which saturated), sugar and salt, as shown in table 29.5.

Healthy eating

Only registered dieticians should give evidence-based dietary advice beyond the guidance of the government

Balance of Good Health from the Food Standards Agency. (See the government-produced booklet *The Eatwell Guide* from the Food Standards Agency food.gov.uk/sites/default/files/media/document/eatwell-guide-master-digital.pdf, as shown in fig. 29.1.)

Note: The Eatwell Guide is subject to Crown copyright. Source: OHID in association with the Welsh Government, Food Standards Scotland and the Food Standards Agency in Northern Ireland

THE EATWELL GUIDE

The Eatwell Guide is a visual method used to educate the public about healthy eating and the fact that no single food contains required nutrient amounts, which

Table 29.6	FOOD GROUP RECOMMENDATIONS ADAPTED FROM THE FOOD STANDARDS AGENCY			
	What's included	**Main nutrient**	**Message**	**Recommendations**
Bread, other cereals and potatoes	Other cereals mean foods such as breakfast cereals, pasta, rice, oats, noodles, maize, millet and cornmeal. This group also includes yams and plantains. Beans and pulses can be eaten as part of this group.	Carbohydrate, fibre, some calcium and iron, B vitamins	Eat lots.	Try to eat wholemeal, wholegrain, brown or high-fibre versions where possible. Try to avoid: • having them fried too often (e.g. chips) • adding too much fat • adding rich sauces and dressings (e.g. cream or cheese sauce on pasta)
Fruit and vegetables	Fresh, frozen and canned fruit and vegetables and dried fruit. A glass of fruit juice also counts. Beans and pulses can be eaten as part of this group.	Vitamin C, carotenes, folates, fibre and carbohydrate	At least five portions a day. Fruit juice, beans and pulses count as only one portion, however much you have in a day.	Eat a wide variety of fruit and vegetables. Try to avoid: • adding fat or rich sauces to vegetables • adding sugar or syrupy dressings to fruit
Milk and dairy foods	Milk, cheese, yoghurt and fromage frais. This group does not include butter, eggs and cream.	Calcium, protein, vitamins B12, A and D	Eat or drink moderate amounts and choose lower-fat versions whenever you can.	Lower-fat versions mean semi-skimmed or skimmed milk, low-fat (0.1% fat) yoghurts or fromage frais, and lower-fat cheeses (e.g. Edam, half-fat cheese and Camembert). Check the amount of fat by looking at the nutrient information on the labels.

Table 29.6	**FOOD GROUP RECOMMENDATIONS ADAPTED FROM THE FOOD STANDARDS AGENCY (cont.)**			
	What's included	**Main nutrient**	**Message**	**Recommendations**
Meat, fish and alternatives	Meat (includes bacon and salami and meat products such as sausages, beefburgers and pâté), poultry, fish, eggs, nuts, beans and pulses. Fish includes frozen and canned fish such as sardines and tuna, fish fingers and fishcakes (at least one portion of oily fish such as sardines and salmon each week).	Iron, protein, B vitamins, especially B12, zinc	Eat moderate amounts and choose lower-fat versions whenever you can.	Lower-fat versions mean things like meat with the fat cut off, poultry without the skin and fish without batter. Cook these foods without added fat. Beans and pulses are good alternatives to meat as they are naturally very low in fat.
Foods containing fat; foods and drinks containing sugar	Foods containing fat: margarine, butter, other spreading fats and low-fat spreads, cooking oils, oil-based salad dressings, mayonnaise, cream, chocolate, crisps, biscuits, pastries, cakes, puddings, ice cream, rich sauces and gravies. Foods and drinks containing sugar: soft drinks, sweets, jam and sugar.	Fat, including essential fatty acids. Some products also contain salt or sugar.	Eat foods containing fat sparingly and look out for the low-fat alternatives. Foods and drinks containing sugar should not be eaten too often, as they can contribute to tooth decay.	Some foods containing fat will be eaten every day, but should be kept to small amounts, for example, margarine and butter, other spreading fats (including low-fat spreads), cooking oils, oil-based salad dressings and mayonnaise. Foods containing fat such as cakes, biscuits, pastries and ice cream should be limited and low-fat alternatives chosen where available. All foods and drinks containing sugar should be eaten mainly at mealtimes to reduce the risk of tooth decay.

means that a mixture of foods should be consumed. Table 29.6 provides Food Standards Agency recommendations relating to the five food groups.

As the guide shows, more foods should be eaten from the potatoes, bread, rice and pasta group and the fruit and vegetables group compared to other groups, whereas oils and spreads should be eaten sparingly. The guide also includes advice on foods to eat less often, hydration, and food labelling as follows:

- **Foods to eat less often and in small amounts** – Foods that should be consumed occasionally and in small amounts include food and drinks high in fat and sugar such as cakes, biscuits, chocolate, sweets, puddings, pastries, ice cream, jam, honey, crisps, sauces, butter, cream and mayonnaise.
- **Hydration** – Have the equivalent of 6–8 glasses of fluid a day. Water, lower-fat milk and sugar-free drinks including tea and coffee are acceptable. Limit fruit juice and/or smoothies to a total of 150ml (5fl oz) a day.
- **Food labelling** – Colour-coded labels on the front of packs can help people choose between foods that are lower in calories, fat, saturated fat, sugar and salt.

PORTION SIZE

Controlling the amount of food is important, as people often underestimate what they eat by up to 50%. The Balance of Good Health does not include information relating to portion sizes apart from fruit and vegetables but the hand guide shown in figure 29.2 can be a useful tool to help regulate portion sizes.

Cultural and religious dietary practices

Cultural and religious practices must be considered when assessing nutritional needs. For example,

Fist	Full hand	Cupped hand	Palm	Thumb
Serving size: 1 cup	Serving size: 20cm	Serving size: ½ cup	Serving size: 80 grams	Serving size: 1 tablespoon
Food examples: • Cereal • Rice • Beans • Soups • Fruit	Food examples: • Breads • Sandwich • Pizza	Food examples: • Pasta • Potatoes • Nuts	Food examples: • Meat • Fish • Poultry	Food examples: • Mayonnaise • Dressing • Ketchups • Cream

Figure 29.2 Hand guide for portion size control

Hinduism forbids the taking of life for food and therefore follows a vegetarian diet. Those who follow the Muslim religion only eat the flesh of ruminant animals (those that digest plant-based foods), excluding pork, and fast for 4 weeks of every year during a period known as Ramadan when they only eat during the hours of darkness.

Nutritional //deficiencies

The areas covered in this chapter are:

- Typical nutritional deficiencies and their associated health problems

- Health issues associated with common dieting behaviours

- The various groups at risk from nutritional deficiencies

- The characteristics and potential negative effects of common eating disorders

Introduction

Building on the foundations of nutrition that were detailed in the previous chapter, this chapter will provide detailed insights into nutritional deficiencies and common fad diets that S&C practitioners should be aware of. In addition, practitioners should be aware of how these issues may impact a client's ability to train and recover from the associated training load.

Nutritional deficiencies

A diet in which the intake of nutrients is less than the estimated average requirements is called nutritional inadequacy, whereas a severe restriction of one or more nutrients is known as nutritional deficiency, which can alter bodily functions and increase the risk of a range of diseases. It is possible to get most nutrients from a healthy balanced diet, which is considered to be a combination of macro- and micronutrients. Unfortunately, nutrient deficiencies are common. The reasons for lower nutrient status are complex and can include factors such as poor-quality food, low quantity, increased dietary requirements, decreased digestion and food availability. Table 30.1 identifies common groups at risk of nutritional deficiencies and the typical problems related to these.

Dieting dangers

The word 'diet' is often perceived to mean a type of caloric restriction to lose weight. Prolonged fasting and diets that severely restrict caloric intake can be dangerous, as they can result in the loss of large amounts of water, electrolytes, minerals, glycogen stores, lean-mass and fat-free tissue. There are many health issues associated with a range of common diets, as can be seen in table 30.2.

Table 30.1	GROUPS AT RISK OF NUTRITIONAL DEFICIENCIES AND ASSOCIATED PROBLEMS
Group at risk	**Associated problems**
Those on severely energy restricted diets.	As well as missing many essential vitamins and minerals, low-carbohydrate diets can cause an effect known as ketoacidosis, which can result in decreased insulin secretion. This would be an issue for clients who generally require an increase in energy intake.
Those who exclude animal products from their diets, such as vegetarians and vegans.	There are no reported health problems associated with those who follow a diet that includes all essential amino acids and essential fats, but supplementation of vitamin B12, vitamin D, iron and calcium is often advised for the general population whereas supplementation of creatine and beta-alanine is recommended for clients involved in strength training or high-intensity exercise.
Those who are pregnant or lactating.	Do not set weight loss goals during pregnancy (on average add an extra 300Kcals/day). Constipation is common, so advise fibre-rich foods. Avoid high-sodium foods that increase water retention. Excessive intake of vitamin A can be toxic. No alcohol, caffeine, liver, soft cheese, pâté, raw eggs, certain fish (due to risk of mercury intake).
Older people.	One of the main concerns for older people is osteoporosis. Ensure sufficient intake of calcium and vitamin D for bone strength and carbohydrate to support the exercise required.

Eating disorders

Even though the area of eating disorders can be sensitive, it is important that the practitioner has a level of understanding, as having an eating disorder is associated with significant mortality. It is also widely acknowledged that there is an association between sports participation and eating disorders and that those who have eating disorders have shorter careers. Eating disorders include *anorexia nervosa* (AN), *bulimia nervosa* (BN) and eating disorders not otherwise specified (EDNOS).

- **Anorexia nervosa** – This is a condition characterised by extreme dieting, a refusal to maintain a normal weight for age and height (less than 85% of expected), a body image distortion, amenorrhea (menstrual irregularities, in women) and a fear of gaining weight that usually develops during adolescence.

- **Bulimia nervosa** – This is an eating disorder characterised by binge eating, excessive exercise, and purging (often by vomiting or the use of laxatives that occurs on average at least twice per week for 3 months).
- **EDNOS** – This is similar to AN and BN but may not meet all the criteria, even though there is a general decrease in level of functioning.

The literature also refers to a category of anorexia athletica (AA), which has different criteria. For example, there is no criterion for the 85% cut-off, as many clients who suffer from eating disorders have a greater lean body mass and may not be below this cut-off point.

It is difficult to quantify the number of individuals with eating disorders for many reasons, such as inaccurate measurement tools and under-reporting. Factors

Table 30.2 COMMON DIETS AND ASSOCIATED HEALTH ISSUES

Marketing claim	Associated health issue
Low-carb diets **(i.e. the Atkins diet or ketogenic diets)**	
Claims that fat will be used more readily if no carbs are available, and that appetite is suppressed due to **ketones**.	Fat content in the diet is often high, leading to increased lipid levels and high caloric content. Acidosis often occurs due to ketones, leading to potential kidney problems. Loss of lean tissue due to protein used as main fuel. Side effects include nausea, vomiting and fatigue.
Food-combining diets	
Suggests it is better not to mix carbs and protein in the same meal because enzymes work better in isolation.	Little scientific evidence to support claims. Not feasible to maintain for long periods.
Severe low-calorie (fasting) diets	
Claims that severe calorie restriction will help to break dietary habits and promote quick weight loss, such as the 5:2 diet.	Weight loss can be severe and nutrient intake depleted, leading to a range of health issues. Lean tissue loss is also common, as is reduced insulin sensitivity.
High-fibre diets	
Based on the concept of fibre expanding and creating a feeling of being full, thus reducing appetite.	High fibre intake can reduce mineral absorption and cause bowel discomfort. High water intake is needed to help passage through the colon.
Food-focused diets **(i.e. grapefruit, cabbage soup, Paleo etc.)**	
• Claims that certain foods can increase fat metabolism and are low in caloric content. • The Paleo diet (also known as the hunter-gatherer diet) has a focus on foods believed to have been consumed by our ancestors and claims a range of benefits, such as weight loss and improved blood sugar control, reduced inflammation and improved gut health.	• Severe lack of many essential nutrients as well as many other side effects, such as fainting, which can all occur quickly into the diet. • The following have been linked to the Paleo diet: high saturated fat intake, nutrient deficiencies and increased LDL cholesterol levels.

Table 30.3	**CHARACTERISTICS AND POTENTIAL EFFECTS OF ANOREXIA NERVOSA AND BULIMIA NERVOSA**
Characteristics	**Potential effects**

Anorexia nervosa

Characteristics	Potential effects
Physical: • Extreme weight loss (85% less of expected) • Growth retardation, delay in puberty • Increase in facial and body hair • Constantly restless **Psychological:** • Fear of weight gain • Denial of condition • Low self-esteem and self-worth • Depression, anxiety • Distorted body image (think they are bigger) **Behavioural:** • Obsessive behaviour (i.e. exercise, calorie counting) • Social withdrawal • Poor appetite	• Amenorrhoea (menstrual irregularities) • Reduced performance (aerobic/anaerobic and strength) • Increased risk of infection due to compromised immune system • Greater risk of osteoporosis due to decrease in bone density • Dehydration (lack of water content in foods) • Electrolyte (i.e. sodium and potassium) imbalance, which can lead to conditions such as cardiac arrhythmias (irregular heartbeat) and hypotension (low blood pressure) • Effects such as gastrointestinal problems, thin, brittle hair and itchy skin • Reduced **basal metabolic rate** • Hepatic steatosis – fatty infiltration of the liver

Bulimia nervosa

Characteristics	Potential effects
Physical: • Food bingeing followed by vomiting • Laxative abuse • Visible tooth decay • Facial swelling • Regular weight fluctuations **Psychological:** • Guilt after food bingeing • Low self-esteem and self-worth • Depression and often anger • Distorted body image (think they are bigger) **Behavioural:** • Impulsive • Obsessive exercise behaviour • Frequent weighing	• Amenorrhoea (menstrual irregularities) due to hormonal disruption • Enamel erosion as a result of acid reflux during vomiting leading to tooth decay and gum disease • Dehydration as a result of regular vomiting leading to gastrointestinal and bowel problems • Electrolyte (i.e. sodium and potassium) imbalance, which can lead to cardiac problems and hypotension (low blood pressure) • Fainting due to lack of energy • Visual indications include swollen glands and bags under the eyes • Inflammation of the oesophagus

Anorexia athletica

Characteristics	Potential effects
Fear of weight gain (even if lean): Restricted calorie intake: Excessive or compulsive exercise:	• Weight is 5% or more below expected • Weight is above anorexic threshold due to muscular development • Distorted body image • Interspersed with planned binges • Usually with other weight control strategies • Menstrual dysfunction, which may include delayed puberty • Gastrointestinal issues

that promote performance excellence can also overlap with those that increase the risk of eating disorders. In the general population the majority of those with AN tend to be younger females, although it is thought that approximately 1 in 20 males have the condition. Similarly, there are males with BN, but the majority are still females.

It is useful to be aware of the common characteristics of both conditions (as shown in table 30.3) so that informed referral to a suitably qualified practitioner can take place. For guidelines on how to approach a client who may have an eating disorder, the reader is directed to the work of Johnson (1994) and Garner (1998). Many sports nutrition textbooks also include a section on eating disorders. The practitioner must therefore be mindful to adopt practices that can reduce risk, identify problems early and facilitate appropriate referral.

Take-home messages

- Dietary issues can be sensitive (e.g. yo-yo dieting; eating disorders).

- There are potential health and performance implications of severe energy restriction and weight loss.

- Practitioners should recognise the signs and symptoms of disordered eating and awareness of healthy eating patterns and be familiar with guidance on managing users with suspected eating disorders.

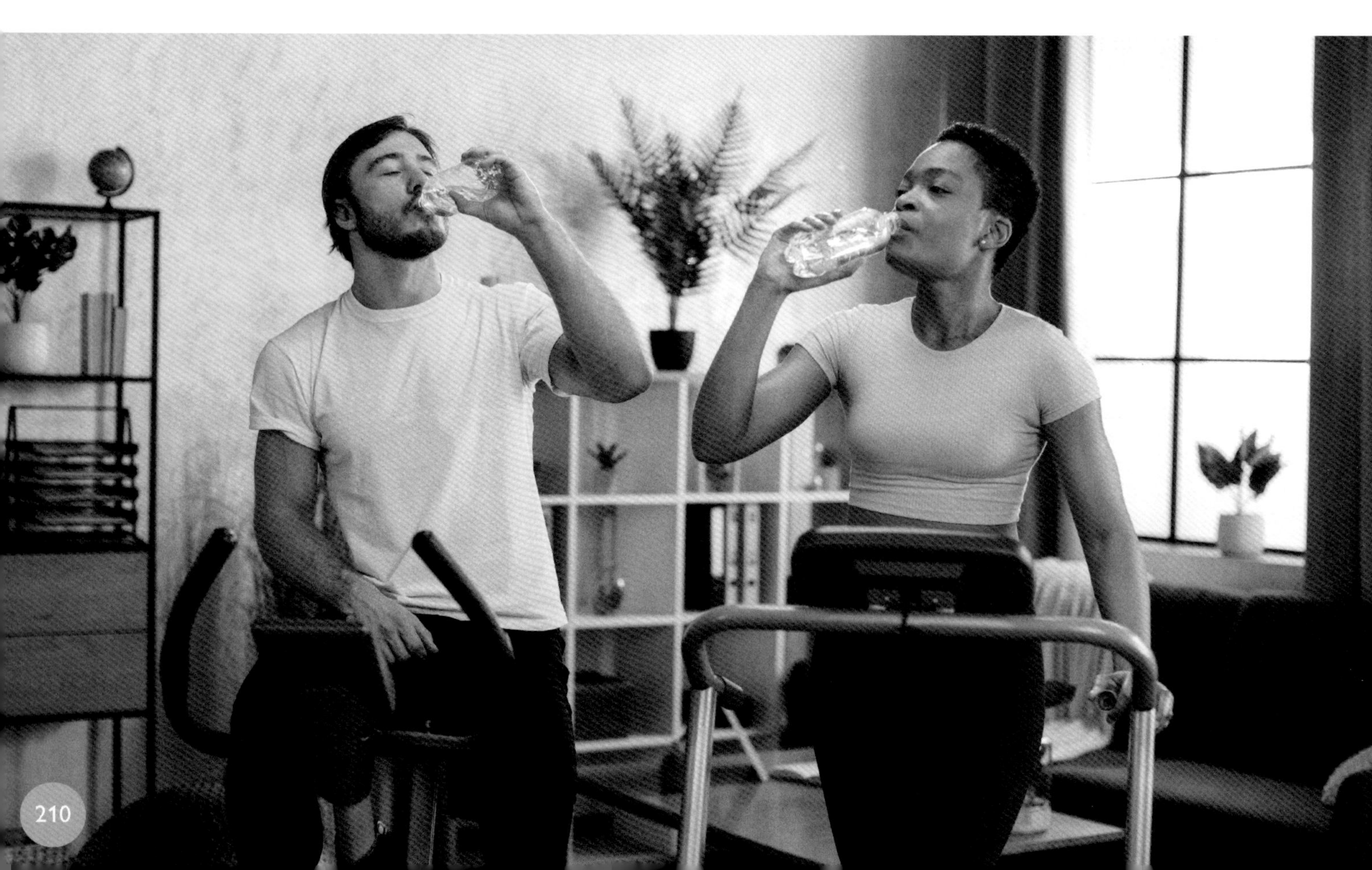

//Energy balance

Introduction

When providing diet plans or offering nutritional advice, S&C practitioners must understand energy balance and the relationship between input (diet) and output (homeostatic function + exercise expenditure). Moreover, practitioners may be required to calculate diet plans based on this so they must understand the key components in regard to energy expenditure.

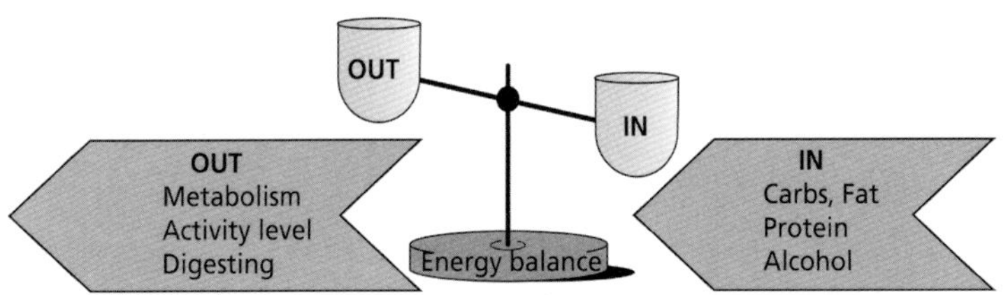

Figure 31.1 The energy balance equation

Energy balance

Energy balance is a complex topic but generally describes the balance between energy intake (in the form of food) and energy expenditure (in terms of energy stores used for normal function and activity). In simplistic terms, if the amount of energy taken in daily is greater than the amount of energy expended then it is likely that the excess energy will result in weight gain. This is known as a positive energy balance. Having a positive energy balance does not always result in weight gain, though, so practitioners should use energy balance estimations with a degree of caution. Having said that, small changes in energy intake and expenditure can arrest weight gain in the majority of people. Energy output and energy input can be estimated in units of calories.

ESTIMATING ENERGY OUTPUT

To determine the daily amount of energy required (calories from food) you will need to estimate how many calories might be used (known as energy output

STEP A – Active metabolic rate

Select one of the options for the level of daily exercise of the client (*see below for level descriptions*):

Sedentary	Lightly active	Moderate active	Very active	Extremely active
M F	**M F**	**M F**	**M F**	**M F**
1.3 1.3	1.6 1.5	1.7 1.6	2.1 1.9	2.4 2.2

STEP B – Basal metabolic rate

Calculate the BMR found in the table below (in Kcals):

Age range	Males	Females
10–17 yrs	(17.7 × W) + 657	(13.4 × W) + 692
18–29 yrs	(15.1 × W) + 692	(14.8 × W) + 487
30–59 yrs	(11.5 × W) + 873	(8.3 × W) + 846
60–74 yrs	(11.9 × W) + 700	(9.2 × W) + 687
75+ yrs	(8.4 × W) + 821	(9.8 × W) + 624

W = *weight in kg.*

STEP C – Consumption of food

Digestion of food requires a certain amount of energy, therefore add an extra 10% of the total from steps A and B. **Total energy expenditure = (Step A × Step B) + (0.1 × Step A × Step B)**

Client name:		Date:	
Step A =	Step B =	A × B =	+ 10% of A × B =

TEE = ... **Kcals**

Figure 31.2 Estimated TEE record sheet (adapted from Schofield, 1985)

or energy expenditure). Energy expenditure calculated on a daily basis is known as total energy expenditure (TEE). TEE is made up of three components.

1. **Active metabolic rate** – The amount of energy your body uses during physical activity.
2. **Basal metabolic rate** – The amount of energy your body uses at rest to maintain essential functions.
3. **Consumption of food** – Also known as the thermic effect of food (TEF), this is the amount of energy you use to digest and process the food you eat.

There are many methods used to estimate TEE, such as that adapted from Schofield's work in 1985. This can be done by following steps A to C shown in figure 31.2. Level descriptions for step A are as follows:

- **Sedentary** – Physically inactive in both work and leisure.
- **Lightly active** – Daily routine includes some walking, or intense exercise once or twice per week.
- **Moderate active** – Intense exercise lasting 20–45 minutes at least three time per week, or a job with a lot of walking, or a moderate-intensity job.
- **Very active** – Intense exercise lasting at least an hour per day, or a heavy physical job.
- **Extremely active** – Such as a sportsperson or a person with a very physically demanding job.

Note: There are other prediction equations that can be used to estimate energy expenditure at rest, such as the Harris–Benedict equation (where weight is in kg, height is in cm and age is in years):

Men: BMR (Kcals) = 66.47 + 13.75(weight) + 5.0(height) − 6.75(age)

Women: BMR (Kcals) = 665.09 + 9.56(weight) + 1.84(height) − 4.67(age)

ESTIMATING ENERGY INPUT

Since estimating energy input requires collection of client information it is essential that confidentiality is addressed when collecting and storing the information. One method of gathering nutritional information is using food diaries, such as the one shown in figure 31.3. The minimum time recommended for keeping a food diary is 7 days, as dietary habits can change throughout the week. When interpreting food diaries, it is important that they include detailed information, such as:

- Snacks
- How the food was cooked, e.g. fried, boiled, grilled
- Sauces and spreads, such as cream, tomato-based and butter
- Alcohol, as this contains calories
- Detail, i.e. what exactly was in a salad and what type of milk was used on cereal

To estimate the average daily intake, the calorie content of the food must be recorded in the diary for each 24-hour period. It is therefore important to instruct clients to keep (or photograph) labels from food wrappers and containers. For foods that do not have this information there are many websites that offer information on the energy content of specific food items. There will always be errors in this type of estimation, as not all software is developed using evidence-based knowledge (and could be biased by suppliers who sponsor the software).

DAILY FOOD DIARY

Time of day	Food or fluid consumed	Food group	Amount (g) or portion size	Kilocals
Morning				
Midday				
Evening				
			Total Kcal =	
Client name:		Date:		
Activity level:				

Figure 31.3 Typical daily food diary (for a blank template, please visit: bloomsbury.com/uk/complete-guide-to-strength-and-conditioning-training-9781399421362)

Take-home messages

- Practitioners should understand the components of energy expenditure and the energy balance equation and know how to determine basal metabolic rate (BMR).

- Practitioners should know how to determine daily energy requirements based on physical activity levels.

APPENDICES

APPENDIX 1
Template for needs analysis and training session considerations

CLIENT ANALYSIS				
Client status	**Training history**	**Training frequency (per week)**	**Training intensity**	**Training type**

SPORT/EVENT ANALYSIS				
Sport details	**Kinematics**	**An/aerobic**	**Power**	**Muscular**

Steps	Category information
Space	
Time/task	
Equipment	
People/players	
Specificity	

APPENDIX 2

Sample programmes of hybrid sports that require the training of multiple components.

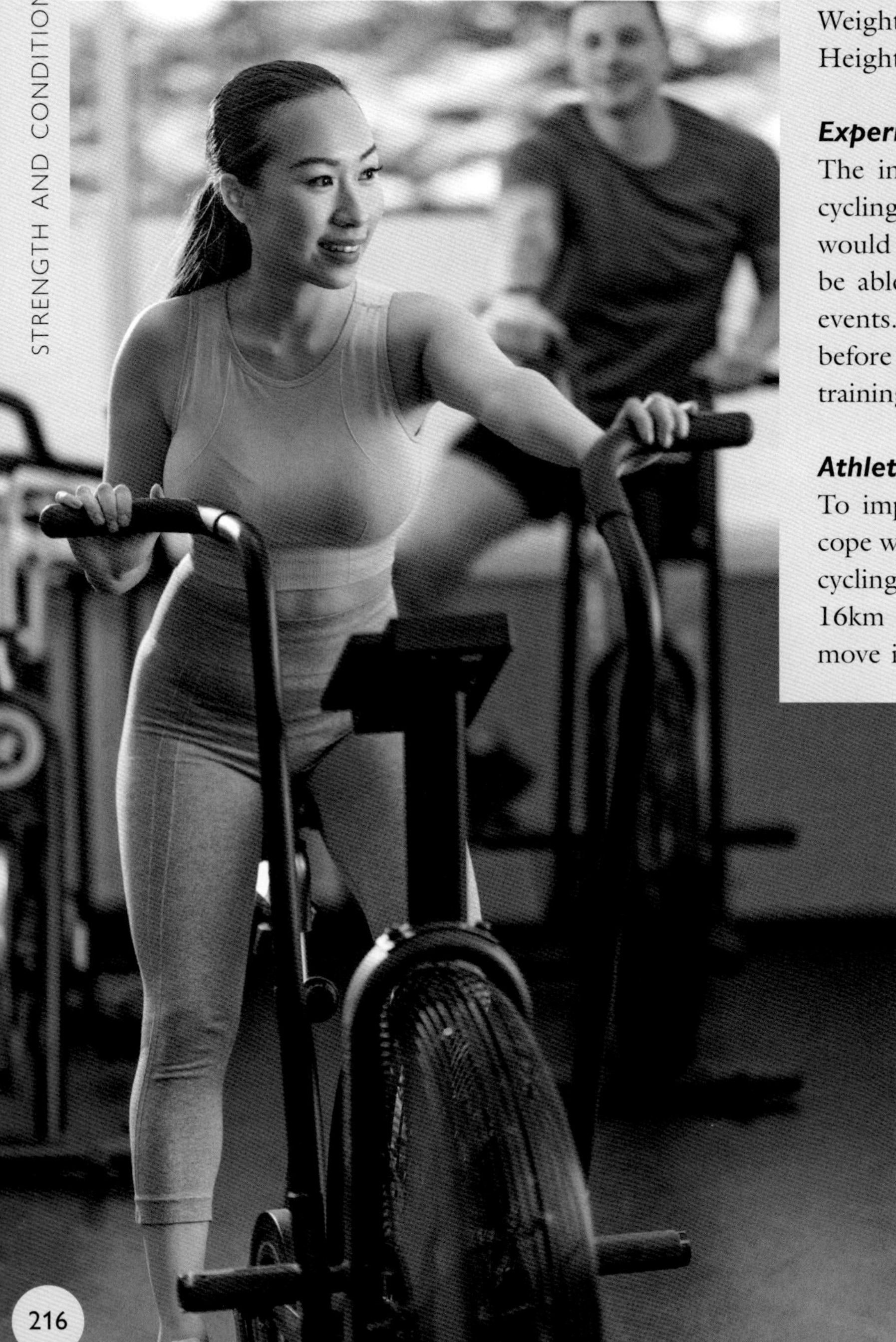

Aerobic endurance programme – amateur road cyclist

Athlete details:
Gender: Male
Age: 30
Weight: 70kg
Height: 175cm

Experience:
The individual has competed in amateur road cycling time trial events for over 10 years but would like to develop his aerobic capacity to be able to compete in longer endurance-based events. He has not had a periodised training plan before and is enthusiastic about developing his training to help him compete in longer events.

Athlete goals:
To improve their aerobic capacity so they can cope with the demands of long endurance-based cycling races. The athlete currently trains for 16km (10-mile) time-trial events but wants to move into competing in longer events.

Training plan:

MACROCYCLE

Main goals: Increase aerobic endurance while maintaining force and power production. Develop upper-body strength and core stabilisation to improve force transfer. Maintain flexibility and body composition.
Tests: VO_2max (aerobic endurance). 5RM (strength). TA contraction (core stability). Sit and reach (flexibility). Skinfolds (body composition).

Jan				Feb				March				April			
Week				Week				Week				Week			
1	2	3	4	1	2	3	4	1	2	3	4	1	2	3	4

MESOCYCLES

Foundation	Development	Conditioning	Performance
• Baseline testing. • Introduce core stabilisation. • Introduce cardio (aerobic). • Assess resistance training ability. • Use light weights to develop ligament strength.	• Increase the volume of core stability exercises. • Increase the cardio (aerobic) volume and intensity. • Build up the volume and intensity of weights for strength endurance.	• Re-test at the end of week 4. Increase the challenge of core stability exercises. • Introduce anaerobic exercises to support the aerobic programme. • Increase the intensity and volume (weights).	• Progress to using a stability ball as the bench and introduce plyometric upper-body exercises. • Increase the intensity of anaerobic and aerobic endurance training. • Maintain the intensity and volume of strength endurance training.

MICROCYCLES

Wk 1	Wk 2	Wk 3	Wk 4	Wk 1	Wk 2	Wk 3	Wk 4	Wk 1	Wk 2	Wk 3	Wk 4	Wk 1	Wk 2	Wk 3	Wk 4
CS1	CS1	CS1	CS1	CS2	CS2	CS2	CS2	CS3	CS3	CS3	CS3	CS4	CS4	CS4	CS4
WB1	WB1	WB1	WB1	WB2	WB2	WB2	WB2	WB2	WB2	WB2	WB2	WB3	WB3	WB3	WB3
LB1	LB1	LB1	LB1	CS3	CS3	CS3	CS3	CS4	CS4	CS4	CS4	CS5	CS5	CS5	CS5

CS = Cardio session   LB = Lower body   WB = Whole body

Specificity = ✓	Adaptation = ✓	Overload = ✓	Progression = ✓	Regression = ✓	Individuality = ✓	Recovery = ✓

MICROCYCLE (CARDIOVASCULAR)

Client name:

Mesocycle: **Microcycle week:**

	Exercise	Duration	Intensity (RM)	Comment
Cardio 1	Warm-up – light cycle	10 mins	RPE 2–3	
	HR zone 2 cycling	45 mins	RPE 3–5	A pace that can be maintained comfortably.
	HR zone 3 cycling	10 mins	RPE 6–7	Maintain cycling technique and trunk control.
	HR zone 2 cycling	45 mins	RPE 3–5	A pace that can be maintained. comfortably.
	HR zone 3 cycling	10 mins	RPE 6–7	Maintain cycling technique and trunk control.
	Cool-down – light cycle	10 mins	RPE 2–3	
Cardio 2	Warm-up – light cycle	10 mins	RPE 2–3	
	HR zone 2 cycling	45 mins	RPE 3–5	A pace that can be maintained comfortably.
	HR zone 3 cycling	30 mins	RPE 6–7	Maintain cycling technique and trunk control.
	HR zone 2 cycling	45 mins	RPE 3–5	A pace that can be maintained comfortably.
	Cool-down – light cycle	10 mins	RPE 2–3	
Cardio 3	Warm-up – light cycle	10 mins	RPE 2–3	Warm-up – light cycle.
	HR zone 2 cycling	45 mins	RPE 3–5	A pace that can be maintained comfortably.
	HR zone 3 cycling	30 mins	RPE 6–7	Maintain cycling technique and trunk control.

Cardio 3 *(cont.)*	HR zone 4 cycling	5 mins	RPE 8+	Focus on speed maintenance.
	HR zone 2 cycling	5 mins	RPE 3–5	A pace that can be maintained comfortably.
	HR zone 4 cycling	5 mins	RPE 8+	Focus on speed maintenance.
	Cool-down – light cycle	10 mins	RPE 2–3	Cool-down – light cycle.
Cardio 4	Warm-up – light cycle	10 mins	RPE 2–3	Warm-up – light cycle.
	HR zone 2 cycling	45 mins	RPE 3–5	A pace that can be maintained comfortably.
	HR zone 4–5 cycling	5 mins	RPE 8+	Focus on speed maintenance.
	HR zone 2 cycling	5 mins	RPE 3–5	A pace that can be maintained comfortably.
	HR zone 4–5 cycling	5 mins	RPE 8+	Focus on speed maintenance.
	HR zone 2 cycling	5 mins	RPE 3–5	A pace that can be maintained comfortably.
	HR zone 4–5 cycling	5 mins	RPE 8+	Focus on speed maintenance.
	HR zone 2 cycling	5 mins	RPE 3–5	A pace that can be maintained comfortably.
	HR zone 4–5 cycling	5 mins	RPE 8+	Focus on speed maintenance.
	Cool-down – light cycle	10 mins	RPE 2–3	Cool-down – light cycle.
Cardio 5	Warm-up – light cycle	10 mins	RPE 2–3	Warm-up – light cycle.
	HR zone 2 cycling	45 mins	RPE 3–5	A pace that can be maintained comfortably.
	HR zone 3 cycling	45 mins	RPE 6–7	Maintain cycling technique and trunk control.
	HR zone 2 cycling	15 mins	RPE 3–5	A pace that can be maintained comfortably.
	Cool-down – light cycle	10 mins	RPE 2–3	Cool-down – light cycle.

Anaerobic endurance programme – grass hockey player – anaerobic capacity training

Athlete details:

Gender: Female
Age: 25
Weight: 70kg
Height: 170cm

Experience:

The athlete is an accomplished field hockey player who is aiming to move to a team in a higher league. The league is more physically demanding and is played at a higher pace and requires the athlete to cover more running distance at higher running speeds.

Athlete goals:

The athlete would like to develop their ability to perform repeated high-speed runs and sprints in preparation for moving to their new team in the upcoming season. This will include developing the athlete's anaerobic capacity to enable them to be able to perform repeated high-speed runs with minimal time for recovery between efforts.

Training plan:

MACROCYCLE

Main goals: Increase anaerobic endurance. Increase repeated sprint and high-speed running capacity.
Tests: Onset blood lactate (anaerobic endurance). Intermittent fitness tests – 30–15 IFT/Yo-yo, lower-body strength tests (specifically posterior chain).

June				July				August				September			
Week				Week				Week				Week			
1	2	3	4	1	2	3	4	1	2	3	4	1	2	3	4

MESOCYCLES

Foundation	Development	Conditioning	Performance
• Baseline testing. • Introduce core stabilisation and flexibility exercises. • Introduce HIIT-style anaerobic cardio. • Assess resistance training ability. • Use light weights to develop ligament strength.	• Increase the volume of core stability exercises. • Increase the anaerobic HIIT cardio volume and intensity. • Build up the volume and intensity of weights for strength endurance.	• Re-test at the end of week 4. • Increase the challenge of core stability exercises. • Increase anaerobic HIIT cardio volume. Introduce repeated sprint training. • Increase the intensity/decrease the volume – eccentric posterior chain focus.	• Introduce plyometric lower-body exercises. • Increase the intensity of repeated sprint training. Maintain the intensity/decrease the volume – eccentric posterior chain focus.

MICROCYCLES

Wk 1	Wk 2	Wk 3	Wk 4	Wk 1	Wk 2	Wk 3	Wk 4	Wk 1	Wk 2	Wk 3	Wk 4	Wk 1	Wk 2	Wk 3	Wk 4
CS1	CS1	CS1	CS1	CS1/2	CS1/2	CS1/2	CS1/2	CS2/3	CS2/3	CS2/3	CS2/3	CS2/3	CS2/3	CS2/3	CS2/3
UB1	UB1	UB1	UB1	WB1	WB1	WB1	WB1	WB2	WB2	WB2	WB2	WB3	WB3	WB3	WB3
LB1	LB1	LB1	LB1	CS1/2	CS1/2	CS1/2	CS1/2	CS2/3	CS2/3	CS2/3	CS2/3	CS2/3	CS2/3	CS2/3	CS2/3

CS = Cardio session UB = Upper body LB = Lower body WB = Whole body

Specificity	Adaptation	Overload	Progression	Regression	Individuality	Recovery
= ✓	= ✓	= ✓	= ✓	= ✓	= ✓	= ✓

MICROCYCLE (CARDIO – ANAEROBIC/REPEATED SPRINT)

Client name:

Mesocycle: **Microcycle week:**

	Exercise		**Intensity (RM)**		**Comment**
Cardio 1	Warm-up Ground-based movements + 10 mins' light jogging	2	Sets	2 × 10m per exercise	Bear crawls, walkouts, Spiderman crawls, deep squats, lunges (forwards, backwards, lateral).
	HIIT set 1	1	Sets	30/30 secs work/rest × 10 reps	Linear running (on a pitch or treadmill) @50–60% max speed.
	HIIT set 2	1	Sets	15/15 secs work/rest × 10 reps	Linear running (on a pitch or treadmill) @60–70% max speed.
	HIIT set 3	1	Sets	15/15 secs work/rest × 10 reps	Linear running (on a pitch or treadmill) @60–70% max speed.
	HIIT set 4	1	Sets	20/10 secs work/rest × 10 reps	Linear running (on a pitch or treadmill) @60–70% max speed.
	Mobility and flexibility	3	Sets	30-sec holds for static stretches 8–12 reps for dynamic stretches	Focus on main lower-body muscle groups – hamstrings, quadriceps, glutes, adductors and abductors, calves. Start with dynamic stretches and finish with static stretches.
Cardio 2	Warm-up Ground-based movements + 10 mins' light jogging + acceleration drills to prepare for sprints	2	Sets	2 × 10m per exercise	Bear crawls, walkouts, Spiderman crawls, deep squats, lunges (forwards, backwards, lateral). A skips, B skips, rolling 10m accelerations × 2, rolling 20m accelerations × 2.
	HIIT set 1	1	Sets	20/10 secs work/rest × 10 reps	Linear running (on a pitch or treadmill) @60–70% max speed.

Cardio 2 (*cont.*)	Sprint exposure	1	Sets	2 × 20m sprints 2 × 30m sprints	The athlete should aim for 90% of max speed exposure during these sprints – with an aim of increasing this to a max sprint later in the mesocycle. The rest between each sprint should allow for full recovery. This may require 1–2 mins' rest between reps depending on the profile of the athlete – practitioners should assess this with their client.
	HIIT set 2	1	Sets	20/10 secs work/rest × 10 reps	Linear running (on a pitch or treadmill) @60–70% max speed.
	HIIT set 3	1	Sets	15/15 secs work/rest × 10 reps	Linear running (on a pitch or treadmill) @70–80% max speed.
	HIIT set 4	1	Sets	15/15 secs work/rest × 10 reps	Acceleration and deceleration circuit (on a pitch) while dribbling a hockey ball – practitioner to design a specific circuit to represent cutting and turning movements that may mimic what the athlete would do during a hockey match.
	Mobility and flexibility	3	Sets	30-sec holds for static stretches 8–12 reps for dynamic stretches	Focus on main lower-body muscle groups – hamstrings, quadriceps, glutes, adductors and abductors, calves. Start with dynamic stretches and finish with static stretches.
Cardio 3	Warm-up Ground-based movements + 10 mins' light jogging + acceleration drills to prepare for sprints	2	Sets	2 × 10m per exercise	Bear crawls, walkouts, Spiderman crawls, deep squats, lunges (forwards, backwards, lateral). A skips, B skips, rolling 10m accelerations × 2, rolling 20m accelerations × 2.
	Sprint exposure	1	Sets	2 × 20m sprints 2 × 30m sprints	The athlete should aim for 95%+ of max speed exposure during these sprints. The rest between each sprint should allow for full recovery. This may require 1–2 mins' rest between reps depending on the profile of the athlete – practitioners should assess this with their client.

Cardio 3 (*cont.*)	HIIT set 1	1	Sets	20/10 secs work/rest × 10 reps	Linear running (on a pitch or treadmill) @60–70% max speed.
	HIIT set 2	1	Sets	20/10 secs work/rest × 10 reps	Linear running (on a pitch or treadmill) @60–70% max speed.
	HIIT set 3	1	Sets	15/15 secs work/rest × 10 reps	Acceleration and deceleration circuit (on a pitch) while dribbling a hockey ball – practitioner to design a specific circuit to represent cutting and turning movements that may mimic what the athlete would do during a hockey match.
	HIIT set 4	1	Sets	15/15 secs work/rest × 10 reps	Acceleration and deceleration circuit (on a pitch) while dribbling a hockey ball – practitioner to design a specific circuit to represent cutting and turning movements that may mimic what the athlete would do during a hockey match.
	Mobility and flexibility	3	Sets	30-sec holds for static stretches 8–12 reps for dynamic stretches	Focus on main lower-body muscle groups – hamstrings, quadriceps, glutes, adductors and abductors, calves. Start with dynamic stretches and finish with static stretches.

Note: Practitioners should allow for adequate recovery between each set of HIIT and sprints. The duration of rest will differ depending on the current fitness levels of the athlete and the intensity of the previous set of exercise. A rest of 2–3 minutes between sets would be considered as a normal period of time within these high-intensity training sessions.

It is important for practitioners to consider the condition of the athlete before prescribing sprint training. Within the foundation block of training, before the athlete has sprint exposure prescribed within their training, the practitioner should consider programming exercises that target force and power development in the posterior chain muscles and specifically the glutes and hamstrings. Eccentric hamstring and glute exercises such as hip thrusts, Romanian dead lifts and Nordic hamstring exercises have been shown to reduce hamstring injury risks. Therefore, this will help to minimise the risks of injury caused by sprinting for the athlete.

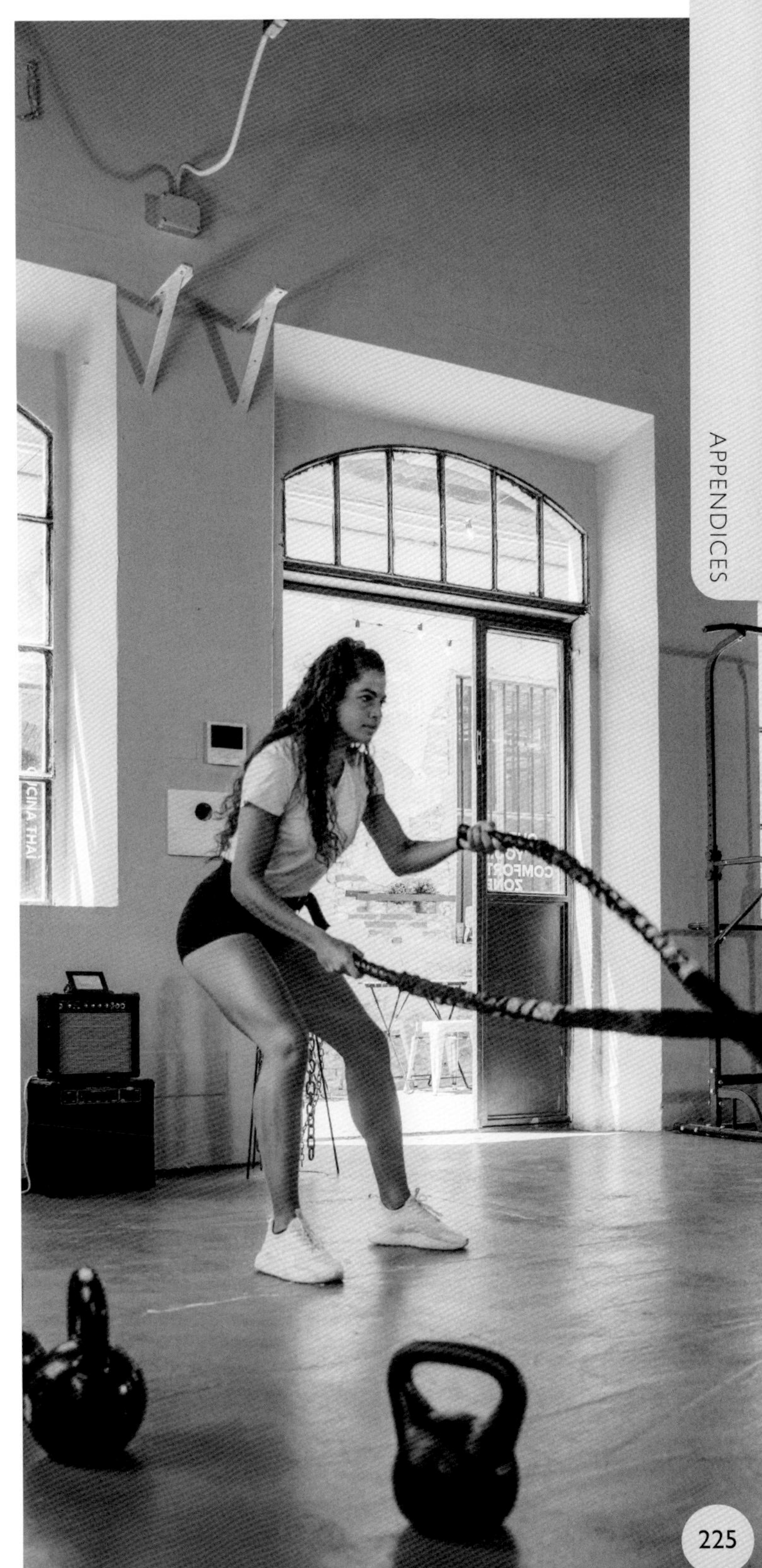

Core stabilisation programme
– amateur tennis player

Athlete details:
Gender: Male
Age: 19
Weight: 80kg
Height: 180cm

Experience:
The client is a regional-level amateur tennis player with no prior experience of S&C training.

Athlete goals:
The athlete and their coach feel that they have good lower- and upper-body strength but have weak core stabilisation and lack the ability to transfer power through the core during tennis actions such as serving, forehand and backhand striking. Therefore, the athlete would like a programme that will further increase their whole-body strength and power outputs but will also focus on strengthening their core and increasing their ability to transfer strength and power through this system for tennis.

Training plan:

<table>
<tr><td colspan="16" align="center">MACROCYCLE</td></tr>
<tr><td colspan="16">Main goals: Increase whole-body strength and power outputs. Develop core stability and rotation.
Tests: 5RM (strength). Power tests. TA contraction (core stability). Sorenson test.</td></tr>
<tr><td colspan="4" align="center">January</td><td colspan="4" align="center">February</td><td colspan="4" align="center">March</td><td colspan="4" align="center">April</td></tr>
<tr><td colspan="4" align="center">Week</td><td colspan="4" align="center">Week</td><td colspan="4" align="center">Week</td><td colspan="4" align="center">Week</td></tr>
<tr><td>1</td><td>2</td><td>3</td><td>4</td><td>1</td><td>2</td><td>3</td><td>4</td><td>1</td><td>2</td><td>3</td><td>4</td><td>1</td><td>2</td><td>3</td><td>4</td></tr>
</table>

<table>
<tr><td colspan="4" align="center">MESOCYCLES</td></tr>
<tr><td>Foundation</td><td>Development</td><td>Conditioning</td><td>Performance</td></tr>
<tr>
<td>
<ul>
<li>Baseline testing.</li>
<li>Introduce core stabilisation and flexibility exercises.</li>
<li>Assess resistance training ability.</li>
<li>Use light weights to develop ligament strength.</li>
</ul>
</td>
<td>
<ul>
<li>Increase the volume of core stability exercises.</li>
<li>Build up the volume and intensity of weights for hypertrophy.</li>
</ul>
</td>
<td>
<ul>
<li>Re-test at the end of week 4.</li>
<li>Increase the challenge of core stability exercises with a focus on rotational exercises.</li>
<li>Increase the intensity/decrease the volume to develop power outputs.</li>
</ul>
</td>
<td>
<ul>
<li>Maintain the intensity and the challenge of core stability exercises with a focus on tennis-specific movements (e.g. lateral rotation and bracing).</li>
</ul>
</td>
</tr>
</table>

<table>
<tr><td colspan="16" align="center">MICROCYCLES</td></tr>
<tr><td>Wk 1</td><td>Wk 2</td><td>Wk 3</td><td>Wk 4</td><td>Wk 1</td><td>Wk 2</td><td>Wk 3</td><td>Wk 4</td><td>Wk 1</td><td>Wk 2</td><td>Wk 3</td><td>Wk 4</td><td>Wk 1</td><td>Wk 2</td><td>Wk 3</td><td>Wk 4</td></tr>
<tr><td>WB1</td><td>WB1</td><td>WB1</td><td>WB1</td><td>WB2</td><td>WB2</td><td>WB2</td><td>WB2</td><td>WB3</td><td>WB3</td><td>WB3</td><td>WB3</td><td>WB4</td><td>WB4</td><td>WB4</td><td>WB4</td></tr>
<tr><td>CS1</td><td>CS1</td><td>CS1</td><td>CS1</td><td>CS2</td><td>CS2</td><td>CS2</td><td>CS2</td><td>CS2/3</td><td>CS2/3</td><td>CS2/3</td><td>CS2/3</td><td>CS3</td><td>CS3</td><td>CS3</td><td>CS3</td></tr>
</table>

WB = Whole body CS = Core Stabilisation

Specificity = ✓	Adaptation = ✓	Overload = ✓	Progression = ✓	Regression = ✓	Individuality = ✓	Recovery = ✓

MICROCYCLE (CORE STABILISATION AND ROTATION)				
Client name:				
Mesocycle:				**Microcycle week:**
	Exercise	**Intensity (RM)**		**Comment**
CS1	Warm-up – mobility and flexibility	2	Sets	8–10 reps of dynamic mobility exercises to develop core rotation and mobility	Press-up scapula shrugs, cat/cows, Spiderman rotations, Supermans, kneeling thoracic rotations against a wall, shoulder internal and external rotation.
	Dead bugs	3	Sets	6–8 reps per side	Alternate hands and feet extending from neutral position.
	Palof press (cable)	3	Sets	5 reps per side	The exercise is designed to teach core bracing – cue to not allow the resistance on the cable to cause rotation.
	Plank to lateral plank transfers	3	Sets	5 per side	Transferring from a plank to a lateral plank through controlled core stabilisation and rotation. Cue to keep the body and legs in line – don't allow the hips to drop.
	Farmer's walk – single-arm dumbbell	3	Sets	2 × 20m per arm	Self-selected weight. Keep the core stable and the body aligned with the load on one side of the body.
	Medicine ball slams	3	Sets	8–10 reps per side	Cue to slam the medicine ball through the floor from an overhead position. This helps the athlete to understand force transfer through the body – encourage knees to bend as the ball is slammed into the floor.
CS2	Warm-up – mobility and flexibility	2	Sets	8–10 reps of dynamic mobility exercises to develop core rotation and mobility	Press-up scapula shrugs, cat/cows, Spiderman rotations, Supermans, kneeling thoracic rotations against a wall, shoulder internal and external rotation.
	Static bear crawl arm raises	3	Sets	5–8 per arm	Maintain neutral core position without rotation during arm raises.
	Cable or banded core rotations	3	Sets	6–8 per side	This exercise should closely relate to the release phase of a tennis backhand – as the core laterally rotates, the athlete simultaneously drives the hands from hip height across the body.

CS2 (*cont.*)	Bilateral box drop landing with perturbations	3	Sets	5 drop landings	Instruct the athlete to jump from a box (30–40cm) and land on both feet. As they land, the practitioner uses a Swiss ball to apply pressure to the body. The athlete must brace to remain stable in their landing position.
	Press-up position single-arm resistance band row	3	Sets	5 reps per side	Self-select the strength of the resistance band. Maintain neutral core position throughout the exercise.
	Single-arm, standing dumbbell shoulder press	3	Sets	8–10 reps	Ensure core stability during this exercise – the single-arm press will challenge the core to remain activated and aligned during the press.
	Medicine balls lateral rotation throws	3	Sets	6 throws per side	Cue to 'throw the ball through the wall' and to drive from the core rotation.
CS3	Warm-up – mobility and flexibility	2	Sets	8–10 reps of dynamic mobility exercises to develop core rotation and mobility	Press-up scapula shrugs, cat/cows, Spiderman rotations, Supermans, kneeling thoracic rotations against a wall, shoulder internal and external rotation.
	Barbell landmine core rotations with single-arm shoulder press	3	Sets	6 reps per side (12 core rotations)	Focus on the intent of the shoulder press – drive the barbell quickly and use the core as a stable base to generate power. Self-select a weight that does not limit the speed of the shoulder drive.
	Barbell core roll-outs	3	Sets	6–8 reps	Ensure the back is not extending during this exercise, so that the core remains activated and stable throughout.
	Resisted dead bugs	3	Sets	8–10 reps per side	Use a resistance band – held in both hands and pulled back by the coach while the legs extend out maximally one at a time.
	Bear crawls	3	Sets	2 × 10m per set	Maintain neutral core position during the crawl.
	Unilateral box drop landing with perturbations	3	Sets	5 drop landings per side	Instruct the athlete to jump from a box (30–40cm) and land on one foot. As they land, the practitioner uses a Swiss ball to apply pressure to the body. The athlete must brace to remain stable in their landing position.

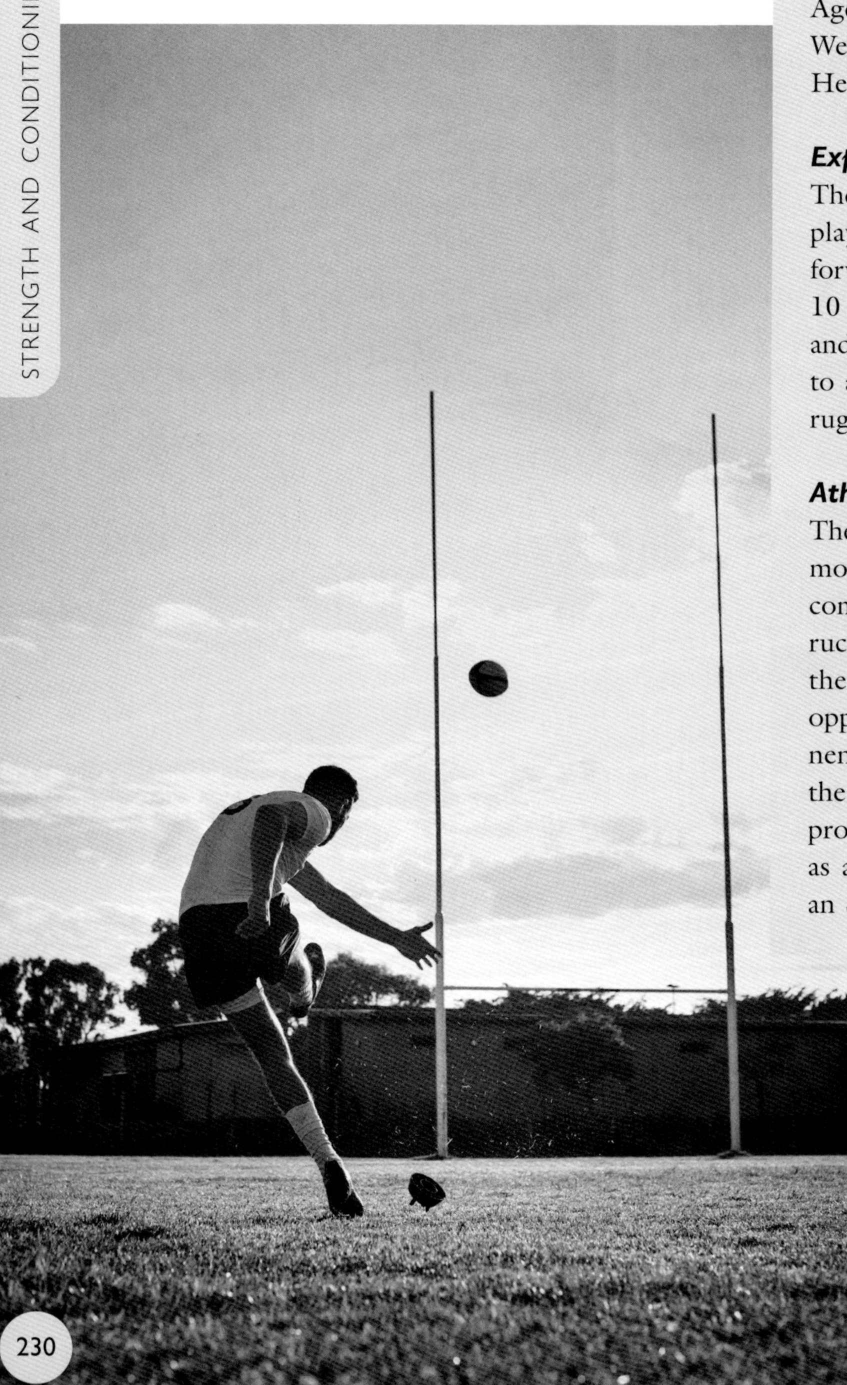

Strength programme
– semi-professional rugby player

Athlete details:
Gender: Male
Age: 23
Weight: 90kg
Height: 185cm

Experience:
The athlete is a semi-professional rugby union player who plays in the second row of the forward pack. They have played rugby for over 10 years and have some experience of strength and conditioning but would like to fully commit to an S&C programme to prepare for the next rugby season.

Athlete goals:
The athlete feels they need to be stronger and more powerful to be more effective during common rugby actions such as tackles, scrums, rucks and mauls. They feel they do not have the same strength capacity as some of their opponents and want to develop this component. They have done some S&C training in the past but have never fully committed to a programme and would like to use the off-season as an opportunity to fully immerse themself in an S&C periodised training programme.

Training plan:

MACROCYCLE

Main goals: Increase holistic strength and power outputs. Develop upper-body strength and core stabilisation.
Tests: 5RM (strength). TA contraction (core stability). Sorenson test (core endurance).

July				August				September				October			
Week				Week				Week				Week			
1	2	3	4	1	2	3	4	1	2	3	4	1	2	3	4

MESOCYCLES

Foundation	Development	Conditioning	Performance
• Baseline testing. • Introduce core stabilisation and flexibility exercises. • Assess resistance training ability. • Use light weights to develop ligament strength.	• Increase the volume of core stability exercises. • Build up the volume and intensity of weights for hypertrophy. • Introduce functional rugby-specific strength and power sessions.	• Re-test at the end of week 4. • Increase the challenge of core stability exercises. • Increase the intensity/ decrease the volume (weights) to develop strength. • Develop rugby-specific strength/power training.	• Progress to using a stability ball as the bench and introduce plyometric upper-body exercises. • Increase the intensity/ decrease the volume further to develop power. • Maintain rugby-specific strength/power training.

MICROCYCLES

Wk 1	Wk 2	Wk 3	Wk 4	Wk 1	Wk 2	Wk 3	Wk 4	Wk 1	Wk 2	Wk 3	Wk 4	Wk 1	Wk 2	Wk 3	Wk 4
WB1	WB1	WB1	WB1	WB2	WB2	WB2	WB2	WB2	WB2	WB2	WB2	WB3	WB3	WB3	WB3
UB1	UB1	UB1	UB1	RS1	RS1	RS1	RS1	RS2	RS2	RS2	RS2	RS3	RS3	RS3	RS3
LB1	LB1	LB1	LB1	LB2	LB2	LB2	LB2	LB2	LB2	LB2	LB2	LB3	LB3	LB3	LB3

UB = Upper body LB = Lower body WB = Whole body RS = Rugby-specific

Specificity = ✓	Adaptation = ✓	Overload = ✓	Progression = ✓	Regression = ✓	Individuality = ✓	Recovery = ✓

MICROCYCLE (RUGBY-SPECIFIC)

Client name:

Mesocycle:

Microcycle week:

	Exercise	Intensity (RM)			Comment
Rugby-specific 1	Warm-up – ground-based movements	2	Sets	2 × 10m per exercise	Bear crawls, walkouts, Spiderman crawls, deep squats, lunges (forwards, backwards, lateral).
	Standing single-arm shoulder press (dumbbell)	3	Sets	6–8 reps per side	Self-selected weight.
	French contrast anterior press – TRX press-ups Press-ups to box	3	Sets	8–12 reps per exercise	Targets strength, power and plyometric development. Start with a very low box (5–10cm).
	Single-arm dumbbell row from a bear crawl stance	3	Sets	6–8 reps per side	Focus on core stabilisation throughout the exercise.
	Resisted sprints – sled pulls/ prowler pushes	4	Sets	2 × 20m sprints	Ensure prolonged rest (>90 secs between sets) to allow for recovery. Self-selected weight. Cue to drive knees into the ground.
	Hip thrusts – barbell or resistance machine	3	Sets	8–12 reps	This exercise is to increase robustness of the posterior chain to minimise injury risks from high-speed running/sprinting.
	Dead bugs	3	Sets	8–12 reps	Maintain neutral spine – make sure the back is not arching from the floor.
Rugby-specific 2	Warm-up – ground-based movements	2	Sets	2 × 10m per exercise	Bear crawls, walkouts, Spiderman crawls, deep squats, lunges (forwards, backwards, lateral).
	Barbell landmine core lateral rotations (bilateral) to single-arm shoulder press	3	Sets	6–8 reps per side	Self-selected weight.
	French contrast anterior press – bench press superset with bench press med ball throws	3	Sets	10 reps per exercise	Targets strength, power and plyometric development.

Rugby-specific 2 (*cont.*)	Resisted sprints – sled pulls/ prowler pushes	4	Sets	2 × 20m sprints	Ensure prolonged rest (>90 secs between sets) to allow for recovery. Increase weight from rugby-specific 1. Cue to drive knees into the ground.
	French contrast posterior chain – split-stance RDL to banded tantrums	3	Sets	8 reps per side RDL 30 secs' max effort tantrums	This exercise is to increase robustness of the posterior chain to minimise injury risks from high-speed running/sprinting.
	Dead bugs	3	Sets	8–12 reps	Maintain neutral spine – make sure the back is not arching from the floor.
Rugby-specific 3	Warm-up – ground-based movements	2	Sets	2 × 10m per exercise	Bear crawls, walkouts, Spiderman crawls, deep squats, lunges (forwards, backwards, lateral).
	Resistance-banded horizontal jumps and vertical jumps	3	Sets	10 horizontal 10 vertical	Minimise ground contact time for vertical jumps.
	Bear crawls with perturbations (pushes and pulls from the coach)	3	Sets	1-minute continuous crawls	Maintain trunk control.
	Weighted dead bugs	3	Sets	8–12 reps	Maintain neutral spine – make sure the back is not arching from the floor. Use a dumbbell held in the hands or, if available, an aqua bag to create instability.
	Barbell front squat with shoulder press	3	Sets	4–6 reps	Focus on rate of force development and speed of movement – use a lower weight if speed is slow.
	Hip thrusts – barbell or resistance machine	3	Sets	4–6 reps	This exercise is to increase robustness of the posterior chain to minimise injury risks from high-speed running/sprinting. Focus on speed of lift – reduce the weight if speed is slow.
	Single-arm dumbbell row from a bear crawl stance	3	Sets	6–8 reps per side	Focus on core stabilisation throughout the exercise.

Speed – rugby player converting from 15s to 7s

Athlete details:
Gender: Female
Age: 21
Weight: 75kg
Height: 175cm

Experience:
The athlete has played rugby union (15s) during their time at university for the last 3 years as a centre. She will continue her studies at the university during the next academic year but will convert from rugby 15s to rugby 7s for the next season.

Athlete goals:
The athlete understands the game of rugby 7s is much faster and requires more high-speed running and sprint running distances than rugby 15s. Therefore, she would like to develop her ability to complete repeated bouts of high-intensity running efforts and sprints while minimising the increased injury risks of increasing high-speed running and sprint distances.

Training plan:

<table>
<tr><td colspan="16" align="center">MACROCYCLE</td></tr>
</table>

Main goals: Increase aerobic and anaerobic endurance. Increase repeated sprint and high-speed running capacity.
Tests: VO_2max (aerobic endurance). Onset blood lactate (anaerobic endurance). Intermittent fitness tests – 30–15 IFT/Yo-yo, lower-body strength tests (specifically posterior chain).

June				July				August				September			
Week				Week				Week				Week			
1	2	3	4	1	2	3	4	1	2	3	4	1	2	3	4

<table>
<tr><td colspan="16" align="center">MESOCYCLES</td></tr>
</table>

Foundation	Development	Conditioning	Performance
<ul><li>Baseline testing.</li><li>Introduce core stabilisation and flexibility exercises.</li><li>Introduce HIIT-style aerobic cardio.</li><li>Assess resistance training ability.</li><li>Use light weights to develop ligament strength.</li></ul>	<ul><li>Increase the volume of core stability exercises.</li><li>Increase aerobic and anaerobic HIIT cardio volume.</li><li>Build up the volume and intensity of weights for hypertrophy.</li></ul>	<ul><li>Re-test at the end of week 4.</li><li>Increase the challenge of core stability exercises.</li><li>Increase aerobic and anaerobic HIIT cardio volume.</li><li>Introduce repeated sprint training.</li><li>Increase the intensity/ decrease the volume – eccentric posterior chain focus.</li></ul>	<ul><li>Introduce plyometric lower-body exercises.</li><li>Increase the intensity of repeated sprint training. Maintain the intensity/decrease the volume – eccentric posterior chain focus.</li></ul>

<table>
<tr><td colspan="16" align="center">MICROCYCLES</td></tr>
</table>

Wk 1	Wk 2	Wk 3	Wk 4	Wk 1	Wk 2	Wk 3	Wk 4	Wk 1	Wk 2	Wk 3	Wk 4	Wk 1	Wk 2	Wk 3	Wk 4
CS1	CS1	CS1	CS1	CS1/2	CS1/2	CS1/2	CS1/2	CS2/3	CS2/3	CS2/3	CS2/3	CS2/3	CS2/3	CS2/3	CS2/3
UB1	UB1	UB1	UB1	LB1/2	LB1/2	LB1/2	LB1/2	LB2/3	LB2/3	LB2/3	LB2/3	LB2/3	LB2/3	LB2/3	LB2/3
LB1	LB1	LB1	LB1	CS1/2	CS1/2	CS1/2	CS1/2	CS2/3	CS2/3	CS2/3	CS2/3	CS2/3	CS2/3	CS2/3	CS2/3

CS = Cardio session UB = Upper body LB = Lower body

Specificity = ✓	Adaptation = ✓	Overload = ✓	Progression = ✓	Regression = ✓	Individuality = ✓	Recovery = ✓

MICROCYCLE (RUGBY-SPECIFIC)				
Client name:				
Mesocycle:			**Microcycle week:**	
	Exercise	**Intensity (RM)**		**Comment**
Cardio 1	Warm-up – ground-based movements + 10 mins' light jogging	2 Sets	2 × 10m per exercise	Bear crawls, walkouts, Spiderman crawls, deep squats, lunges (forwards, backwards, lateral).
	HIIT set 1	1 Sets	30/30 secs work/rest × 10 reps	Linear running (on a pitch or treadmill) @50–60% max speed.
	HIIT set 2	1 Sets	30/30 secs work/rest × 10 reps	Linear running (on a pitch or treadmill) @50–60% max speed.
	HIIT set 3	1 Sets	15/15 secs work/rest × 10 reps	Linear running (on a pitch or treadmill) @60–70% max speed.
	HIIT set 4	1 Sets	15/15 secs work/rest × 10 reps	Linear running (on a pitch or treadmill) @60–70% max speed.
	Mobility and flexibility	3 Sets	30-sec holds for static stretches 8–12 reps for dynamic stretches	Focus on main lower-body muscle groups – hamstrings, quadriceps, glutes, adductors and abductors, calves. Start with dynamic stretches and finish with static stretches.
Cardio 2	Warm-up – ground-based movements + 10 mins' light jogging + acceleration drills to prepare for sprints	2 Sets	2 × 10m per exercise	Bear crawls, walkouts, Spiderman crawls, deep squats, lunges (forwards, backwards, lateral). A skips, B skips, rolling 10m accelerations × 2, rolling 20m accelerations × 2.
	HIIT set 1	1 Sets	30/30 secs work/rest × 10 reps	Linear running (on a pitch or treadmill) @60–70% max speed.
	HIIT set 2	1 Sets	30/30 secs work/rest × 10 reps	Linear running (on a pitch or treadmill) @60–70% max speed.

Cardio 2 (*cont.*)	Sprint exposure	1	Sets	2 × 20m sprints 2 × 30m sprints	The athlete should aim for 90% of max speed exposure during these sprints – with an aim of increasing this to a max sprint later in the mesocycle.
	HIIT set 3	1	Sets	15/15 secs work/rest × 10 reps	Linear running (on a pitch or treadmill) @70–80% max speed.
	HIIT set 4	1	Sets	15/15 secs work/rest × 10 reps	Linear running (on a pitch or treadmill) @70–80% max speed.
	Mobility and flexibility	3	Sets	30-sec holds for static stretches 8–12 reps for dynamic stretches	Focus on main lower-body muscle groups – hamstrings, quadriceps, glutes, add and abductors, calves. Start with dynamic stretches and finish with static stretches.
Cardio 3	Warm-up – ground-based movements + 10 mins' light jogging + acceleration drills to prepare for sprints	2	Sets	2 × 10m per exercise	Bear crawls, walkouts, Spiderman crawls, deep squats, lunges (forwards, backwards, lateral). A skips, B skips, rolling 10m accelerations × 2, rolling 20m accelerations × 2.
	Sprint exposure	1	Sets	2 × 20m sprints 2 × 30m sprints	The athlete should aim for 95%+ of max speed exposure during these sprints.
	HIIT set 1	1	Sets	30/15 secs work/rest × 10 reps	Linear running (on a pitch or treadmill) @60–70% max speed.
	HIIT set 2	1	Sets	30/15 secs work/rest × 10 reps	Linear running (on a pitch or treadmill) @60–70% max speed.
	HIIT set 3	1	Sets	19/11 secs work/rest × 10 reps	Linear running (on a pitch or treadmill) @70–80% max speed.
	HIIT set 4	1	Sets	19/11 secs work/rest × 10 reps	Linear running (on a pitch or treadmill) @70–80% max speed.
	Mobility and flexibility	3	Sets	30-sec holds for static stretches 8–12 reps for dynamic stretches	Focus on main lower-body muscle groups – hamstrings, quadriceps, glutes, adductors and abductors, calves. Start with dynamic stretches and finish with static stretches.

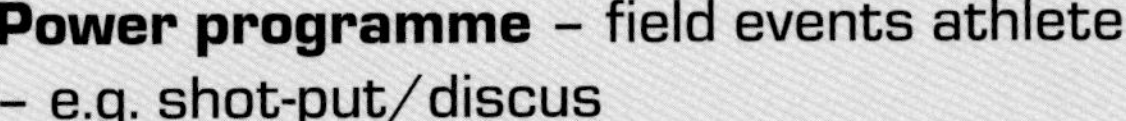

Power programme – field events athlete – e.g. shot-put/discus

Athlete details:
Gender: Female
Age: 23
Weight: 80kg
Height: 175cm

Experience:
The client is a regional-level amateur field events athlete who specialises in the shot-put but also competes in the discus. She has limited experience of S&C training but understands the importance of it and knows that it could elevate her performance.

Athlete goals:
The athlete would like to invest some time into an S&C programme to develop her power output with the aim for pushing towards qualifying for national competitions within the next season. The client would like to focus on the shot-put, as this is her preferred event.

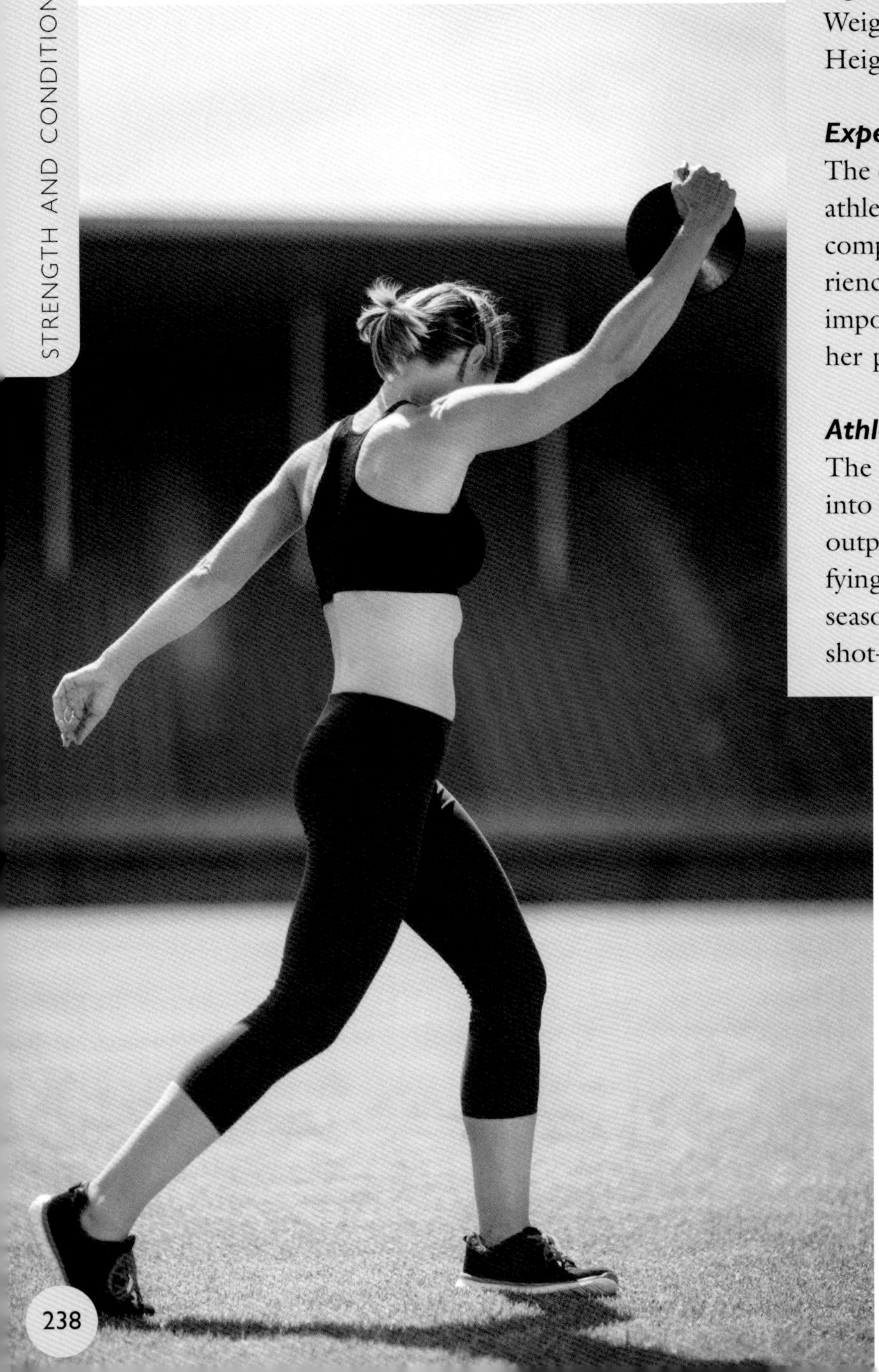

Training plan:

<table>
<tr><td colspan="16" align="center">MACROCYCLE</td></tr>
</table>

Main goals: Increase whole-body strength and power outputs. Develop core stability and rotation.
Tests: 5RM (strength). Power tests. TA contraction (core stability). Sorenson test.

January				February				March				April			
Week				Week				Week				Week			
1	2	3	4	1	2	3	4	1	2	3	4	1	2	3	4

<table>
<tr><td colspan="16" align="center">MESOCYCLES</td></tr>
</table>

Foundation	Development	Conditioning	Performance
• Baseline testing. • Introduce core stabilisation and flexibility exercises. • Assess resistance training ability. • Use light weights to develop ligament strength.	• Increase the volume of core stability exercises. • Build up the volume and intensity of weights for hypertrophy.	• Re-test at the end of week 4. • Increase the challenge of core stability exercises. • Increase the intensity/ decrease the volume to develop power outputs. • Introduce upper-body plyometric exercises.	• Maintain the intensity/ decrease the volume to maximise power output – it's important to focus on the intent of the exercises: aim for speed of lifts to develop power.

<table>
<tr><td colspan="16" align="center">MICROCYCLES</td></tr>
</table>

Wk 1	Wk 2	Wk 3	Wk 4	Wk 1	Wk 2	Wk 3	Wk 4	Wk 1	Wk 2	Wk 3	Wk 4	Wk 1	Wk 2	Wk 3	Wk 4
WB1	WB1	WB1	WB1	WB2	WB2	WB2	WB2	SS1	SS1	SS1	SS1	SS2	SS2	SS2	SS2
UB1	UB1	UB1	UB1	UB2	UB2	UB2	UB2	WB3	WB3	WB3	WB3	WB3	WB3	WB3	WB3
LB1	LB1	LB1	LB1	LB2	LB2	LB2	LB2	WB4	WB4	WB4	WB4	WB4	WB4	WB4	WB4

UB = Upper body LB = Lower body WB = Whole body, Sport-specific = SS

Specificity = ✓	Adaptation = ✓	Overload = ✓	Progression = ✓	Regression = ✓	Individuality = ✓	Recovery = ✓

MICROCYCLE (SPORT-SPECIFIC POWER DEVELOPMENT)

Client name:

Mesocycle: **Microcycle week:**

	Exercise	Intensity (RM)			Comment
SS1	Warm-up Fundamental movement skills – focus on core stability	2	Sets	2 × 10m per exercise	Bear crawls, walkouts, Spiderman crawls, deep squat, lunges (forwards, backwards, lateral).
	Barbell landmine core rotations with single-arm shoulder press	3	Sets	6 reps per side (12 core rotations)	Focus on the intent of the shoulder press – drive the barbell quickly and use the core as a stable base to generate power. Self-select a weight that does not limit the speed of the shoulder drive.
	French contrast training – anterior chain – barbell bench press + bench press medicine ball throws	3	Sets	6–8 reps bench press 6–8 medicine ball throws	Post-activation potentiation – strength/power exercise followed by an upper-body plyometric exercise. Cue to repeatedly throw the medicine ball with minimal time being held (e.g. catch and throw away immediately).
	Medicine ball lateral rotation throws	3	Sets	6 throws per side	Cue to 'throw the ball through the wall' and to drive from the core rotation.
	Pull-ups	3	Sets	4–6 reps	Use resistance bands if a full pull-up cannot be achieved without support.
	Resisted dead bugs	3	Sets	8–10 reps per side	Use a resistance band – held in both hands and pulled back by the coach while the legs extend out maximally one at a time.

SS2	Fundamental movement skills – focus on core stability	2	Sets	2 × 10m per exercise	Bear crawls, walkouts, Spiderman crawls, deep squats, lunges (forwards, backwards, lateral).
	Barbell single-leg RDL – step-up to a box – bilateral shoulder press	3	Sets	4 per side (RDL and step-up) with 8 shoulder press reps per set	Similar to other exercises – allow for controlled RDL and then cue to be explosive for the step-up into shoulder press.
	Cable or banded core rotations – low to high arm trajectory	3	Sets	6–8 per side	This exercise should closely relate to the release phase of a shot-put throw – as the core laterally rotates, the athlete simultaneously drives the hands from hip height across the body to above the head.
	Barbell core roll-outs	3	Sets	6–8 reps	Ensure the back is not extending during this exercise, so that the core remains activated and stable throughout.
	Box jumps	3	Sets	10 reps	Self-select box jump height and aim to increase the height in subsequent sessions.
	Single-arm, standing dumbbell shoulder press	3	Sets	8–10 reps	Ensure core stability during this exercise – the single-arm press will challenge the core to remain activated and aligned during the press.
	Mobility and flexibility	3	Sets	30-sec holds for static stretches 8–12 reps for dynamic stretches	Focus on all main muscle groups but specifically those that are involved in rotation of the hips and upper body. Hip mobility exercises such as 90/90 rotations, lying knee rotations, latissimus dorsi, deltoid and scapula mobility and stability are key areas to target.

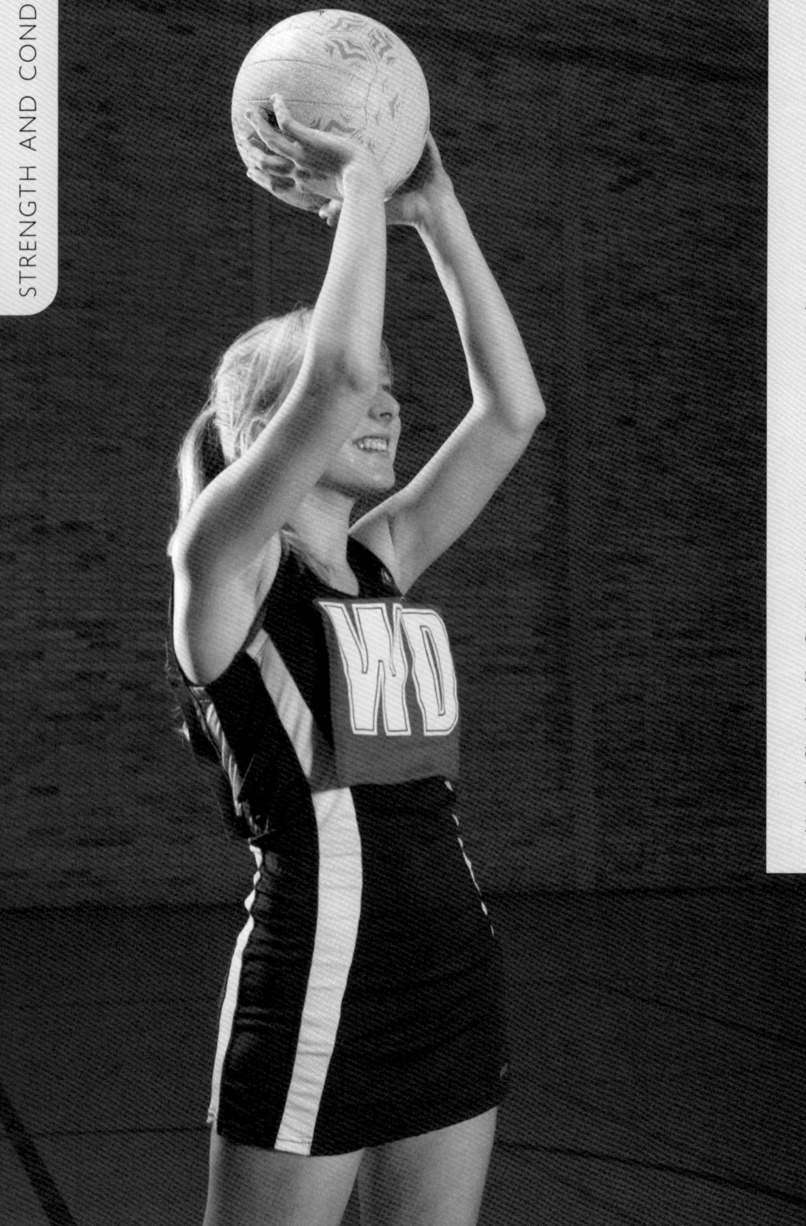

Agility programme – amateur netballer

Athlete details:
Gender: Female
Age: 18
Weight: 70kg
Height: 170cm

Experience:
The athlete has trained and competed in netball for over 10 years at a regional level but will be making the transition from competing in junior leagues into an adult league next season, which commences in 4 months.

Athlete goals:
The athlete plays as a goal defence and would like to develop her ability to accelerate and decelerate more quickly to give her a greater capacity to react to the stimulus of the game in order to better mark opponents, cope with a faster game, increase the number of successful interceptions and to turn the ball over to her team more quickly. While the development of netball-specific agility (reacting to a netball-specific stimulus) will need to take place within netball training sessions, this programme will aim to improve the athlete's physical capacity to accelerate, decelerate and change direction more quickly.

Training plan:

MACROCYCLE

Main goals: Increase the ability to accelerate, decelerate and change direction. Develop upper-body strength and core stabilisation.

Tests: 5-0-5 change of direction test, Illinois change of direction test. 5RM (strength). TA contraction (core stability).

July				August				September				October			
Week				Week				Week				Week			
1	2	3	4	1	2	3	4	1	2	3	4	1	2	3	4

MESOCYCLES

Foundation	Development	Conditioning	Performance
• Baseline testing. • Introduce core stabilisation. • Assess resistance training ability. • Use light weights to develop ligament strength.	• Increase the volume of core stability exercises. • Introduce netball-specific acceleration, deceleration and change of direction exercises. • Build up the volume and intensity of weights for hypertrophy.	• Re-test at the end of week 4. • Increase the challenge of core stability exercises. • Increase the intensity of netball-specific training with reactive stimuli. • Increase the intensity/decrease the volume (weights).	• Progress to using a stability ball as the bench and introduce plyometric upper-body exercises. • Progress netball-specific training to reflect game intensity with reactive stimuli. • Maintain the intensity of weights training.

MICROCYCLES

Wk 1	Wk 2	Wk 3	Wk 4	Wk 1	Wk 2	Wk 3	Wk 4	Wk 1	Wk 2	Wk 3	Wk 4	Wk 1	Wk 2	Wk 3	Wk 4
WB1	WB1	WB1	WB1	WB2	WB2	WB2	WB2	NS2	NS2	NS2	NS2	NS4	NS4	NS4	NS4
LB1	LB1	LB1	LB1	LB2	LB2	LB2	LB2	WB3	WB3	WB3	WB3	WB4	WB4	WB4	WB4
WB2	WB2	WB2	WB2	NS1	NS1	NS1	NS1	NS3	NS3	NS3	NS3	NS5	NS5	NS5	NS5

LB = Lower body WB = Whole body NS = Netball-specific conditioning

Specificity = ✓	Adaptation = ✓	Overload = ✓	Progression = ✓	Regression = ✓	Individuality = ✓	Recovery = ✓

MICROCYCLE (NETBALL-SPECIFIC)

Client name:

Mesocycle:				**Microcycle week:**
	Exercise		**Intensity (RM)**	**Comment**
Netball-specific 1–5	Warm-up – ground-based movements	2 Sets	2 × 10m per exercise	Bear crawls, walkouts, Spiderman crawls, deep squats, lunges (forwards, backwards, lateral).
	Speed development	3 Sets	Repeat each exercise 3 times	Pogo jumps (uni- and bilateral), A skips, B skips, unilateral bounds, horizontal broad jumps.
	Acceleration development	3 Sets	Repeat each exercise 3 times	Accelerations from split stance, drop step and cross step – reacting to different stimuli (voice commands, coloured codes etc).
	Deceleration development	3 Sets	Repeat each exercise 3 times	Deceleration progressions – force absorption during penultimate steps, resistance band braking body position and trunk control.
	Change of direction development	3 Sets	Repeat each exercise 3 times	5-0-5 drills, multidirectional runs to stimuli (voice commands, coloured cones), T and Y running drills. Focus on core stabilisation during the turn.
	Flexibility and mobility	3 Sets	30-sec holds for static stretches	Focus on main lower-body muscle groups – hamstrings, quadriceps, glutes, adductors and abductors, calves.
			8–12 reps for dynamic stretches	Start with dynamic stretches and finish with static stretches.

Netball-specific session will progress in intensity, volume and how challenging they are from session 1–5.

Ways in which the exercises will develop:

- Resistance will be added to acceleration, deceleration and speed exercises using resistance bands placed around the waist of the athlete and fixed to a harness or held by an S&C coach.
- Time constraints will be added to change of direction and reactivity drills to increase the rate of decision making and reactions the athlete requires.
- Multiple stimuli will be introduced and distracting 'false' stimuli (stimuli designed to distract the athlete but should not deter the athlete's decision making – e.g. a mannequin that should not be passed to) will be used to reflect what the athlete may experience during a competitive netball match.
- During the first sessions, running, acceleration, deceleration and change of direction drills will take place at slower speeds so the athlete can focus on optimising the correct technique and core control required for each exercise. The speed the athlete performs these drills and exercises will then increase and progress to maximum as the training sessions progress.

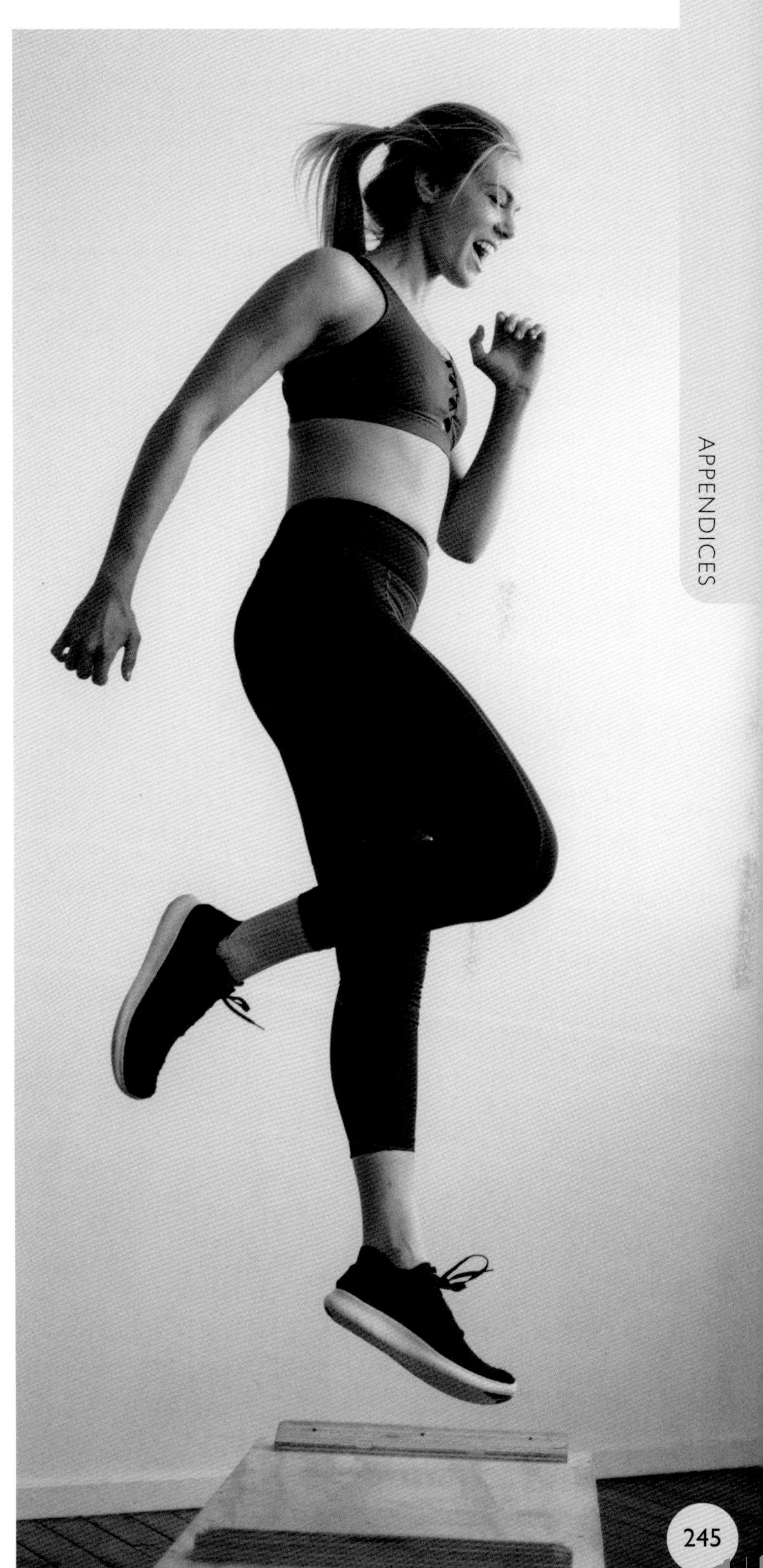

APPENDIX 3

HEALTH AND FITNESS ASSESSMENT CONSENT FORM

The purpose of this health and fitness assessment is to provide the practitioner with a physiological profile that will inform the design of an individualised exercise programme. All exercise programmes have an element of risk (as do assessments) but the assessment is designed to minimise or identify any potential risks. The assessment involves various tests that are outlined below. All tests will be explained beforehand, but you are free to ask questions at any time. You may become uncomfortable during the test, therefore you are free to withdraw from the test at any time, especially if you feel undue pain or discomfort. If you feel you should not take part because of any injury that might be aggravated, then please inform the practitioner.

(practitioners should give a brief description of ALL tests below)

(Please tick)

I confirm that I have read and understood the assessment information and, by signing below, consent to participate in the chosen tests. ☐

I understand I am free to withdraw at any point in time, without the need to give a reason and without my medical care or legal rights being affected. ☐

Client's name:

Client's signature: Date: /   /

Witnessed by: Date: /   /

Print name:

APPENDIX 4

ACCIDENT/INCIDENT REPORT FORM

Use this form to report accidents, injuries, medical situations and criminal activities.
If possible, complete it within 24 hours of the event.

PERSON FILING REPORT

Full name: ....

Title/job role: ....

Signature: ....

Date: ....

EVENT DETAILS

Date of event: ....

Time: ....

Location: ....

Incident description: ....

....

....

PERSON(S) INVOLVED

Full name: ....

Contact: ....

Address: ....

....

Full name: ....

Contact: ....

Address: ....

....

WITNESSES

Full name: ....

Contact: ....

Address: ....

....

Full name: ....

Contact: ....

Address: ....

....

POLICE/MEDICAL SERVICES

Police notified? .... Yes No

If yes, was a report filed? .... Yes No

Was medical treatment given? .... Yes No Refused

ACTION

Report received by: ....

Date: ....

Follow-up action: ....

ADDITIONAL COMMENTS:

....

....

GLOSSARY

Acceleration The rate of change in velocity.

Adaptation Change due to repeated stimuli such as resistance training.

Adenosine triphosphate (ATP) Main energy currency of the cell.

Adrenaline A neurotransmitter that can stimulate the breakdown of fat and glycogen.

Aerobic In the presence of oxygen.

Aerobic capacity The total amount of energy that can be produced aerobically during a bout of exercise (also known as cardiovascular endurance).

Aerobic fitness The ability to deliver oxygen to the working muscles and use it during exercise.

Agility A rapid whole-body movement with change of velocity or direction in response to a stimulus.

Agonist Refers to a muscle or muscle group responsible for the main action.

Alveoli Air sac in the lungs.

Amino acid Small molecules that act as the building blocks of any cell needed for growth and repair.

Anaerobic In the absence of oxygen.

Anaerobic capacity The total amount of energy that can be produced aerobically during a bout of exercise.

Anaerobic power The maximal rate at which energy can be produced.

Anaerobic threshold The point at which the energy demand of the exercise being carried out can no longer be met by the aerobic system.

Anorexia nervosa An eating disorder characterised by immoderate food restriction and irrational fear of gaining weight.

Antagonist Refers to a muscle or muscle group responsible for opposing the main action.

Anthropometry The science relating to the measurement of body mass and proportions of the human body.

Atherosclerosis Narrowing and hardening of the arteries.

Autonomic nervous system Neurons that are not under conscious control.

Basal metabolic rate The rate at which the body uses energy at rest and is measured in Kilocalories.

Blood pressure The force of the blood on the artery walls.

Body composition This refers to the ratio of fat to lean tissue in an individual.

Body mass index (BMI) Weight/height^2.

Bulimia nervosa Eating disorder characterised by binge eating and purging.

Calorie The amount of energy needed to increase the temperature of 1 gram of water by 1°C.

Capillary The smallest type of blood vessel.

Carbohydrate An organic compound that consists only of carbon, hydrogen and oxygen.

Cardiac output The amount of blood pumped out of each ventricle per minute.

Cardiovascular disease Disease of the heart (and related vessels).

Cerebral palsy Brain lesions leading to movement and speech problems.

Cholesterol A fat-like steroid used to form cell membranes.

Concentric contraction A muscular contraction against a resistance in which the muscle length shortens.

Contraction Electrical stimulation of muscle to shorten it.

Correlation Relationship between two data sets.

Criterion measure Considered the gold standard for a particular method of measurement.

Dehydration Water loss from a state of normal amounts of body water.

Delayed onset muscle soreness (DOMS) Perception of post-exercise soreness.

Diaphragm Muscle used to aid breathing.

Dorsiflexion Ankle movement where the foot and toes are pulled upwards towards the shin.

Eccentric contraction A muscular contraction against a resistance in which the muscle lengthens.

Endocrine system An integrated system of organs, glands and tissues that involve the release of extra-cellular signalling molecules known as hormones.

Energy The capacity to do work.

Energy system A term used to describe the source or pathway of producing ATP.

Enzymes Proteins that can speed up chemical reactions.

Euhydration A state of water balance in the body.

Eversion Movement of the sole of the foot away from the midline of the body (results in sole facing outwards).

Experimental error Main source of variation to affect test reliability.

Expired air Air that is breathed out.

Extension Movement at a joint in which the joint angle increases.

Extrinsic motivation The task leads to a reward.

Fascia Type of connective tissue.

Fast twitch Type of muscle fibre associated with strength and speed.

Flexibility The available range of motion around a specific joint.

Flexion Movement at a joint in which the joint angle decreases.

Gland A group of cells that release hormones.

Glycaemic index (GI) A ranking of foods from 0 to 100, based on the rate at which a carbohydrate is broken down

Golgi tendon organs Proprioceptors in tendons sensing force and stretch.

Goniometry Measurement of joint angles.

Haemoglobin Part of a red blood cell that caries oxygen or carbon dioxide.

Heart rate (HR) The number of heart beats per minute.

Heart rate recovery Ability of the heart to return to near resting levels after exercise.

High-density lipoprotein Cholesterol transporters often referred to as the 'good cholesterol' by transporting cholesterol to the liver to be broken down and excreted.

Homeostasis The ability of the body to maintain a regular environment

Hormone A chemical messenger in the body.

Hyperplasia Increase in number of muscle fibres.

Hypertension High blood pressure.

Hypertrophy Enlargement of an organ such as muscle.

Hypotension Low blood pressure.

Insertion The site where the muscle and bone are attached and move during contraction.

Insulin A hormone secreted by the pancreas, which reduces blood sugar levels.

Intensity A measurement of the difficulty level or 'hardness' of the exercise.

Internal rotation Rotation of a part of the body towards the mid-point.

Intrinsic motivation The task itself brings about the reward.

Inversion Movement of the sole of the foot towards the midline of the body (results in sole facing inwards).

Ketones Chemicals in the body regarded as toxins.

Lactic acid A waste product as a result of glycogen breakdown without the presence of oxygen.

Ligament Tissue in the body that connects bone to bone, used for support.

Lipid A broad term used for naturally occurring molecules such as fats, waxes and sterols.

Low-density lipoprotein Known as the 'bad cholesterol'. Tends to deposit cholesterol on blood vessel walls.

Metabolic rate The amount of energy expended at a given time.

Mineral A naturally occurring substance that is solid at room temperature.

Mitochondria The 'power cell' or site of aerobic energy production.

Molecule Two or more atoms joined together.

Muscular endurance The ability of a muscle or muscle group to perform repeated contractions against a resistance over a period of time.

Muscular strength The maximum amount of force a muscle or muscle group can generate.

Neural Relating to the nervous system.

Neuromuscular Relating to the muscular and associated nervous system.

Neurotransmitter A chemical substance released from a nerve ending.

Obesity The percentage body fat at which the risk of disease to the individual is increased.

Origin The attachment point of a muscle to a bone nearest to the midline of the body.

Osteoporosis A condition of reduced bone density.

Outcome goals Goals concerned only with the ultimate outcome.

Overtraining Where a person exceeds the body's ability to recover from exercise.

Pancreas Organ in the body that secretes insulin.

PAR-Q Physical Activity Readiness Questionnaire.

Perceived exertion A subjective measurement of exercise intensity.

Phosphocreatine A high-energy molecule that is stored in muscles and mainly used for rapid ATP production.

Plantarflexion Ankle movement where the foot and toes point downwards away from the shin.

Plyometric Rapid eccentric loading followed by a brief isometric phase and explosive rebound using stored elastic energy and powerful concentric contractions.

Power The product of force and velocity.

Prone Lying on the front.

Proprioception Sense of position in space.

Protein Chains of individual amino acids.

Reciprocal inhibition Where muscles on one side of a joint relax to allow contraction of muscles on the opposite side.

Repetition maximum (RM) The maximum amount of weight that can be lifted for a prescribed number of repetitions.

Resting heart rate (RHR) The heart rate at resting levels measured in beats per minute (bpm).

Risk stratification Process of categorising risk.

Saccharide Simplest form of carbohydrate.

Self-efficacy Self-confidence in one's ability to succeed.

Skinfold Indirect method of assessing body composition.

Slow twitch Type of muscle fibre associated with endurance.

Stability A body's resistance to the disturbance of equilibrium.

Standard deviation How data points are clustered around the mean.

Stretch-shortening cycle Muscle contraction response to a rapid stretch.

Stroke volume The amount of blood ejected from one ventricle per heartbeat.

Supine Lying on the back.

Tendon Connective tissue that surrounds muscle fibres.

Testosterone A hormone that is responsible for muscle growth.

Tissue A collection of cells with a physiological function.

Training load The interaction between volume, intensity and frequency of training.

Transversus abdominis Muscle of the core, involved in forced expiration.

Triglyceride Type of fat used for fuel in the body (glycerol backbone with three fatty acid chains attached).

Validity (test) Purported to specifically measure what the tester or testing team is investigating.

Velocity Movement per unit time with direction.

Venous return The amount of blood that enters the heart from the venous circulation.

Ventilatory threshold The point at which the flow of air in and out of the alveoli surpasses normal rate.

Vestibular system A sensory system providing information relating to position and movement of the head.

Vitamin An organic compound required by an organism as a vital nutrient in limited amounts.

VO$_2$ The amount of oxygen that is delivered and used by the working muscles ($mlO_2.kg^{-1}.min^{-1}$).

VO$_2$max The maximum amount of oxygen that is delivered and used by the working muscles.

Watt The rate of doing work.

REFERENCES

Chapter 1 Screening

American College of Sports Medicine (2025) *ACSM's Guidelines for Exercise Testing and Prescription (12th ed)*, Lippincott, Williams & Wilkins.

Coulson, M. (2021) *The Fitness Practitioners Handbook (4th ed)*, Bloomsbury.

Chapter 2 Needs analysis

Bishop, C., & Turner, A. (2024) Undertaking a needs analysis to inform fitness testing and program design. In *Conditioning for Strength and Human Performance* (229–245), Routledge.

Scroggs, K., & Simonson, S.R. (2021) Writing a needs analysis: Exploring the details. *Stren & Cond J*, 43(5):87–95.

Johnson, D.L., & Bird, M.D. (2022) Performance profiling in strength and conditioning. *Stren & Cond J*, 44(4): 62–69.

Chapter 3 Goal setting

Locke, E.A., & Latham, G.P. (1990) *A Theory of Goal Setting and Task Performance*, Prentice Hall.

Locke, E.A., Shaw, K.N., Saari, L.M., & Latham, G.P. (1981) Goal setting and task performance: 1969–1980. *Psychological Bulletin*, 90(1):125.

Burton, D., & Weiss, C. (2008) The fundamental goal concept: The path to process and performance success. In T. Horn (Ed.). *Advances in Sport Psychology (3rd ed.)*, 339–375, Human Kinetics.

Williamson, O., et al., (2024) The performance and psychological effects of goal setting in sport: A systematic review and meta-analysis. *Int Rev of Sport and Exerc Psych*, 17:2, 1050–1078.

Atkinson, R., & Hilgard, E.R. (2014) *Introduction to Psychology (16th ed.)*, Wadsworth Publishing.

Butler, R.J. (2000) *Sport Psychology in Performance*, Oxford University Press.

Cox, R.H. (2011) *Sport Psychology Concepts and Applications (7th ed.)*, Brown & Benchmark.

Weinberg, R., & Gould, D. (2014) *Foundations of Sport and Exercise Psychology (6th ed.)*, Human Kinetics.

Chapter 4 The Components and principles of fitness

Coulson, M. (2021) *The Fitness Practitioners Handbook (4th ed)*, Bloomsbury.

American College of Sports Medicine (2025) *ACSM's Guidelines for Exercise Testing and Prescription (12th ed)*, Lippincott, Williams & Wilkins.

Baechle, R.T. (2016) *Essentials of Strength Training and Conditioning (4th ed.)*, Human Kinetics.

Chapter 5 Aerobic endurance

Fares, R., Vicente-Rodríguez, G., & Olmedillas, H. (2022) Effect of active recovery protocols on the management of symptoms related to exercise-induced muscle damage: A systematic review. *Strength and Cond J*, 44(1): 57–70.

Cole, C.R., et al., (1999) Heart-rate recovery immediately after exercise as a predictor of mortality. *N Engl J Med*, 341(18):1351–1357.

Cygankiewicz, I., & Zareba, W. (2013) Heart rate variability. *Handbook of Clinical Neurology*, 117:379–393.

Buchheit, M., & Laursen, P.B. (2013) High-intensity interval training, solutions to the programming puzzle: Part I: cardiopulmonary emphasis. *Sports Med*, 43(5):313–338.

Chapter 6 Anaerobic endurance

Sandford, G.N., Laursen, P.B., & Buchheit, M. (2021) Anaerobic speed/power reserve and sport performance: scientific basis, current applications and future directions. *Sports Med*, 51(10):2017–2028.

Ghosh, A.K. (2004) Anaerobic threshold: Its concept and role in endurance sport. *Malay J of Med Sci: MJMS*, 11(1):24.

Short, K.R., & Sedlock, D.A. (1997) Excess postexercise oxygen consumption and recovery rate in trained and untrained subjects. *J of Appl Phys*, 83(1):153–159.

Gaesser, G.A., & Brooks, C.A. (1984) Metabolic bases of excess post-exercise oxygen. *Med Sci Sports Exerc*, 16(1):29–43.

Laursen, P.B., & Buchheit, M. (2019) *Science and Application of High-intensity Interval Training*, Human Kinetics.

Chapter 7 Stabilisation

Panjabi, M.M. (1992) The stabilizing system of the spine. Part I. Function, dysfunction, adaptation, and enhancement. *J Spinal Disord*, 5:383–389.

Panjabi, M.M. (1992) The stabilizing system of the spine. Part II. Neutral zone and instability hypothesis. *J Spinal Disord*, 5:390–396.

Behm, D.G., et al., (2010) The use of instability to train the core musculature. *Appl Physiol Nutr Metab*, 35(1):91–108.

Bergmark, A. (1989) Stability of the lumbar spine: A study in mechanical engineering. *Acta Orthop Scand Suppl*, 230:1–54.

Colston, M. (2012) Core stability, part 1: Overview of the concept. *Int J Athl Ther Train*, 17(1):8–13.

Colston, M. (2012) Core stability, part 2: The core-extremity link. *Int J Athl Ther Train*, 17(2):10–15.

Gibbons, S.G.T., & Comerford, M.J. (2001) Strength versus stability: part 1. Concepts and terms. *Orthop Division Rev*, 2:21–27.

Konin, J.G. (2003) Facilitating the serape effect to enhance extremity force production. *Athl Ther Today*, 8(2):54–56.

Cook, G., Burton, L., & Hoogenboom, B. (2006) Pre-participation screening: The use of fundamental movements as an assessment of function. Part 1. *N Am J Sports Phys Ther*, 1(2):62–72.

Akuthota, V., & Nadler, S.F. (2004) Core strengthening. *Arch Phys Med Rehabil*, 85(3)(suppl 1):S86–S92.

Niederer, D., & Mueller, J. (2020) Sustainability effects of motor control stabilization exercises on pain and function in chronic nonspecific low back pain patients: A systematic review with meta-analysis and meta-regression. *PLOS One*, 15(1):e0227423.

Era, P., Konttinen, N., Mehto, P., Saarela, P., & Lyytinen, H. (1996) Postural stability and skilled performance -3 a study on top-level and naive rifle shooters. *J. Biomech*, 29:301–306.

Lang, D., & Zhou, A. (2021) Relationships between postural balance, aiming technique and performance in elite rifle shooters. *Eur. J. Sport Sci*, doi: 10.1080/17461391.2021.1971775.

Opala-Berdzik, A., Głowacka, M., & Juras, G. (2021) Postural sway in young female artistic and acrobatic gymnasts according to training experience and anthropometric characteristics. *BMC Sports Sci. Med. Rehabil*, 13:11.

Jadczak, Ł, Grygorowicz, M., Dzudzi´nski, W., & Sliwowski, R. (2019a) Comparison of static and dynamic balance at different levels of sport competition in professional and junior elite soccer players. *J. Strength Cond Res*, 33:3384–3391.

Szafraniec, R., Bartkowski, J., & Kawczyński, A. (2020) Effects of short-term core stability training on dynamic balance and trunk muscle endurance in novice olympic weightlifters. *J Hum Kinet*, 74:43–50.

Chapter 8 Muscular strength and endurance

Baumgartner, R.N., et al., (1998) Epidemiology of sarcopenia among the elderly in New Mexico. *Amer J of Epidem*, 147(8):755–763.

Mitchell, W.K., et al., (2012) Sarcopenia, dynapenia, and the impact of advancing age on human skeletal muscle size and strength: A quantitative review. *Front Physiol*, 3:260.

Newman, A.B., et al., (2006) Strength, but not muscle mass, is associated with mortality in the health, aging and body composition study cohort. *J Gerontol Biol Sci Med Sci,* 61:72–7.

Mang, Z.A. et al., (2022) Aerobic adaptations to resistance training: The role of time under tension. *Int J of Sports Med,* 43(10):829–839.

Seiler, S., Joranson, K., Oleson, B.V., & Hetlelid, K.J. (2011) Adaptations to aerobic interval training: interactive effects of exercise intensity and total work duration. *Scand J of Med and Sci in Sports,* 23:74–83.

Macinnes, M.J., & Gibala, M. (2016) Physiological adaptations to interval training and the role of exercise intensity. *J of Phys,* 595(9):2915–2930.

Rivera-Brown, A.M., & Frontera, W.R. (2012) Principles of exercise physiology: Responses to acute exercise and long-term adaptations to training. *J of Injury, Funct and Rehab,* 4:797–804.

Athanasiou, N., Bogdanis, G.C., & Masterakos, G. (2022) Endocrine responses of the stress system to different types of exercise. *Reviews in Endo and Met Dis,* 24:251–266.

Kotwal, N., Bansal, N., & Kumar, S. (2020) Aerobic vs resistance exercise – the endocrine perspective. *J of Med Acad,* doi:10.5005/jp-journals-10070-0057.

Skarabot, J., et al., (2020) The knowns and unknowns of neural adaptations to resistance training. *Euro J of Appl Phys,* 121:675–685.

Fleck, S.J., & Kraemer, W.J. (2004) *Designing Resistance Training Programmes (2nd ed.).* Human Kinetics.

Chapter 9 Speed

Alcaraz, P.E., Carlos-Vivas, J., & Martinez-Rodriguez, A. (2018) The effectiveness of resisted sled training (RST) for sprint performance: A systematic review and meta-analysis. *Sports Med,* 48:2143–2165.

Paradisis, G.P., Bissas, A., & Cooke, C.B. (2015) Effect of combined uphill-downhill sprint training on kinematics and maximum running speed in experienced sprinters. *Int J of Sports Sci and Coach,* 10(5):887–897.

Bertochi, G.F.A., Tasinafo Jnr, M.F., Santos, I.A., et al., (2024) The use of wearable resistance and weighted vest for sprint performance and kinematics: A systematic review and meta-analysis. *Scient Repor,* 14:5453.

Cecilia-Gallego, P., Odriozola, A., Beltran-Garrido, J.V., & Alvarez-Herm, J. (2022) Acute effects of overspeed stimuli with towing system on athletic sprint performance: A systematic review with meta-analysis. *J of Sports Sci,* 40(6):704–716.

Delecluse, C. (1997) Influence of strength training on sprint running performance. *Sports Med.* 24:148–156

Chapter 10 Power

Kirby, T.J., Erickson, T., & McBride, J.M. (2010) Model for progression of strength, power, and speed training. *Strength Cond J,* 32:86–90.

Bompa, T.O., & Haff, G.G. (2009) *Periodization: Theory and Methodology of Training,* Human Kinetics.

Harris. G.R., Stone, M.H., O'Bryant, H.S., Proulx, C.M., & Johnson, R.L. (2000) Short-term performance effects of high power, high force, or combined weight-training methods. *J Strength Cond Res,* 14:14–20.

Komi, P.V., & Buskirk, E.R. (1972) Effects of eccentric and concentric muscle conditioning on tension and electrical activity of human muscle. *Ergonomics,* 15:417–434.

Wisløff, U., Castagna, C., Helgerud, J., Jones, R., & Hoff, J. (2004) Strong correlation of maximal squat strength with sprint performance and vertical jump height in elite soccer players. *Br J Sports Med,* 38:285–288.

Keiner, M., et al., (2022) The influence of maximum squatting strength on jump and sprint performance: A cross-sectional analysis of 492 youth soccer players. *Int J of Environ Res and Pub Health,* 19:5835.

Skratek, J., Kadlubowski, B., & Keiner M. (2024) The effect of traditional strength training on sprint and jump performance in 12- to 15-year-old elite soccer players: A 12-month controlled trial. *J of Strength and Cond Res,* 38(11):1900–1910.

de Salles Painelli, V. Risks and Recommendations for

Resistance Training in Youth Athletes: A Narrative Review with Emphasis on Muscular Fitness and Hypertrophic Responses. *J. of Sci. in Sport and Exercise* (2023). https://doi.org/10.1007/s42978-023-00251-y

Dobbs, I.J., et al., (2021) Effects of a 4-week neuromuscular training programme on movement competency during the back-squat assessment in pre- and post-peak height velocity male individuals. *J Strength Cond Res*, 1:35(10):2698–2705.

Davies, G., Riemann, B.L., & Manske, R. (2015) Current concepts of plyometric exercise. *Int J Sports Phys Ther*, 10(6):760–86.

Weakley, J., et al., (2021) The validity and reliability of commercially available resistance training monitoring devices: A systematic review. *Sports Med*, 51(3):443–502.

Nevin, J. (2019) Autoregulated resistance training: Does velocity-based training represent the future? *Strength Cond J*, 41(4):34–39.

Weakley, J., et al., (2021) Velocity-based training: From theory to application. *Strength Cond J*, 43(2):31–49.

Chapter 11 Agility

Sheppard, J.M., & Young, W.B. (2006) Agility literature review: Classifications, training and testing. *J of Sports Sci*, 24(9):919–932.

Cureton, T.K. (1942) *Physical Fitness Workbook: Fit for democracy—Fit to fight*, Stipes.

Turner, A.N., Read, P., Maestroni, L., Chavda, S., Yao, X., Papadopoulos, K., & Bishop, C. (2022) Reverse engineering in strength and conditioning: Applications to agility training. *Stren & Cond J*, 44(4):85–94.

Dawes, J. (Ed.). (2019) *Developing Agility and Quickness*, Human Kinetics Publishers.

The Royal Society for the Prevention of Accidents. rospa.com/home-safety/falls-prevention (accessed 16.06.25).

Chapter 12 Flexibility

Alter, M.J. (1996) *Science of Flexibility (2nd ed.),* Human Kinetics.

Chaabene, H., Behm, D.G., Negra, Y, & Granacher, U. (2019) Acute effects of static stretching on muscle strength and power: An attempt to clarify previous caveats. *Front in Phys*, 10:1468.

Mašić, S., Čaušević, D., Covic, N., Spicer, S., & Doder, I. (2024) The benefits of static stretching on health: A systematic review. *J of Kines and Exerc Sci*, 33:1–7.

Knudson, D. (2010) Programme stretching after vigorous physical training. *J Stren and Cond*, 32:55–57.

Opplert, J., & Babault, N. (2018) Acute effects of dynamic stretching on muscle flexibility and performance: An analysis of the current literature. *Sports Med*, 48:299–325.

Chapter 13 Body composition

American College of Sports Medicine (2002) *ACSM's Exercise Management for Persons with Chronic Diseases and Disabilities*, Human Kinetics.

Heyward, V.H. (1996) *Advanced Fitness Assessment & Exercise Prescription*, Human Kinetics.

National Institute for Health and Clinical Excellence (2006) *Obesity: The prevention, identification, assessment and management of overweight and obesity in adults and children*, NICE.

Andreoli, A., Garaci, F., Cafarelli, F.P., & Guglielmi, G. (2016) Body composition in clinical practice. *Euro J of Radiol*, 85(8):1461–1468.

Chapter 14 Performance assessment

Baumgartner, T.A., Strong, C.H., & Hensley, L.D. (2002) *Conducting and Reading Research in Health and Human Performance*, McGraw Hill.

Gratton, C., & Jones, I. (2004) *Research Methods for Sport Studies*, Routledge.

Graziano, A. & Raulin, M. (2003) *Research Methods: A process of inquiry (5th ed.)*, Pearson.

Morin, J.B., Jiménez-Reyes, P., Brughelli, M., & Samozino, P. (2019) When jump height is not a good indicator of lower limb maximal power output: Theoretical demonstration, experimental evidence and practical solutions. *Sports Med*, 49:999–1006.

Rudisill, S.S., Varady, N.H., Kucharik, M.P., Eberlin, C.T., & Martin, S.D. (2023) Evidence-based hamstring injury prevention and risk factor management: A systematic review and meta-analysis of randomized controlled trials. *Amer J of Sports Med*, 51(7):1927–1942.

Thomas, J.R., & Nelson, J.K. (2001) *Research Methods in Physical Activity (4th ed.)*, Human Kinetics.

Hopkins, W., Marshall, S., Batterham, A., & Hanin, J. (2009) Progressive statistics for studies in sports medicine and exercise science. *Med and Sci in Sports and Exerc*, 41:3.

Chapter 15 Aerobic endurance testing

Léger, L., et al., (1984) Aerobic capacity of 6 to 17-year-old Quebecois--20-meter shuttle run test with 1-minute stages. *J Canad des Sciences Appl au Sport*, 9(2):64–69.

Brouha, L., Heath, C.W., & Ashton, G. (1943) Step test simple method of measuring physical fitness for hard muscular work in adult men. *Rev Canad Biol*, 2:86–91.

Zhang, Y. et al. (1991) Effects of exercise testing protocol on parameters of aerobic function. *Med and Sci in Sports and Exerc*, 23(5):625–630

Shephard, R.J. (1984) Tests of maximum oxygen intake: A critical review. *Sports Med*, 1:99–124

Buchheit M. (2008) The 30–15 intermittent fitness test: Accuracy for individualizing interval training of young intermittent sport players. *J Strength Cond Res*, 22:365–374.

Cooper, K.H. (1968). A means of assessing maximum oxygen intake. *JAMA*, 203:135–138.

Kline, G., Porcari, J., Hintermeister, R., Freedson, P., Ward, A., McCarron, R., Ross, J., & Rippe, J. (1987) Estimation of vo_2max from a 1-mile track walk, gender, age, and body weight. *Med Sci Sports Exerc*, 19:253–259.

Bangsbo, J., Iaia F.M., & Krustrup, P. (2008) The Yo-Yo intermittent recovery test: A useful tool for evaluation of physical performance in intermittent sports. *Sports Med*, 38(1):37–51.

Buchheit, M., & Brown, M. (2020) Pre-season fitness testing in elite soccer: Integrating the 30–15 Intermittent Fitness Test into the weekly microcycle. *J of Sport Perf and Sci*, 111(1):1–3.

Chapter 16 Anaerobic endurance testing

Baker, J., Ramsbottom, R., & Hazeldine, R. (1993) Maximal shuttle running over 40 m as a measure of anaerobic performance. *Brit J of Sports Med*, 27:228–236

Gaskill, S.E., et al., (2001) Validity and reliability of combining three methods to determine ventilatory threshold. *Med Sci in Sports Exer*, 33(11):1841–1848.

Binder, R.K., Wonisch, M., Corra, U., Cohen-Solal, A., Vanhees, L., Saner, H., & Schmid, J.P. (2008) Methodological approach to the first and second lactate threshold in incremental cardiopulmonary exercise testing. *Euro J of Prev Card*, 15(6):726–734.

Dotan, R., & Bar-Or, O. (1983) Load optimization for the Wingate anaerobic test. *Euro J of Appl Phys and Occ Phys*, 51(3):409–417.

Andrade, V.L., et al., (2015) Running-based anaerobic sprint test as a procedure to evaluate anaerobic power. *Int J Sports Med*, 36:1–7

Chapter 17 Stabilisation testing

Richardson, et al. (1999) *Therapeutic Exercises for Spinal Segmental Stabilisation in Low Back Pain*. Churchill, Livingstone.

Biering-Sorensen, F. (1984) Physical measurements as risk indicators for low-back trouble over a one-year period. *Spine*, 9:106–119.

McGill, S.M., Childs, A., & Liebenson, C. (1999) Endurance times for low back stabilization exercises: Clinical targets for testing and training from a normal database. *Arch Phys Med Rehabil*, 80:941–944.

Guilhem, G., et al., (2014) Validity of trunk extensor and flexor torque measurements using isokinetic dynamometry. *J of Electromyog and Kines*, 24:986–993.

Greene, P.F., Durall, C.J., & Kernozek, T.W. (2012) Intersession reliability and concurrent validity of isometric endurance tests for the lateral trunk muscles. *J of Sport Rehab*, 21(2):161–166.

Chapter 18 Muscular strength and endurance testing

Minisian, R.A., Kuschner, S.H., & Lane, C.S. (2022) A review of handgrip strength and its role as a herald of health. *Open Ortho J*, 16:3–8.

Diener, M.H., Golding, L.A., & Diener, D. (1995) Validity and reliability of a one-minute half sit-up test of abdominal strength and endurance. *Sport Med Train and Rehab*, 6:105–119.

Golding, et al., (1986) *The Y's Way to Physical Fitness: The Complete Guide to Fitness Testing and Instruction (3rd ed.)*, Human Kinetics, 113–124.

Thompson, S.S., et al., (2021) A novel approach to 1RM prediction using the load-velocity profile: A comparison of models. *Sports*, 9:88.

Jidovtseff, B., et al., (2011) Using the load-velocity relationship for 1RM prediction. *J of Strength and Cond Res*, 25(1):267–270.

Brzycki, M. (1993) Strength testing – Predicting a one-rep max from reps-to-fatigue. *JOPERD*, January:88–90

Baumgartner, T.A., Oh, S., Chung, H., & Hales, D. (2002) Objectivity, reliability, and validity for a revised push-up test protocol. *Measurement in Physical Education and Exercise Science*, 6(4): 225–242.

Clemons, J. (2019) Construct validity of two different methods of scoring and performing push-ups. *J of Str & Cond Res*, 33(11)2971–2980.

Chapter 19 Speed testing

Chu, D.A. (1996) *Explosive Power and Strength*, Human Kinetics.

Davis, B., et al., (2000) *Physical Education and the Study of Sport (4th ed.)*, Harcourt Publishers, 125.

Karavelioğlu, M.B., Başkaya, G., & Aydın, S. (2023) Investigation of 30 meter sprint performances with and without finish line in athletes in terms of personality traits. *CBÜ Beden Eğitimi ve Spor Bilimleri Dergisi*, 18(1):311–323.

Chapter 20 Power testing

Ruben, R.M., et al., (2010) The acute effects of an ascending squat protocol on performance during horizontal plyometric jumps. *J Strength Cond Res*, 24:358–369.

Sargent, D.A. (1921) The physical test of a man. *American Phys Ed Rev*, 26:188–194.

Sato, K., Sands, W.A., & Stone, M.H. (2012) The reliability of accelerometery to measure weightlifting performance. *Sports Biomech*, 11(4):524–531.

Canavan, P.K., & Vescovi, J.D. (2004) Evaluation of power prediction equations: Peak vertical jumping power in women. *Med and Sci in Sports and Exer*, 36(9):1589–1593

Chapter 21 Agility testing

Roozen, M. (2004) Illinois agility test. *NSCA's Performance Training Journal*, National Strength and Conditioning Association, 3(5):5–6.

Draper, J., & Lancaster, M. (1985) The 505 test: A test for agility in the horizontal plane. *Austr J of Sci and Med in Sport*, 17(1):15–18.

Hoffman, J. (2006) *Norms for Fitness, Performance, and Health*, Human Kinetics.

Lesch, K.J., Tuomisto, S., Tikkanen, H.O., & Venojärvi, M. (2024) Validity and reliability of dynamic and functional balance tests in people aged 19–54: A systematic review. *Int J Sports Phys Ther*, 19(4):381–393.

Plisky, P.J., et al., (2009) The reliability of an instrumented device for measuring components of the star excursion balance test. *N Am J Sports Phys Ther*, 4(2):92–99.

Schell, J., & Leelarthaepin, B. (1994) *Physical Fitness Assessment in Exercise and Sports Science (2nd ed)*, Leelar Biomedisience Services, 327.

Ryan, C., Uthoff, A., McKenzie, C., & Cronin, J. (2022) Traditional and modified 5-0-5 change of direction test: Normative and reliability analysis. *Strength & Cond J*, 44(4):22–37.

Plisky, P., Schwartkopf-Phifer, K., Huebner, B., Garner, M.B., & Bullock, G. (2021) Systematic review and meta-analysis of the Y-balance test lower quarter: Reliability, discriminant validity, and predictive validity. *Int J of Sports Phys Ther*, 16(5):1190.

Olivier, B., Martin, C., Zumana, N., & Godlwana, L. (2019) Intra-rater and inter-rater reliability of six musculoskeletal preparticipatory screening tests. *South Afric J of Physio*, 75(1):1–10.

Chapter 22 Flexibility testing

Heyward, V.H. (2006) *Advanced Fitness Assessment and Exercise Prescription (5th ed.)*, Human Kinetics.

Wells, K.F., & Dillon, E.K. (1952) The sit and reach. A test of back and leg flexibility. *Research Quarterly. Amer Ass for Health, Phys Ed and Rec*, 23(1):115–118.

Miller, J. (2023) Injury risk assessment including flexibility. In *Laboratory Manual for Strength and Conditioning*, Routledge, 25–51.

Chapter 23 Body composition testing

Drinkwater, D.T., Martin, A.D., Ross, W.D., & Clarys, J.P. (1984) Validation by cadaver dissection of Matiegka's equations for the anthropometric estimation of anatomical body composition in adult humans. In J.A.P. Day, ed. *The 1984 Olympic Scientific Congress Proceedings-Perspectives in Kinanthropometry*, Human Kinetics, 221–227.

Durnin, J.V.G.A., & Womersley, J. (1974) Body fat assessed from total body density and its estimation from skinfold thickness: Measurements on 481 men and women aged from 16 to 72 years. *Brit J of Nutr*, 32:77.

Lukaski, H.C., Bolonchuk, W.W., Hall, C.B., & Siders, W.A. (1986) Validation of tetrapolar bioelectric impedance method to assess human body composition. *J of Appl Phys*, 60:1327–1332.

Martin, A.D., Ross, W.D., Drinkwater, D.T., & Clarys, J.P. (1985) Prediction of body fat by skinfold calliper: Assumptions and cadaver evidence, *Int J of Obes*, 9:31–39.

Marra, M., et al., (2019) Assessment of body composition in health and disease using bioelectrical impedance analysis (BIA) and dual energy x-ray absorptiometry (DXA): A critical overview, *Contr Med and Molec Imag*, 2019:1–9.

Dana, L., et al., (2008) Body composition methods: Comparisons and interpretation. *J of Diabetes Sci and Technol*, 2(6):1139–1146.

Heyward, V. (2001) ASEP methods recommendations: Body composition assessment. *JEP online*, 4(4):1–12.

Nickerson, B.S., Esco, M.R., Bishop, P.A., Fedewa, M.V., Snarr, R.L., Kliszczewicz, B.M., & Park, K.S. (2018) Validity of BMI-based body fat equations in men and women: A 4-compartment model comparison. *J of Stren & Cond Res*, 32(1):121–129.

Barrios, P., Martin-Biggers, J., Quick, V., & Byrd-Bredbenner, C. (2016) Reliability and criterion validity of self-measured waist, hip, and neck circumferences. *BMC Med Res Methodology*, 16:1–12.

Chapter 24 Manipulation of training variables

McCrary, J.M., Ackermann, B.J., & Halaki, M. (2015) A systematic review of the effects of upper body warm-up on performance and injury. *Br J Sports Med*, 49:935–942.

McGowan, C.J., Pyne, D.B., Thompson, K.G., & Rattray, B. (2015) Warm-up strategies for sport and exercise: Mechanisms and applications. *Sports Med*, 45:1523–1546.

Bishop, D. (2003) Warm up II: Performance changes following active warm up and how to structure the warm up. *Sports Med*, 33:483–498.

Van Hooren, B., & Peake, J.M. (2018) Do we need a cool-down after exercise? A narrative review of the psycho-physiological effects and the effects on performance, injuries and the long-term adaptive response. *Sports Med*, 48:1575–1595.

Borg, G. (1961) Interindividual scaling and perception of muscular work. *Kungl Fys Salisk Forh Lund*, 117–125.

Weston, M., et al., (2015) The application of differential ratings of perceived exertion to Australian Football League matches. *J of Sci and Med in Sport*, 18(6):704–708.

Baechle, R.T. (2016) *Essentials of Strength Training and Conditioning (4th ed.)*, Human Kinetics

Bompa, T.O. (2009) *Periodisation Theory and Methodology of Training (5th ed.)*, Human Kinetics.

Chapter 25 Fatigue and recovery strategies

McNair, et al., (1971) *Manual for the Profile of Mood States*, Educational and Industrial Testing Service.

Halson, S. L., Appaneal, R. N., Welvaert, M., Maniar, N., & Drew, M. K. (2022) Stressed and Not Sleeping: Poor Sleep and Psychological Stress in Elite Athletes Prior to the Rio 2016 Olympic Games. *International journal of sports physiology and performance*, 17(2), 195–202. https://doi.org/10.1123/ijspp.2021-0117

Gleeson, M. (2002) Biochemical and immunological markers of over-training. *Sports Sci and Med*, 1:31–41.

Phillips, R.O. (2015) A review of definitions of fatigue–And a step towards a whole definition. *Traffic Psychol Behav*, 29:48–56.

Aragon, A.A., & Schoenfeld, B.J. (2013) Nutrient timing revisited: Is there a post-exercise anabolic window? *J Int Soc Sports Nutr*, 10(1):5.

Tipton, K., & Wolfe, R.R. (2001) Exercise, protein metabolism, and muscle growth. *Int J Sport Nutr Exerc Metab*, 11(1):109–132.

Dattilo, M. et al., (2011) Sleep and muscle recovery: Endocrinological and molecular basis for a new and promising hypothesis. *Med Hypotes*, 77(2):220–222.

Allan, R., & Mawhinney, C. (2017) Is the ice bath finally melting? Cold water immersion is no greater than active recovery upon local and systemic inflammatory cellular stress in humans. *J of Physiol*, 595(6):1857.

Bieuzen, F., Bleakley, C.M., & Costello, J.T. (2013) Contrast water therapy and exercise induced muscle damage: A systematic review and meta-analysis. *PLOS One*, 8(4):62356.

Light, K.E., Nuzik, S., Personius, W., & Barstrom, A. (1984) Low-load prolonged stretch vs. high-load brief stretch in treating knee contractures. *Phys Ther*, 64(3):330–333.

Herbert RD, de Noronha M, Kamper SJ. Stretching to prevent or reduce muscle soreness after exercise. Cochrane Database of Systematic Reviews 2011, Issue 7. Art. No.: CD004577. DOI: 10.1002/14651858.CD004577.pub3. (accessed 05.08.25).

Mueck-Weymann, M., Janshoff, G., & Mueck, H. (2004) Stretching increases heart rate variability in healthy individuals complaining about limited muscular flexibility. *Clin Auto Res*, 14:15–18.

Mohr, A.R., Long, B.C., & Goad, C.L. (2014) Effect of foam rolling and static stretching on passive hip-flexion range of motion. *J of Sport Rehab*, 23(4):296–299.

Wiewelhove, T., et al., (2019) A meta-analysis of the effects of foam rolling on performance and recovery. *Front in Physiol*, 10:376.

Hendricks, S., den Hollander, S., Lombard, W., & Parker, R. (2020) Effects of foam rolling on performance and recovery: A systematic review of the literature to guide practitioners on the use of foam rolling. *J of Body and Move Ther*, 24(2):151–174.

Vella, L.D., & Cameron-Smith, D. (2010) Alcohol, athletic performance and recovery. *Nutrients*, 2(8):781–789.

Rose, C., Edwards, K.M., Siegler, J., Graham, K., & Caillaud, C. (2017) Whole-body cryotherapy as a recovery technique after exercise: A review of the literature. *International Journal of Sports Medicine*, 38(14):1049–1060.

McGorm, H., Roberts, L.A., Coombes, J.S., & Peake, J.M. (2018) Turning up the heat: An evaluation of the evidence for heating to promote exercise recovery, muscle rehabilitation and adaptation. *Sports Med*, 48(6)1311–1328.

Howatson, G., Leeder, K., & Van Someren, K. (2016) The BASES expert statement on athletic recovery strategies. *Sport Exerc Sci*, 48:6–7.

Dupuy, O., Douzi, W., Theurot, D., Bosquet, L., & Dugué, B. (2018) An evidence-based approach for choosing post-exercise recovery techniques to reduce markers of muscle damage, soreness, fatigue, and inflammation: A systematic review with meta-analysis. *Frontiers in physiology*, 403.

Chapter 26 Practitioner skills

Mehrabian, A. (1971) *Silent Messages (1st ed.)*, Wadsworth.

Bugdayci, S., & Demir, H. (2023) The examination of communication skills and self-efficacy of coaches. *Turk J of Sport and Exer*, 25(3):423–432.

Khan, A., Butt, M.Z.I., & Jamil, M. (2022) Communication is a key determinant of successful coaching. *Gomal Uni J of Res*, 38(2):205–213.

Purnomo, E., et al., (2021) Profile: Interpersonal communication skills for future coaches. *Int J of Hum Move and Sports Sci*, 9(5):964–972.

LaPlaca, D.A., & Schempp, P.G. (2020) The characteristics differentiating expert and competent strength and conditioning coaches. *Res Quart for Exerc and Sport*, 91(3):488–499.

Carson, F., Blakey, M., Foulds, S.J., Hinck, K., & Hoffmann, S.M. (2022) Behaviors and actions of the strength and conditioning coach in fostering a positive coach-athlete relationship. *J of Stren & Cond Res*, 36(11):3256–3263.

Chapter 27 Motivation

Keller. J.M. (1987) Development and use of the ARCS model of instructional design. *J of Instruct Develop*, 10:2–10.

Deci, Edward & Olafsen, Anja & Ryan, Richard. (2017). Self-Determination Theory in Work Organizations: The State of a Science. *Annual Review of Organizational Psychology and Organizational Behavior*. 4. 10.1146/annurev-orgpsych-032516-113108. Bandura, A. (1986) *Social foundations of thought and action: A social cognitive theory*, Prentice-Hall.

Di Maio, S., Keller, J., Hohl, D.H., Schwarzer, R., & Knoll, N. (2021). Habits and self-efficacy moderate the effects of intentions and planning on physical activity. *Br J of Health Psychol*, 26:50–66.

Radcliffe, J.N., Comfort, P., & Fawcett, T. (2015) Psychological strategies included by strength and conditioning coaches in applied strength and conditioning. *J of Stren & Cond Res*, 29(9):2641–2654.

Chapter 28 Legal and ethical considerations

American College of Sports Medicine (2025) *ACSM's Guidelines for Exercise Testing and Prescription (12th ed)*, Lippincott, Williams & Wilkins.

Coulson, M. (2021) *The Fitness Practitioners Handbook (4th ed)*, Bloomsbury.

The Management of Health and Safety at Work. hse.gov.uk/managing/index.htm (accessed 16.06.25)

Control of substances hazardous to health (COSHH). hse.gov.uk/coshh (accessed 16.06.25).

Children Act 1989. legislation.gov.uk/ukpga/1989/41/contents (accessed 16.06.25)

Chapter 29 Nutrients

Public Health England (2016) *Protecting and Improving the Nation's Health*. PHE publications gateway number: 2016202.

Shang, X., et al., (2016) Dietary protein intake and risk of type 2 diabetes: Results from the Melbourne Collaborative Cohort Study and a meta-analysis of prospective studies. *Am J Clin Nutr*, 104:1352–1365.

Hellmann, J., Zhang, M.J., Tang, Y., Rane, M., Bhatnagar, A., & Spite M. (2013) Increased saturated fatty acids in obesity alter resolution of inflammation in part by stimulating prostaglandin production, *J Immunol*, 191:1383–1392.

Sears, B., & Perry, M. (2015) The role of fatty acids in insulin resistance. *Lipids Health Dis*, 14:121.

Briggs, M.A., Petersen, K.S., & Kris-Etherton, P.M. (2017) Saturated fatty acids and cardiovascular disease: Replacements for saturated fat to reduce cardiovascular risk. *Health*, 5:E29.

Cordain L, et al., (2005) Origins and evolution of the Western diet: Health implications for the 21st century. *Am J Clin Nutr*, 81:341–354.

Abdullah, S.M., Defina, L.F., Leonard, D., et al., (2018) Long-term association of low-density lipoprotein cholesterol with cardiovascular mortality in individuals at low 10-year risk of atherosclerotic cardiovascular disease. *Circulation*, 138:2315–2325.

Strippoli, G.F., Craig, J.C., Rochtchina, E., et al., (2011) Fluid and nutrient intake and risk of chronic kidney disease. *Nephrology (Carlton)*, 16:326–334.

Charkoudian, N., Halliwill, J.R., Morgan, B.J., et al., (2003) Influences of hydration on post-exercise cardiovascular control in humans. *J Physiol*, 552:635–644.

Maughan, R.J., & Shirreffs, S.M. (2010) Development of hydration strategies to optimize performance for individuals in high-intensity sports and in sports with repeated intense efforts. *Scand J Med Sci Sports*, 20(2):59–69.

Cian, C., Barraud, P.A., Melin, B, et al., (2001) Effects of fluid ingestion on cognitive function after heat stress or exercise induced dehydration. *Int J Psychophysiol*, 42:243–251.

Grandjean, A.C., Reimers, K.J. & Buyckx, M.E. (2003) Hydration: Issues for the 21st century. *Nutr Rev*, 61:261–271.

Jequier, E., & Constant, F. (2010) Water as an essential nutrient: The physiological basis of hydration. *Eur J Clin Nutr*, 64:115–123.

Chouraqui, J.P. (2023) Children's water intake and hydration: A public health issue. *Nutr Rev*, 81(5):610–624.

Chapter 30 Nutritional deficiencies

Kiani, A.K., et al., (2022) Main nutritional deficiencies. *J Prev Med Hyg*, 63(3):E93–E101.

Deemer, S.E., Plaisance, E.P., & Martins, C. (2020) Impact of ketosis on appetite regulation: A review. *Nutr Res*, 77:1–11.

Rogerson, D. (2017) Vegan diets: Practical advice for individuals and exercisers. *J Int Soc Sports Nutr*, 14:36.

Williamson, C.S. (2006) Nutrition in pregnancy: Briefing paper. British Nutrition Foundation. *Nutr Bull*, 31:28–59.

Sunyecz, J.A. (2008) The use of calcium and vitamin D in the management of osteoporosis, *Therap and Clin Risk Manage*, 4(4):827–836.

Aldrich, N.D., Perry, C., Thomas, W., Raatz, S.K. & Reicks, M. (2013) Perceived importance of dietary protein to prevent weight gain: A national survey among midlife women. *J. Nutr. Educ. Behav*, 45:213–221.

Vergnaud, A.C., et al., (2013) Macronutrient composition of the diet and prospective weight change in individuals of the EPIC-PANACEA study. *PLOS One*, 8:E57300.

Markova, M., et al., (2018) Rate of appearance of amino acids after a meal regulates insulin and glucagon secretion in patients with type 2 diabetes: A randomized clinical trial. *Am J Clin Nutr*, 108:279–291.

El-Salhy, M., et al., (2017) Dietary fibre in irritable bowel syndrome (review). *Int J Mol Med*, 40:607–613.

Currie, A., & Morse, E.D. (2005) Eating disorders in individuals: Managing the risks. *Clinics in Sport Med*, 24:871–883.

Beals, K.A., & Manore, M.M. (1994) The prevalence of eating disorders in elite female individuals. *Int J Sport Nutr*, 4(2):175–195.

Sundgot-Borgen, J. (1994) Eating disorders in female individuals. *Sports Med*, 17(3):176–188.

Johnson, M.D. (1994) Disordered eating in active and athletic women. *Clin Sport Med*, 13(2):255–269.

Garner, D.M., Rosen, L.W., & Barry, D. (1998) Eating disorders among individuals. Research and recommendations. *Child Adolesc Psychiatr Clin N Am*, 7(4):839–857.

Chapter 31 Energy balance

Hill, J.O., & Commerford R. (1996) Physical activity, fat balance, and energy balance. *Int J Sport Nutr*, 6:80–92.

Hill, J.O., Wyatt, H.R., & Peters, J.C. (2013) The importance of energy balance. *Eur Endocrinol*, 9(2):111–115.

Schofield, W.N. (1985) Predicting basal metabolic rate, new standards and review of previous work. *Hum Nutri: Clin Nutr*, 39(1):5–41.

We would like to give a special thank you to Caroline Hewlett and Holly Jarrald for their much-appreciated guidance and attention to detail in what we feel is a comprehensive practical guide to strength and conditioning for a range of readers. Thanks also to Leah, Courtney and Owen for their excellent video demonstrations.

INDEX